Non-Toxic

DR. WEIL'S HEALTHY LIVING GUIDES

Andrew Weil, MD, Series Editor

Integrative Medicine is healing-oriented medicine that takes account of the whole person, including all aspects of lifestyle. It emphasizes the therapeutic relationship between practitioner and patient, is informed by evidence, and makes use of all appropriate therapies.

Published and forthcoming titles:

Optimal Men's Health by Myles Spar
Non-Toxic: Guide to Living Healthy in a Chemical World by Aly Cohen and Frederick vom Saal
Optimal Aging by Mikhail Kogan and Len Sherp
Optimal Skin Health by Robert Norman
Optimal Wellness by Farshad Marvasti and Richard Carmona

ADVANCE PRAISE FOR
NON-TOXIC

"The idea that our home environment and product choices can make us sick is a powerful motivator for cleaner living. Drs. Cohen and vom Saal reveal the dangers lurking within our food, water, clothing, personal care products, household products, and cellular technology, and share practical, cost-effective, tips and recommendations to battle the challenges of 'clean' living in a world without meaningful regulations. This is an important and timely guide to understanding our toxic world and what we can all do to protect our bodies from harmful exposures and their chronic health consequences."

—Mark Hyman MD, best-selling author of numerous books, including *Food Fix: How to Save Our Health, Our Economy, Our Communities, and Our Planet One Bite at a Time*

"What could be more important than the health of our brain! *Non-Toxic* shares practical information to help reduce harmful brain exposures—from pregnancy all the way through old age—and empowers readers to take control of the chemical world around them."

—Dhru Pirohit, creator/host of *Broken Brain* podcast

"*Non-Toxic* reveals the vast extent our ever-increasing exposure to toxins coupled with the failure of governmental agencies to intervene for our protection. The text not only makes it clear that to protect our health we have to serve as our own advocates, but also provides clear strategies enabling us to accomplish this goal. This is a clear and eloquent presentation of where we are, how we got here, and what we can do moving forward to offset some of the most important health threats of our modern world."

—David Perlmutter, MD, Author, #1 *New York Times* bestsellers, *Grain Brain* and *Brain Wash*

"As the founder of the Cancer Schmancer Movement and an ardent believer that how you live equals how you feel, I can speak firsthand that Dr. Aly Cohen, who is one of our medical advisors, is the real deal! Read this book and learn how to live well, be well, and stay well!

—Fran Drescher, Actor, Producer, Author, Health Activist, and Public Diplomacy Envoy on Health, US State Department

"*Non-Toxic* is the blueprint for staying healthy in an increasingly complex environment. You CAN reduce harmful exposures without turning your whole life upside down or breaking the bank. When misinformation abounds, a scientifically based resource with practical recommendations for making safer choices for everything from food to home furnishings, is truly a treasure. I will be recommending this book to all my patients and colleagues."

—Tieraona Low Dog, MD, Pecos, NM, Integrative Physician and Author, *Healthy at Home*

"If your doctor has never told you how important it is to reduce toxic chemical exposures in your food, water and home, you might need a new doctor. You definitely need *Non-Toxic*, a book so indispensable to good health its purchase ought to be covered by insurance. Dr. Aly Cohen and Professor Fred vom Saal lucidly explain how toxic chemicals hurt you and prescribe practical steps you can take to get them out of your life."

—Ken Cook, President, Environmental Working Group

"Every day I witness increasing concern for both personal health and planetary ecological health, especially as humanity experiences global interconnectedness in real time. In *Non-Toxic*, the authors provide rigorously researched assessments of what we're faced with as well as practical actions to protect ourselves and others. As more of us make these changes, our collective impact will be a reduced toxics burden for all life. I enthusiastically recommend *Non-Toxic* as a superb guide to meaningful personal and global action."

—Shana S. Weber, Ph.D., Director, Office of Sustainability Princeton Environmental Institute, Princeton University

"An authoritative and accessible guide to how we got into the chemical pickle we are in, what it means for your health, and how you can take positive, practical action to navigate through the chemical onslaught that comes at us every day."

—Pete Myers, Ph.D., co-author *Our Stolen Future*

Non-Toxic

Guide to Living Healthy
in a Chemical World

Aly Cohen MD, FACR
Frederick vom Saal, Ph.D.

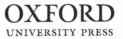

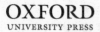

OXFORD
UNIVERSITY PRESS

Oxford University Press is a department of the University of Oxford. It furthers
the University's objective of excellence in research, scholarship, and education
by publishing worldwide. Oxford is a registered trade mark of Oxford University
Press in the UK and certain other countries.

Published in the United States of America by Oxford University Press
198 Madison Avenue, New York, NY 10016, United States of America.

Library of Congress Cataloging-in-Publication Data
Names: Cohen, Aly, 1973– author. | Vom Saal, Frederick S. author.
Title: Non-toxic : guide to living healthy in a chemical world /
by Aly Cohen MD, FARC, Frederick vom Saal, Ph.D.
Description: New York, NY : Oxford University Press, [2020] |
Series: Dr. Weil's healthy living guides | Includes bibliographical references and index. |
Identifiers: LCCN 2020013831 (print) | LCCN 2020013832 (ebook) |
ISBN 9780190082352 (paperback) | ISBN 9780190082376 (epub) |
ISBN 9780190082369 (pdf)
Subjects: LCSH: Environmental toxicology—Popular works. |
Environmental health—Popular works.
Classification: LCC RA1226 .C63 2020 (print) | LCC RA1226 (ebook) | DDC 615.9/02—dc23
LC record available at https://lccn.loc.gov/2020013831
LC ebook record available at https://lccn.loc.gov/2020013832

9 8 7 6 5

Printed by LSC Communications, United States of America

God, grant me the serenity to accept the things I cannot change,
Courage to change the things I can,
And wisdom to know the difference.

—Serenity Prayer, by Reinhold Niebuhr (1892–1971)

Contents

Series Foreword

Andrew Weil, MD
Series Editor

The authors of this book, Drs. Aly Cohen and Frederick vom Saal, a clinician and a researcher, collaborated previously on an academic text, *Integrative Environmental Medicine,* published by Oxford University Press in 2017 as part of the Weil Integrative Medicine Library series. It addressed a serious deficiency in the training of physicians and allied health professionals: lack of education about environmental causes of illness and what to do about them. Many people today are rightly concerned about toxic exposures, air and water pollution, chemicals in food and household products, and the dangers of cell phones and other electronic devices. Too often, doctors have been unable to answer their questions or help them navigate the confusing and often contradictory data available.

Now, Drs. Cohen and vom Saal have produced a book for the reading public, a volume in Oxford's *Dr. Weil's Healthy Living Guides*. It not only summarizes the best evidence about environmental toxins, it gives practical advice about what you can do to reduce the risk of being harmed by them.

I have long stressed the basic elements of healthy living: good nutrition, regular physical activity, adequate rest and sleep, practices to neutralize harmful effects of stress and optimize mental and emotional wellness, and wise use of preventive medical services. Sad to say, I must now add to that list: awareness of environmental toxins and hazards and ways to protect yourself from them. This book gives you the information you need.

Tucson, Arizona
February 2020
Andrew Weil MD

Introduction

The Story of Truxtun,
Aly's Golden Retriever

Truxtun was like every golden retriever you've probably ever met. A fluffy ball of love, wildly flirtatious, filled with boundless energy, and just plain gorgeous to look at. So it came as a bit of a surprise when, shortly after turning 4 and a half, he started to huff and puff and peter out after just a few rounds of catch in the yard. Even Sir Commodore Thomas Truxtun, the 18th-century naval officer and commander of the USS *Constitution* (now docked in Baltimore Harbor), for whom he was named, would have had enough energy to climb a simple flight of stairs—especially in his home built on land once visited by Sir Commodore Thomas Truxtun himself! But Truxtun was a good sport, so even while resting comfortably on the carpeted floor, at the feet of his two human brothers, he feigned a healthy appearance and smiled with delight.

Between diaper changes for our second son, who was around 6 months at the time, and chasing our older son (who was then 2 and a half) around the house, Truxtun, our "first born," was no longer the sole recipient of our attention. He dealt with it rather gracefully, entertaining himself more outdoors, sitting in the sun, holding that red plastic toy solidly in his jaw, waiting patiently for his turn at affection.

The panting was not obvious at first. Between busy work hours, crying babies, and sleepless nights, Truxtun's heavy breathing did not create immediate concern. When he stopped eating his food, and especially his dog treats, my husband, Steve, and I knew something was up and quickly set up an appointment with our vet. Maybe he swallowed a sock? They were among his favorite contraband items to pilfer. Or maybe it was some kind of virus from doggy daycare, where he spent time on occasion. The first vet he saw did not find anything on exam, so I took him home rather frustrated as to why he was still panting. The next day, however, Truxtun had had enough, and he laid down on the kitchen floor, blocking foot traffic, and I just knew: this dog was sick.

I took him back to see another vet at the clinic, and this time the vet pointed to the yellow discoloration (known as jaundice) inside Truxtun's ears, clearly indicating liver problems. I took him to the large-animal hospital for further testing that afternoon, and Steve met me there. Blood was drawn, chest x-ray and ultrasound of his abdomen were performed, and then the doctor came in to talk with us. On ultrasound, Truxtun had a liver the size of a baseball, shrunken and too small to maintain the normal workings of his body. The vet suspected autoimmune liver disease, also seen in humans, but incredibly rare in dogs (especially golden retrievers). With autoimmune liver disease, the body's immune system is somehow triggered to attack its own liver, causing inflammation and dysfunction, and eventually the liver shrinks to a size too small and ineffective to maintain normal function. I gasped. I cried. My heart was broken. As an autoimmune disease doctor for humans (the irony of such a moment!), I fully understood what this meant for Truxtun . . . and for us.

Over the next 4 months of Truxtun's life, our vet, my husband (also a physician), and I treated him as a human. We ordered steroids and medications to "quiet" his body's immune system in order to slow the progression of his liver disease. Using an ultrasound, our vet marked an "X" on Truxtun's belly, indicating the area in his abdomen where enormous amounts of fluid began to build up because the liver was overwhelmed and failing. In the evenings, after putting two babies down for bed, Steve and I would head to the kitchen. We'd unravel intravenous tubing and empty bags, and one of us would reluctantly stick a long needle into the center of the "X" on Truxtun's underbelly, while he stood still and patient, so we could draw thick, amber-colored fluid out of his body. As time went on, a quart of fluid removed from his belly turned into a gallon; Truxtun would immediately begin to breathe more comfortably and we'd all head to bed only slightly relieved. Although I was a young doctor at the time, a few years out of training, there was no patient I had ever worked with whom I loved and cared for more.

Between work, kids, and caregiving for Truxtun, there was not much time to speculate about what might have caused Truxtun to develop liver failure, but obvious questions came to mind. Was his food contaminated? It had not been long since news had spread of dog food contamination in the United States, due to melamine, a toxic industrial chemical. Perhaps we gave him a bad batch of dog food? What about his dog treats? I didn't know much about pesticides at the time, but I knew they couldn't be good for you, and we lived next to about 200 acres of farmland. Could he have gotten sick because of our proximity to the regular pesticide spraying in our backyard? What about his flea and tick medicine, which is also a pesticide? Having no formal knowledge of their health risks, I had a bad feeling every time I squeezed that stinky liquid onto the back of his neck. And that red plastic toy, called a Kong, that he NEVER dropped out of his mouth, except to eat, give it a toss, or lick our faces. After chewing off the actual wood siding of our home at 12 weeks of age, we gave him the Kong to distract him, and it served as the perfect remedy for puppy total home annihilation. Truxtun loved that toy so much, he slept with it in his mouth, dropped it on the baby's lap for a game of catch, and ecstatically dove for it in the pool. No matter how cracked, decayed, discolored, and dirty that Kong was, Truxtun held it proudly in his mouth.

I wasn't trained in toxicology (other than for medications in medical school) and never thought twice about the world around me having any kind of deleterious effects on my body, or Truxtun's for that matter. Hell, I drank Diet Dr Pepper every day for years and had been eating Cheez Wiz and Oreos like they were their own food group. Diet and nutrition were not on my radar, nor had I been taught anything about these topics in medical school (even today, students only get a total of ~5–8 hours of diet/nutrition education over 4 years of medical school)—of course harmful environmental exposures, such as food chemicals, plastic chemicals, personal care product chemicals, cleaning chemicals, fabric chemicals, water contaminants, didn't even cross my mind at the time of Truxtun's illness.

Heartbroken and confused about Truxtun's illness, I decided, in between diaper changes, work, and trying to survive the rigor of young married life, that I would research how a dog might acquire autoimmune liver disease. I read about drinking water, food additives, pesticides, and bug sprays. I read position statements from the World Health Organization and the American Academy of Pediatrics. What about that red plastic toy that was always in Truxtun's mouth? I found a few case reports in the medical literature about young healthy people working in plastics factories who developed autoimmune diseases, including autoimmune liver disease. I discovered vast bodies of medical literature on plastic chemicals such as polyvinyl chloride (vinyl), phthalates, and bisphenol A, and health effects in both animal and human studies. I was shocked. I was enraged. Where were the regulations? The labeling? Where was the appropriate testing to evaluate whether chemicals were safe for humans (and pets!) BEFORE they are allowed in all of our products?

Soon, I started to make changes in my home; I got rid of liquid "plug-in" air fresheners (I had 10 different fragrances stocked in my kitchen drawer), swapped out pungent cleaning products with products that contained ingredients that my grandmother used. I started to eat more "cleanly," reducing processed foods (yes, I gave up Cheez Wiz and Oreos), weaned myself off of my addiction to diet sodas, used fewer cosmetics and personal care products, and invested in a water filter under my kitchen sink. The more I read, the more I realized the problem; we are inundated with literally thousands of chemicals that are untested for human and pet health, and they infiltrate every aspect of our lives. Many of these chemicals, tested by academic researchers and not the manufacturers themselves, mind you, can affect hormone activity, immune system function, brain function and development both inside and outside of the uterus, and contribute to cancer development. What's more, despite the enormous amount of solid, reproducible studies in the Western medical literature, I had learned nothing of this in all my years of schooling. I was pissed.

Truxtun passed away about 6 months after his diagnosis. Steve and I brought him to the hospital when we just knew it was time to relieve his pain. In true form, he gave us each a big wet lick across the face, and then his tired body went limp. I didn't understand at the time that his illness was the start of a journey that would eventually become my life's work: to educate the public about the effects that chemicals and radiation have on the human body. Only now, almost a decade after his death, I realize that, if he had not become ill, I would likely never have ventured into "environmental health." In that, I find some solace in his passing.

Soon after Truxtun's death, I began giving community lectures, sharing information and tips with patients, and spending literally hours in big box stores reading labels. Having read so much about environmental chemicals online, specifically from a group based in Washington, D.C., called the Environmental Working Group (EWG.org), I cold-called them one day to see if they would take a look at my slides and make sure I was "getting it right." This was not really my area of training, and this group is made up of toxicologists, so why not ask for their input? To my genuine surprise, the head scientist at the time, Johanna Congleton, called me back. I remember that *she* sounded rather surprised on the other end of the phone, even stating that she had not come across many medical doctors interested in environmental chemical issues. Soon after, we met in D.C. and began to create an educational lecture for physicians that would qualify physicians to earn Continuing Medical Education or CME credit. It took me a year of reading to understand the basics of low dose exposure, endocrine system disruption, animal versus human studies, epidemiologic studies relating health effects to exposures, reading product labels, and regulatory and legislative issues. Johanna regularly emailed me key scientific articles, and together we created PowerPoint slides and a solid, "evidence-based" program that I could present to doctors in academic and community hospitals across the country.

After three years and 23 lectures at many of the top academic institutions in the United States, I had to slow down. Sadly, I had not received the response I was hoping for from physicians and hospital systems; doctors were unenthusiastic toward the concept of introducing "environmental health" topics into their daily routine and patient care, and hospital systems were uninterested in making changes in purchasing (e.g., swapping out toxic plastics in IV tubing and bags, respiratory care tubing in intensive care units, neonatology intensive care units [NICU], etc., even after the CDC (Centers for Disease Control and Prevention) published data that babies in NICUs were being massively exposed to endocrine-disrupting chemicals leaching from these medical products). It felt like a losing proposition.

Then, one evening while talking with my kids' teenage babysitter in our kitchen, she asked if her lip balm and shampoo might be harming her; all of a sudden, a lightbulb went off in my head. What if I could share this information with high school students, so they could learn key environmental health information *now*, and make healthier, smarter decisions *throughout* their lives? I reached out to my local (very forward thinking) high school principal, Gary Snyder, and high school head of science, Cherry Sprague, and we began to formulate a pilot project to see if the students were interested in and receptive to "environmental health" information. I created several lectures and workshops on topics such as clean drinking water, personal care products, indoor and outdoor air quality (including vaping!), pesticides and bug sprays, mental health and environmental exposures, and safe use of cell phones and cellular technology. I collected data on baseline knowledge, retention of information, and even the number of lifestyle changes students made in the months following the lecture series.

The results were amazing. Not only were the students interested in these topics, they wanted more information and resources! The data showed that THIS is the demographic to educate. These kids get it and are ready and willing to make simple lifestyle changes that will impact their own health and perhaps the health of generations to follow.

Pivotal Moments: Integrative Medicine and Meeting Dr. vom Saal

In 2011, my husband came across an online 2-year program for physicians to train in integrative medicine, a "holistic" way of looking at human health through the use of nutrition, dietary changes, exercise, improved sleep, management of stress, traditional Chinese and Indian (Ayurvedic) medicine techniques, and other non-"medicinal" forms of healing. I was skeptical at first, but I had already seen improvements in my own health (e.g., reduced migraines, increased energy and mood) with dietary changes to remove food chemicals, so I applied for the only scholarship available there was for a rheumatologist, and I was thrilled to be selected. For 2 years I learned from some of the best leaders in this field: Dr. Victoria Maizes, Dr. Tieraona Low Dog, Dr. Randy Horwitz, and of course, the "Father of Integrative Medicine" himself, Dr. Andrew Weil. My tools as a physician grew exponentially. Despite being trained as a "specialist" in rheumatology, I could now share dietary recommendations with patients, help with their sleep problems, work on their stress and mental health issues, and even offer evidence-based supplements to prevent and alleviate a wide variety of health conditions. Now, I could treat my rheumatoid arthritis patient, not just for joint pain, but also for migraine headaches, or high blood pressure, heartburn, or weight gain—and with fewer medications.

Not long after I completed the fellowship, I was given an exciting opportunity by Dr. Weil to write the textbook on "environmental medicine" for his academic Integrative Medicine Library series with Oxford University Press (there are now 14 books in the series). The offer had one condition: I would have to partner with an academic researcher (I was a clinician). So, I began calling a variety of academic researchers, bench scientists, and even a former surgeon general of the United States, to see if we made a good fit for this project. But after a dozen phone calls and half a dozen interviews, I was again back at the beginning. I decided to call one researcher, in particular, whose journal articles I now regularly consulted. It was a longshot in my mind, to see if he would get on board, but I had nothing to lose.

Even though he's not a member of the Avengers or X-Men franchises, Dr. Frederick vom Saal is what I call a real life superhero. In the world of "environmental biology" and toxicology, he is someone who has set the bar for scientific integrity, tenacity, and perseverance. Perhaps he is best known for his work on the hormonal effects that come from exposure to certain chemicals called endocrine disruptors (discussed in chapter 2). Dr. vom Saal was one of the first researchers in the world, in the 1990s, to uncover the risks associated with bisphenol A (BPA), a pervasive industrial chemical used in thousands of consumer products. *He* is "the guy" who painstaking fought to have bisphenol A removed from baby bottles and sports bottles from the US market in 2012. Dr. vom Saal has written over 200 scientific articles, has contributed to dozens of textbooks, and has been instrumental in shaping toxic chemical research and public policy in the United States and abroad. He is the recipient of countless honors and awards for his groundbreaking research, including the prestigious Heinz Award for his work on industrial chemicals. He is an international speaker, is sought after by newspapers and magazines for his expert opinion, has been invited to testify in congressional hearings and by numerous state legislatures, and he has appeared in numerous TV and movie documentaries, as well as on TV news programs such as *20/20, Frontline*, and the *Today Show*.

So, when I picked up the phone to call Dr. vom Saal that fateful day, it was as though I was a singer/songwriter from Topeka, Kansas, picking up the phone to ask Mick Jagger to write an album together. To this day, I can recall our conversation; not only was he excited by the project, he happened to be a huge fan of integrative medicine, and fully understood the role that environmental medicine *should* play in clinical medicine. It was kismet!

Our textbook, *Integrative Environmental Medicine*, published in 2017, was truly a unique collaboration between some of the most renowned researchers in biology, toxicology, environmental sciences, and practicing physicians who treat many of the downstream effects from environmental exposures (e.g., thyroid disease, hormonally sensitive cancers, obesity). Now, Dr. vom Saal and I have come together to create this guidebook, *Non-Toxic*, for the lay person—the person that *I* was just a handful of years ago—when Truxtun's illness set me on this journey.

Why Environmental Health Matters

Our environment has changed profoundly over the past century. While human beings have been evolving for well over 4.5 million years, it is only in the last 100 years that more than 90,000 new chemicals have been seeping into almost every aspect of human life. Not only are these 90,000 chemicals a major part of our day-to-day activities through what we eat, drink, breathe, and lather onto our skin, they have also been absorbed into our flesh and blood; laboratory testing now detects many of these chemicals in our blood, urine, placenta, breast milk, and semen. From the day of conception to the last breath we take, exposure to thousands of harmful chemicals has become the human "womb-to-tomb" experience.

After World War II, industrial chemical production began to explode and was filled with promises of greater convenience, lower cost, reduced need for natural resources, and improved quality of life for all. A virtual explosion of synthetic materials saturated the market: nylon, melamine, rayon, polycarbonate, polyvinyl chloride, styrofoam, naugahyde, plexiglass, pesticides, and solvents, used to create everything from Hula Hoops to food packaging, pesticides to air deodorizers. So primative was our understanding of the effect new chemical inventions might eventually have that the inventor of the toxic pesticide DDT, Swiss chemist Paul Muller, was awarded the Nobel Prize in Physiology and Medicine in 1948. Over a 60-year period, what was once considered extraordinary has evolved into the ordinary, with billions of pounds of synthetic materials created, manufactured, used once, and thrown away with abandon. **We are both responsible for and victims of our own pollution**. Just take a look at the numbers:

- Every day, the United States imports about 45 million pounds of synthetic chemicals.
- Each year, about 1,000 new chemicals are put into use.
- 15 new polymers are patented in the United States every week.
- Over 1000 likely endocrine-disrupting chemicals currently exist—
- BUT only 5 chemicals *have ever been banned* in the United States under the Toxic Substance Control Act (passed in 1976), under the Ford administration. And, the revised Toxic Substances Control Act (passed in mid-2016) has failed to improve the regulatory response to toxic chemicals.

It's not surprising that as the enormous variety and amount of chemicals in our environment has dramatically increased, so have the new cases of many chronic diseases, such as type 2 diabetes, obesity, thyroid disease, asthma, allergy, autoimmune disease, autism, attention deficit hyperactive disorder (ADHD), and several cancers. Evidence from around the world reveals that exposure to chemicals in everyday cleaning and personal care products, air pollution, food, drinks, building materials and furnishings, and food packaging have contributed to many of these health issues. In addition, there are numerous toxic chemicals that can contribute to increased susceptibility to infectious diseases, such as COVID-19, through altering the baseline inflammatory setting created by exposure. It's a chemical "soup" from which we must now extricate ourselves! This toxic chemical soup that is creating a chronic inflammatory state in our bodies is thus putting us into a higher risk of severe illness and death when we encounter infectious diseases.

The public wrongly assumes that chemicals have the same regulatory oversight and safety testing as medications. Most of us assume that "if it's on the shelf, it must be safe," when in fact, to most people's surprise, the vast majority of chemicals in the stuff we love and use every day, lack safety testing of any kind or prior approval from any US regulatory agency, prior to going to market!

To add to the chemical pollution of our planet and health effects on our bodies, radiation sources—such as cell phones, tablets, computers, and a growing world of WIFI, Bluetooth, and sensor technology—are raising serious health concerns; there has been virtually no discussion by any US regulatory agency of the potentially more dangerous levels of EMR (electromagnetic radiation) from 5th generation wireless technology (5G WIFI). Because of its high frequency and short transmission range, 5G requires a huge number of microwave transmitters to be installed in neighborhoods, and everyone will be exposed. Reminiscent of the VHS recorders in the 1980s, newer, cheaper, disposable technology has begun to evolve, pulling in a wider swath of consumers with a younger and younger fan base, only adding to the potential health risk debate.

What Can You Do to Make Changes, Improve Your Health, and Live Longer?

Living in modern times, we love the conveniences that many of these chemicals and technologies have allowed. Throw away, single-use plastics reduce our need to wash dishes, nonstick pans save us the added sweat needed for those caked-on recipes, air fresheners cover smells that just might require extra cleaning, food preservatives and packaging keep the food from spoiling, and pesticides ward off unsightly bugs that may ruin the look of a perfect apple. We have opened a Pandora's box of chemical creations that have the ability to cause great harm to our health, but are we willing to give up short-term conveniences for long-term health gains?

In other words, what's the "buy-in" to change, when we all know change is not easy?

Whether or not each of us develops illness or disease depends on many factors, but our genetic makeup (genes from our parents/grandparents), our lifestyles (e.g., diet, exercise, stress, sleep quality), and our environment (e.g., food chemicals, water contaminants, personal care-product chemicals, radiation exposure, air quality) are among the most well-studied by academic scientists. In addition, our lives are *fluid*; as children we were fed by others with their own ideas of health, but later on as adults we make dietary choices for ourselves, although often prior habits are hard to break. When we are young, we may live for years in a chemically toxic environment, but we may move into a cleaner, safer environment later on in life. Our personal care products often change with time either because of great marketing or our ability to pay for more expensive products (which doesn't mean they are any safer!). With so much moment-to-moment variability of our environment, this book aims to empower you, the reader, to harness control within the areas of your life that you *can* control. By sharing information and recommendations to reduce harmful exposures in the environments and activities you do every day, you'll be armed with the tools to reduce risk for worsening or developing health problems.

Similar to the message of the Serenity Prayer, this book is a tool to open readers' minds to what they can and can't change and to give wisdom to know the difference. This book is designed to embolden and empower you to make changes that are right for you and your family and to embrace prevention in order to avoid downstream health issues and chronic disease. Although prevention in many ways requires faith, the "buy-in" is using scientific information to help shape decisions that may have profound effects on the health and well-being for you and, as new science shows, even generations to follow.

What We CAN DO

Unfortunately, the love affair with harmful chemicals has not ended, and many that were introduced over the past century to improve our day-to-day lives are exactly the same chemicals that need to be eliminated. Effective government policy and oversight in the United States does not currently exist. Fortunately, many consumer advocacy groups such as the Environmental Working Group; Healthy Child, Healthy World; and Moms Across America continue to shine a spotlight on the system's failures and to put pressure on manufacturers to make real and lasting changes to both our chemical laws and product ingredients. Healthcare providers are not formally taught environmental health information in any meaningful way that reaches their patients. *The real work must come from individuals*. No one can make better changes for the health of your body and those you love than an educated consumer . . . YOU!

Key Take-Home Points from This Book

- Don't trust that the government is protecting you from harmful chemicals and radiation.
- Don't wait for others to keep you safe from toxic chemicals, do it yourself.
- Survey your body to see what goes *in, on, and around* it.
- Your nose knows! One of the first indications that you are in a toxic environment may be the smell, so trust your senses and instincts and remove yourself or remove the offending problem as soon as you can.
- Cost of convenience: decide what you can and can't live without.
- The "less is more" approach will always win out.
- Better to be safe than sorry.
- Working to clean out chemicals is a journey and may take some time. No problem! Aim to make reasonable changes in a comfortable and timely manner so behavior and product swaps actually stick.

In keeping with the philosophy of Integrative Medicine (IM), which is healing-oriented medicine that takes account of the whole person (body, mind, spirit), as well as all aspects of lifestyle, our focus is on *prevention* as opposed to just management of symptoms. In doing so, we embrace the Precautionary Principle that states that when an activity raises threats of harm to the environment or human health, precautionary measures should be taken even if some cause-and-effect relationships are not fully established.[1] That means, lack of hard evidence for a cause-and-effect relationship does not mean that risk is not actually present. Our recommendations are based on the best science available, effort level, cost, and plain old common sense.

As a distinguished professor of biology and laboratory researcher (Fred vom Saal Ph.D.), and a physician and clinical researcher (Aly Cohen, MD), we combine our unique life experiences, generational perspectives, research, and training to share with you clear, reasonable, practical recommendations that can be incorporated into your daily routine effortlessly. No matter where on this journey you may find yourself, we hope to partner with you to reduce exposures to environmental health hazards, for a long, healthy life for you, your family. . . . and, of course, your beloved pets.

Reference

1. deFur PL, Kaszuba M. Implementing the precautionary principle. *The Science of the total environment.* 2002;288(1–2):155–165.

1

Overview of Environmental Exposures
How We Got Into This Pickle

Unless someone like you cares a whole awful lot, nothing is
going to get better. It's not.

—Dr. Seuss, *The Lorax (1904–1991)*

Overview

In order to put into perspective where we are *now*, we need to begin by
briefly looking back at human history with regard to the environment
humans evolved in and their sources of food and water. As recently as
10,000 years ago, modern human beings, the *Homo sapiens*, began farming
and domesticating livestock, which gave them the ability to have more control over the availability of food. But, this dramatically altered the types
of foods that humans had evolved eating.[1] Previously, the diet of early

hunter-gatherer humans was very different. Our ancestors ate meat from wild animals that foraged grasses with high nutritional content. They ate wild fish that fed on algae fresh from the ocean, free of mercury and chemicals that are difficult to break down over time such as polychlorinated biphenyls (PCBs), polybrominated biphenyls (PBDEs), and polyfluoroalkyl substances (PFASs), as well as pesticides. Our ancestors did not eat fish with man-made chemicals that bioaccumulate up the food chain, a process in which contaminated small plants and animals are eaten by progressively larger animals, making them more and more contaminated.

Oceans were not filled with tons of plastics that gradually degrade into microplastic particles and end up in food and water that humans consume. Our distant ancestors consumed limited amounts of dairy because cows were not yet domesticated. Mothers provided infants with milk for up to 4 years, in sharp contrast to the current Western norm of a greatly reduced period of breast-feeding (lactation); prolonged breast-feeding also led to appropriate spacing of pregnancies, which not only worked as an extremely effective contraceptive, but significantly improved infant survival.[2]

The diet of early humans was high in fruits, nuts, and berries, and prior to the transition to farming, the human diet was low in grains—wheat, barley, rye, corn—that now, along with the pesticides sprayed on them, dominate our food supply. The foods eaten by hunter-gatherers were high in protein and complex, nutrient-filled carbohydrates (fruits and vegetables), high in magnesium, and extremely low in sodium—contrary to the current standard American diet, often referred to as the SAD diet, which is an appropriate acronym, since the American diet is horribly unhealthy.[3,4] When prehistoric man was not fending off saber-toothed tigers or other predators, they spent their days in the sun, absorbing vitamin D through their uncovered, un–sun-screened skin, breathing clean, unadulterated air, and bathing in freshwater streams.

Food Made Easy: The Agricultural Revolution

Mankind's transition to cultivated farm crops and domesticated farm animals occurred at different times in history in different parts of the world. One of the biggest changes occurred with the invention of better farming equipment along with changes in farming practices, such as crop rotation, which led to the British Agricultural Revolution of the 17th–19th centuries. This brought about greater productivity in farming and a sharp increase in the population, providing the urban labor force for the Industrial Revolution.

Also, new social and hygiene practices developed, leading to less infection and death by pestilence.

In comparison to pre-historic life, no longer did humans have to chase animals for meat or follow growing seasons across a continent to gather fruits and nuts. Humans could collect seeds from plants and grow them right outside of their front door. They could raise animals on farms without having to search all day for the kill or instead, working all day tending to crops and livestock—the Industrial Revolution had begun due to the ability to produce enough food to transport to large populations living in cities.

Today, our food is dramatically different than it was even just 200 years ago. In the United States meat comes from animals reared in concentrated animal feeding operations (CAFOs) housing thousands of animals that are regularly fed antibiotics, a cocktail of growth-stimulating hormones, and genetically modified grains with high levels of pesticide residues, such as glyphosate and other ingredients found in Roundup, all of which end up in the meat. Our strawberries are fumigated by workers in hazmat suits, and our fish are farmed in overcrowded, dirty pens, and are fed food that has been found to be contaminated with highly persistent and toxic PCBs.[5]

We rely on inexpensive, easily available, processed foods that are high in calories, saturated fat, and synthetic sugars, but low in nutrient value, and contain a variety of food chemicals to keep them shelf stable, and to maintain color and flavor, long after natural ingredients would have lasted. We drink artificially colored and flavored drinks such as soda, energy drinks, and juices that raise blood pressure and blood sugar, increasing our risk for obesity, diabetes, stroke, cancer, and a host of other diseases.

Fire Up the Machines: The Industrial Revolution

The Industrial Revolution, which occurred during the eighteenth and nineteenth centuries, was a major period of change for modern-day humans. During this period, new forms of manufacturing developed, with the transition from handheld tools to machines and the use of coal and steam power over other conventional biofuels, such as wood. The spinning wheel allowed for the mass production of textiles, and new chemistry led to the production of dyes. All together, the inventions during this period spurred the creation of factories and thousands of jobs; this was made possible due to the dramatic increase in food production that allowed a massive influx of people into cities to work in the factories. Improved iron making led to metal materials at a lower cost. Among other innovations, tin and steel made food non-perishable, allowing food to ship long distances, reducing waste and cost. With the explosion of factories running on coal energy, coal residue—or "particulate matter" (commonly known as soot), began to fill the air. Soon the skies in England darkened with soot, blocking sunlight, and impacting lung function, leading to lung and related diseases in large industrialized cities. The health consequences of a carbon-based economy on air quality throughout the world (and global warming) is as big an issue in 2020 as it was during the Industrial Revolution. Today, outdoor air pollution is a major cause of the increasing incidence of respiratory diseases in many parts of the world. The COVID-19 pandemic that was recognized in early 2020 demonstrated that having a damaged respiratory and immune-response system was a potential death sentence for those infected with this virus.

New Pollutants

The Industrial Revolution brought many new pollutants. By the mid-1800s, discoveries such as coal tar—a thick, smelly, toxic black wasteproduct of coal burning—led to the development of dyes, aspirin, food sweeteners like Saccharin, perfumes, early plastics, and the explosive TNT.

> "It is not the strongest or the most intelligent who will survive, but those who can best adapt to change."
>
> —*Charles Darwin (1809–1882)*

Skyrocketing use of chemicals led to a special class of pollution we still have today, called persistent organic pollutants (POPs). These include compounds containing chlorine (known as "organochlorines"), used to produce plastic pipes and refrigerants and often added to materials to kill bacteria and viruses. Other POPs include chlorinated pesticides (DDT), perfluorinated chemicals (PFOA and PFOS used on nonstick pans), brominated flame retardants, polychlorinated biphenyls (PCBs), and dioxins (chlorine-containing industrial waste).

POPs linger in the environment, taking decades or centuries to break down. They resist natural degradation from sunlight and soil bacteria and ride long distances on wind and sea currents to the north and south poles and bioaccumulate up the food chain. Pregnant women are warned not to eat large-species delicacies like tuna or swordfish steaks because they are loaded with contaminants that can cross through the placenta and disrupt normal development of a growing fetus, reduce IQ, and cause neuromuscular deficits. Sadly, this was the case for many pregnant mothers eating PCB-contaminated fish that were caught in the Great Lakes between the United States and Canada, which at one time were heavily polluted with POPs.[6]

Today's Synthetic Age

The Synthetic Age, which began during the early 1940s, introduced "chemical marvels" to the home with the invention of polyethylene Hula Hoops, melamine dishes, polycarbonate food containers, polystyrene cups, Teflon pot coatings, Saran Wrap food covering, Formica countertops, polyurethane-foam sofas, nylon stockings, naugahyde upholstery, vinyl flooring, acrylic paints, Gore-Tex, and polyester fabrics. On an industrial scale, the Synthetic Age brought about new chemical solvents for better cleaning, specialty metals like magnesium and aluminum, Plexiglas for lighter weight and increased safety in aircraft, oil additives that prevent machinery from freezing in cold weather, and pesticides that protected troops from disease. In the home, plastics and other synthetics allowed for new types of food storage and preparation, and waterproofing of materials, that made them last longer. Plastics allowed for the creation of cheaper versions of expensive, already existing materials such as gold, steel, and wood. The Age of Plastics brought with it hopes for "Better Living through Chemistry," as famously stated by advertisements for Monsanto, a large chemical corporation in the United States. Between 1940 and 1960, the US output of plastics increased from 300 million to 6 billion pounds (see Figure 1.1). Today, approximately 45 million pounds of chemicals are imported every day. Over the next 25 years, global chemical production is expected to double and be well above a trillion pounds per year.

- Approximately *90,000 compounds* are approved for commercial use right now, but only *a handful* have been tested for neural, reproductive, and developmental toxicity.
- In the United States chemicals are considered safe to use in products until there is clear evidence that they are causing human harm (an impossibly high bar that has paralyzed US regulators).

- The chemical manufacturers, not the US federal regulatory agencies, decide whether to use new chemicals in products, typically declaring them "Generally Regarded as Safe" without any safety testing.
- Every day, the United States imports about 45 million pounds of synthetic chemicals.
- Each year, over *1,000 new chemicals* are put into use.
- 15 new polymers are patented in the United States every week.
- *Only 5* chemicals in commercial use have been banned in the United States under the Toxic Substance Control Act (TSCA) passed in 1976 when Gerald Ford was president. (The new TSCA passed in 2016 was largely written by chemical corporations and is as ineffective as the 1976 TSCA.)

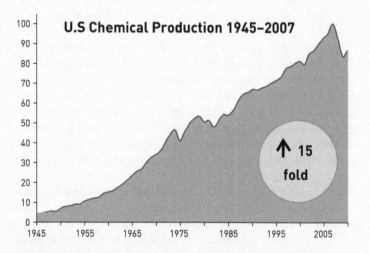

U.S Chemical Production 1945–2007

↑ 15 fold

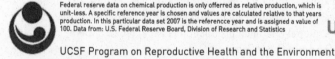

Federal reserve data on chemical production is only offerred as relative production, which is unit-less. A specific reference year is chosen and values are calculated relative to that years production. In this particular data set 2007 is the referencce year and is assigned a value of 100. Data from: U.S. Federal Reserve Board, Division of Research and Statistics

UCSF Program on Reproductive Health and the Environment

University of California
San Francisco

Figure 1.1 Data from the US Federal Reserve Board, Division of Research and Statistics, showing fold change in US Chemical Production 1945–2007. This graph shows the dramatic growth in synthetic chemical production in the US over the last century. Federal reserve data on chemical production is only offered as relative production, which is unit-less.

These astounding numbers bring to mind several questions: Why is the US government devoting so little money to studying the role of toxic chemicals as the cause of disease? Why are public health agencies not responding to the scientific research, conducted by academic scientists, showing a relationship between specific toxins and disease? How could physicians who attended medical school know so little about the relationship of toxic chemicals to the chronic diseases harming the lives of so many people? And, perhaps the most important question, what are these chemicals and new forms of radiation doing not just to our bodies, but our species as a whole, other species, and the global ecosystem?

Chemicals and Radiation Are All Around Us

- Televisions are treated with flame retardants.
- Furniture and carpets are coated with stain guards and water-proofing chemicals.
- Food containers contain plasticizers that leach into food (DEHP and BPA).
- Plastic toys are molded from polyvinyl chloride (PVC).
- Bathrooms are filled with chemical-laden cosmetics and personal care products.
- Drinking water has been found to have many contaminants, such as metals, medications, and industrial chemicals.
- Food is "engineered" with preservatives, coloring, and synthetic flavors.
- Air fresheners, synthetic fragrances, and engine fumes waft through the air.
- Cell phone and tech gadget technology: 2G, 3G, 4G, and now 5G microwave radiation's reach has extended to all corners of our lives.

The Global Web of Pollution

Industrial chemicals are found in surprising quantities, thousands of miles from their source, inside the largest animals in the food chain. Despite their remote location, Eskimos and Canada's Inuit who eat seals and whale, suffer high exposure to chemicals known to be toxic. Whales in the Arctic Circle have been found to carry enormous levels of chemical pollutants such as perfluorocarbons, used on nonstick pans and waterproofing materials, stain guards, and microwave popcorn bags. These chemicals travel on tradewinds, falling to the earth and onto bodies of water and vegetation. They become absorbed into the ecosystem of that environment, bioaccumulating in increasing amounts up the food chain. Many of these chemicals will not break down for a hundred years! Some disrupt the earth's protective ozone layer and allow UVA and UVB light to travel unfiltered to the earth's surface, increasing risks of skin cancer.

How Could the World Become So Polluted?

The short answer to this question is that there has been far too much production of too many chemicals over a relatively short period of time, with limited to no safety testing, limited and ineffective regulation, and not enough forethought for potential harm to humans and wildlife, or the safe and appropriate disposal or recycling of materials.

In the United States, the general assumption among most Americans is that we are lucky to have regulatory agencies that protect us from toxic chemicals in food, water, and air. In fact, there have been some reasonable *attempts* over the past decades by the US Congress to implement effective and appropriate environmental protections: The Food Additives Amendment of 1958, for instance, required the Food and Drug Administration (FDA) to create approaches for testing chemicals in food for safety *before* they enter the US food supply. The Clean Air Act Amendments of 1990 and the Safe Drinking Water Act of 1974 (amended in 1986 and 1996) required the Environmental Protection Agency (EPA) to set national air and water quality standards and to regulate endocrine-disrupting chemicals.

There have been some positive effects of these attempts by Congress to create safety standards. For example, the Clean Air Act has led to the quality of outdoor air in the United States being improved over the past decades, but that has not led to improvement in the quality of the air breathed inside our homes, schools, and businesses. The Safe Drinking Water Act did not end up protecting the residents of Flint, Michigan, and a large number of other communities from toxic levels of lead and other pollutants such as perchlorate (used by the military in explosives) in municipal drinking water. And, in spite of mandates in the Food Additives Amendment of 1958, the vast number (thousands) of chemical additives in the US food supply have never been tested for potential health effects. Moreover, when food additives are actually shown to cause harm, the FDA states that it is unable to take any action! This leads one to wonder if the FDA is ignoring the law due to intense lobbying from chemical corporations.

In the United States, there is a lack of data on potential health effects of the majority of chemicals added either directly to food or indirectly during manufacturing or from packaging. However, the public continues to be assured by the FDA that all of the chemicals in our food and food packaging are safe. The FDA and EPA misrepresent the facts, declaring that safety testing of food, as well as of drinking water and air quality, were performed and results should be trusted by the public, when in fact it is either limited or absent.[29,30] This is a classic example of the maxim, "The absence of *evidence* of harm (due to the absence of any information) is not evidence of an absence of harm."

Then there are chemicals devised by clever chemical companies to substitute for a chemical that has actually been banned from use (although such chemical bans are rare), such as substituting for BPA only in baby bottles and sippy cups while all other uses of BPA are declared safe by the FDA. These substitutes (BPS, BPF, BPSIP, BPZ, etc.) turn out to have the same (or worse) health and safety risks, thus the name, "regrettable substitutions." Flame-retardant chemicals represent a prime example of this whack-a-mole maneuvering; neurotoxic PBDEs replaced neurotoxic PCBs, and are themselves being replaced with a neurotoxic flame-retardant mixture of polybrominated and phosphate compounds, such as Firemaster 550 (see chapter 11). We are essentially on a toxic chemical merry-go-round that no US federal regulatory agency has been able (or willing) to stop.

The Precautionary Principle as the Basis of Chemical Regulation

Many of you reading this may not have heard of the Precautionary Principle, but it is an important concept and one that deserves explanation before moving forward. In 1991, a group of 21 scientists from the United States, Canada, and Europe, gathered at Wingspread, the Johnson Foundation headquarters located in Racine, Wisconsin, and identified the need to apply the Precautionary Principle in managing the risks of toxic chemicals rather than just focusing on corporate profits based on cost-benefit analysis (industry profits vs. the health of people and wildlife). At the 3-day meeting, the Wingspread statement on the Precautionary Principle for regulating endocrine-disrupting chemicals was born. In short, it says: "When an activity raises threats of harm to human health or the environment, precautionary measures should be taken even if some cause and effect relationships are not fully established scientifically."[7] This is an old concept, captured in many traditional aphorisms: "an ounce of prevention is worth a pound of cure," "better safe than sorry," "look before you leap." The Precautionary Principle is also based on the premise that appropriate testing should be required before chemicals are used in products that will result in widespread exposure. In 1992 the United Nations–sponsored "Rio Declaration on Environment and Development" was signed by over 175 countries, including the United States. The declaration endorsed the principle that, "Where there are threats of serious or irreversible damage, lack of full scientific certainty shall not be used as a reason for postponing cost-effective measures to prevent environmental degradation." The Precautionary Principle requires industries and government regulators to weigh the risks to the public rather than primarily the profits of corporations.

Given the importance of this principle, why is precaution a "dirty word" to US regulators but not in most other Western industrialized countries? The unwillingness of US agencies to regulate a large number of man-made chemicals is an example of the dominance of cost-benefit analysis over the Precautionary Principle in the United States. This is a markedly different approach than taken by Europe, where the idea of precaution has been incorporated into environmental laws. Generally, more aggressive action has been taken in Europe to limit exposure to pesticides such as atrazine, which is banned in the European Union (EU); harmful phthalate chemicals in plastic, such as in infant products, are also banned in the EU. France also banned the use of phthalates in medical products (e.g., intravenous tubing, intravenous bags, catheters) used on pregnant women or infants. In Europe, the Precautionary Principle is accepted as the *basis* for chemical regulation.

In the United States, precaution *is* the standard used by the FDA to regulate *drugs*; testing must show drugs to be safe and effective prior to being approved, and the health benefits of the drug must greatly outweigh the potential for harm. However, the division of the FDA that oversees the chemicals used in our *food* (Center for Food Safety and Applied Nutrition; CFSAN) does not follow this approach, allowing for thousands of food chemicals to be used without prior testing.

Example of Where Regulations Have Failed Public Health: Bisphenol A

Bisphenol A (BPA) is made from petroleum. In 1936 it was one of a number of chemicals found to mimic the effects of estrogen, and so was considered for use as a fertility drug. However, in the 1950s chemists found that by linking BPA molecules into chains it became a clear, hard, shatterproof plastic that was named polycarbonate; with some modification it became an epoxy resin that now lines the interior of metal cans used for food and beverages. BPA has become one of the world's highest volume industrial chemicals, with annual production estimated to be almost 9 million tons (over 20 billion pounds). Because of its low cost, industries are reluctant to remove it from thousands of products. Although humans are also exposed to BPA through the skin by exposure to thermal paper (e.g., receipts), dust, and contaminated air,[8] the FDA has primarily been concerned with exposure through ingestion caused by leaching from canned foods and drinks and polycarbonate plastic food containers.[9]

The 1958 Food Additives Amendment was intended "to protect the public health by prohibiting the use of additives in food which have not been adequately tested to establish their safety." The FDA defines "safe" as "a *reasonable certainty* in the minds of competent scientists that the substance is not harmful under its intended conditions of use." However, BPA, along with thousands of other food industry chemicals designated as *generally regarded as safe* (GRAS) were allowed by the FDA to be "grandfathered" into the US food and food packaging system without requirement for safety testing, flagrantly ignoring requirements of the 1958 Food Additives Amendment.[10] Despite the fact that BPA had been shown to have 100% of the efficacy of estrogen produced by women's ovaries, it too was labeled as GRAS and has slowly infiltrated both our food system and our bodies. The FDA has essentially given chemical manufacturers and food corporations complete control of the chemicals added to food, food packaging, and food "washes"[11] since the FDA allows corporations to determine whether chemicals can be declared generally regarded as safe.

Currently, there are over 8,000 published studies reporting health consequences associated with exposure to BPA in both humans and animals: for example, BPA has been identified as a chemical able to disrupt hormones in the human body through interferance not just with estrogen function but also testosterone and thyroid hormone functions. Due to overwhelming international scientific evidence, California placed BPA on its list of enforceable chemicals not allowed in consumer products sold in its state. Also known as Prop 65 or The Safe Drinking Water and Toxic Enforcement Act of 1986, this law provides California to take action to regulate chemicals (such as BPA) that are determined by a state panel to cause cancer (carcinogen) or are determined to be a reproductive or developmental toxin. Canada declared BPA a toxic substance in 2010, and it is both banned for use in baby bottles and considered a chemical of high concern in the EU, Denmark, United Arab Emirates, and China. BPA was banned from use in food-contact packaging in France, and in the EU, BPA is listed as a presumed human carcinogen, mutagen, or reproductive toxicant based on animal studies.

In the United States, despite the overwhelming research on the harmful effects of BPA on humans, it remains in food and beverage containers that are regulated by the food division of the FDA. Although BPA was removed in 2012 from plastic baby bottles and plastic sports bottles in the United States (only after consumers refused to buy these products), dozens of "regrettable substitutes" have since taken its place in products, and research shows that these bisphenol analogues (e.g., BPB, BPF, BPS, BPSIP, BPZ) have similar endocrine-disrupting activity as BPA. So why aren't BPA and its sister chemicals gone from *all* food packaging, when the science shows it leaches from the epoxy coating inside canned foods and from plastic food and drink containers? BPA remains in thousands of US products today, as do its harmful substitutes, due to ineffective regulation by the FDA.

Chemicals in Drinking Water

Lead Contamination

Lead poisoning appears to have been recognized over fifteen hundred years ago as being associated with brain damage and a number of neurologic symptoms (disturbed speech, weak limbs, abnormal gait, tremors, inappropriate laughter, anger, and slobbering). It is possible that the high levels of lead in the pipes that the Romans used to deliver water for drinking and in the pots used for cooking was slowly poisoning people in the Roman Empire. The marvelous new (at the time) technology used aqueducts and lead-based pipes to deliver water to Romans living in cities, and the use of lead-lined cooking pots, was slowly eroding their ability to think.

In the 1960s "lead poisoning" was defined as blood lead levels exceeding 60 µg/dL; at the time, lead was pervasive in a variety of products in the United States. Following extensive research and an uproar from the medical community, who found elevated lead levels in children, regulations went into effect to remove lead from automobile gas, paint, and municipal and household plumbing (and thus drinking water) in the mid-1970s. These regulations resulted in the dramatic decline in blood lead levels of children living in the United States (Figure 1.2).[12]

Over the decades, the "safe level" of lead continued to drop to as low as 10 µg/dL in the 1990s, but it is now accepted by researchers worldwide, and by the American Academy of Pediatrics, that there is *no safe amount of lead*. Despite this consensus, over 500,000 children in the United States are estimated to have blood levels of lead higher than 5 µg/dL (the level

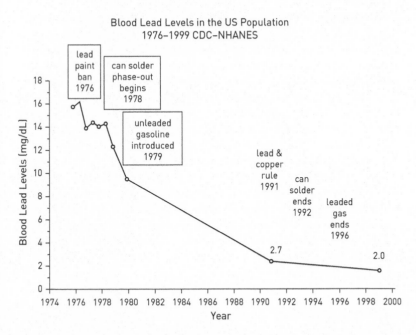

Figure 1.2 Blood levels in the US population over time. There has been a steady decline in blood lead levels since regulation required it to be removed from household paint, gasoline, and other products.

currently deemed safe by the EPA and the level which the CDC recommends public health actions be initiated); these levels cause brain damage and loss of IQ points for the rapidly developing brains of exposed fetuses, infants, and children.

The drinking water contamination in Flint, Michigan, is just one example of a regulatory system gone wrong, in which there were breakdowns at every level of the system. Subsequently, unacceptably high levels of lead in drinking water were found in a large number of other cities. In 2019, it was reported that over 25% of kindergarten students in Cleveland, Ohio, public schools had blood lead levels above 5 µg/dL, and over 90% had detectable lead in their blood.[13] (See chapter 5 for more information on lead in drinking water.)

In the United States, removal of lead from automobile gas, paint, and municipal and household plumbing (and thus from drinking water) was one of the few public health victories of the 20th century in the United States. Legislation was passed despite intense opposition from lead-producing corporations and the Lead Industries Association, the lobbying organization for lead manufacturers. In their book *Deceit and Denial*, Markowitz and Rosner cover the disturbing history of corruption by the Lead Industries Association that resulted in the United States being the last developed country to regulate lead exposure.[14] The history of the corruption by the lead industry offers important insights into how regulatory agencies, members of Congress who accept funding from chemical corporations, and even doctors and scientists who are secretly funded by these corporations, all work together to convince the public that chemicals such as lead are safe at the level established by a regulatory system controlled by corporations that make billions of dollars from the chemical.

Despite this "win," the approach that the US EPA and FDA still take to estimate safe exposure levels is outdated and dominated by decisions designed to protect the interests (profits) of industry, not the health of Americans. Clearly, lead levels that were, and *continue to be,* deemed "safe" (5 µg/dL), are erroneous, and so too are the estimated "safe" levels of many other chemicals used in thousands of products that we are exposed to everyday.

Perchlorate

Perchlorate is one of approximately 10,000 chemicals allowed for use in food and food packaging—and it's also an ingredient in explosives, such as fireworks and rocket fuel. The FDA approved perchlorate for use in plastic packaging and food handling equipment for dry food—like cereal, flour and spices—to reduce the buildup of static charges. Unfortunately, the chemical can migrate from the plastic into food. Perchlorate can also get into food when hypochlorite bleach (used as a disinfectant in food processing and when produce is peeled and washed) is not managed carefully and is allowed to degrade.

The environment on and surrounding military bases is contaminated with perchlorate, which gets into soil and plants and eventually into food and drinking water. Perchlorate is thus a ubiquitous environmental contaminate and it is estimated that virtually everyone in the world is exposed to it at some level.[15]

Perchlorate has been found to have numerous health concerns, but perhaps its effect on the human thyroid gland is the most studied. Perchlorate impairs the thyroid's ability to use iodine in food to make the thyroid hormone T4, which is essential for brain development in fetuses. Thus the presence of perchlorate in the diet and drinking water of pregnant women threatens the maternal ability to produce the thyroid hormone required for normal fetal brain development, and this also subsequently affects brain development and function in young children.

How much perchlorate can fetuses and infants be exposed to without suffering adverse neurobehavioral effects? The US EPA's Office of Solid Waste and Emergency Response (OSWER) set a groundwater preliminary remediation goal (PRG) of 24.5 μg/L to supposedly prevent a level of exposure in a pregnant woman that would affect the fetus. However, this supposed "safe exposure" level by the EPA OSWER actually does not take into account exposure during vulnerable periods of brain development, such as during pregnancy and breast feeding, when higher levels of exposure to perchlorate can lead to brain damage, decreased IQ, and other neurobehavioral effects (more on vulnerable periods in chapter 3). For example, high levels of perchlorate have also been found in the breast milk of nursing mothers.[16]

Because iodine is not made by the human body and must come from the diet, iodine deficiency can make health effects from perchlorate exposure even more severe. Americans used to obtain iodine from enriched bread and from table salt as part of the push for manufacturers to take part in public health measures. But iodine is no longer added to bread and other staple foods, and many Americans no longer consume table salt but opt for sea salt instead; sea salt often does not contain iodine, leaving many people iodine deficient and at increased risk for the development of thyroid abnormalities (hypothyroidism) and leading to poor transfer of iodine from a pregnant woman to a developing fetus, impeding healthy brain development.

Perchlorate is yet another example of an industrial food chemical that was pushed through the system with limited safety testing and designated as GRAS, but which has been found to be harmful to human health. Yet it continues to infiltrate our food system with no end in sight.

Chemicals in Food: Glyphosate and Monsanto's Roundup

Glyphosate is the most widely used weed killer in the United States and around the world as of 2020. The Monsanto Corporation (now owned by the German corporation Bayer) developed and patented the use of glyphosate to kill weeds in the 1970s and first brought it to market in 1974, under the Roundup brand name; it is no longer protected by patent and is marketed under different names by different companies, with glyphosate being combined with different formulations of chemicals (more on glyphosate in chapter 4).[17] In 2015, the World Health Organization's (WHO) International Agency for Research on Cancer (IARC) concluded that glyphosate, the active ingredient in Roundup, is a probable human carcinogen. Despite several high profile civil court cases in 2019 with multimillion dollar awards going to cancer-stricken plaintiffs, the US EPA continues to insist that Roundup is safe. Monsanto's attempts to discredit the IARC conclusion about Roundup are being rejected by juries, but not by government regulators, who continue to allow glyphosate to be used in US farming and food production, as well as for pest control in public and community parks and recreation areas nationwide.

Chemicals in Household Items

Thousands of chemicals have been designed for function (as opposed to for fragrance or for appearance). One group of "functional" chemicals, also known as perfluoroalkyls (PFAS), are used in consumer products such as nonstick pans (Teflon), water-repellent fabrics, firefighting foams, pizza boxes, microwave popcorn bags, stain-resistant carpets, furniture, baby clothes and other baby products, electronics, and other goods. PFAS chemicals are created using the element fluorine, one of the halogens (along with chlorine, bromine, iodine) on the periodic table. Because fluorine bonds tightly to carbons in these molecules, halogens do not break down over time (they persist in the environment and in the bodies of animals and humans, which they enter via migration from everyday materials and by sticking to dust particles) and accumulate in the environment and make their way into the human body. Dust also serves as a source of exposure to other chemicals such as BPA and phthalates that migrate out of plastic, that people are exposed to in their homes.[18] PFAS chemicals, BPA, phthalates, and flame-retardant chemicals containing bromine are linked to neurological deficits in children, developmental problems, impaired fertility, and other health risks (see chapter 11).[19]

Corruption behind US Flame Retardants

Health hazards of perfluorinated compounds, PFAS and PFOA, came to public attention in the United States in 2013, not from the EPA, but from an explosive Pulitzer Prize–winning series of articles in the *Chicago Tribune*. Journalists revealed decades of fraud and corruption by Dupont, which was a main producer of perfluorinated chemicals. The EPA's failure to regulate perfluorinated compounds was also brought into the spotlight. Dupont used product-protection strategies similar to the approaches perfected by the tobacco companies and also used by the Lead Industries Association and BPA industries. This strategy, according to the *Chicago Tribune*, involved buying doctors and scientists to produce fraudulent (completely made up) or clearly flawed research designed to promote the use of these highly persistent and toxic compounds; these fraudulent studies were also used to defend the products in court. The producers of flame retardants engaged in decades of deception to get laws passed mandating the use of what are now known to be highly toxic flame retardants in many household products.

The series of *Chicago Tribune* articles identified a litany of errors in US laws regarding flame-retardant chemicals; the most egregious being that "federal law [1976 Toxic Substances Control Act or TSCA] made it practically impossible to ban hazardous chemicals." The *Chicago Tribune* articles revealed that unscrupulous lawyers wrote legislation protecting flame-retardant manufacturers, lobbyists strong-armed congressional votes, and doctors were paid by the flame-retardant industry to lie under oath about the potential health risks, netting corporations such as Dupont and 3M billions of dollars in profits. Corporations are now facing potentially large judgements in suits, including a lawsuit filed in 2019 by the Attorney

General of New Jersey against Dupont, 3M, and six other manufacturers of flame retardants alleging consumer and environmental fraud.

Hazardous Waste: Where Does It Come From and Where Does It All Go?

Industrial productivity comes with a cost. Worldwide, only a handful of countries are capable of keeping up with waste production efficiently. Recycling programs are costly and typically do not meet expectations and return on investment. Much of the waste generated, be it plastic materials, industrial solvents, or dyes used in textiles, end up in landfills where the materials breakdown and make their way into fresh waterways and oceans. For hazardous waste, such as industrial chemicals, fracking chemicals, and used medical waste, disposal becomes even more complicated due to state and local laws. Our history is rife with stories of unlawful and clandestine disposal practices by chemical companies that led to decades of contamination of soil and water, and the subsequent aftermath of human and wildlife health effects. One of the most well-known examples is the suit brought against Pacific Gas and Electric for contaminating drinking water in Hinkley, California with hexavalent chromium, which resulted in a 333 million dollar verdict against the corporation and made Erin Brockovich famous.

As of June 12, 2019, there were 1344 Superfund sites (hazardous waste material sites) on the National Priorities List (NPL) in the United States.[20] As of 2020, New Jersey has the highest number of Superfund sites (105), with California (97) second, and Pennsylvania third (95). In the early days of the EPA, the agency had a challenging situation in gaining public trust because of the health-related impacts of contaminants reported from some communities. Perhaps the most well known of these hazardous waste sites is the Love Canal site in New York. The site was created from the disposal of more than 21,000 tons of hazardous chemicals from 1942 to 1953 in the abandoned Love Canal Landfill. The landfill was covered with soil and the property was used for the construction of a school and developed into a residential area. Complaints about odors and residues were first reported during the 1960s and these complaints grew with time. As a result of *two* presidential declarations (by President Jimmy Carter), approximately 950 of the more than 1,050 families in the Emergency Declaration Area (EDA), a 10-square-block area surrounding the Love Canal landfill, were evacuated.[21]

The severity of the site's contamination ultimately led to the creation of federal legislation to manage the disposal of hazardous wastes throughout the country. This legislation was titled the Comprehensive Environmental Response, Compensation and Liability Act (CERCLA) (Superfund Law) of 1980. The EPA's Superfund program was established to identify, assess, and clean up the nation's worst hazardous waste sites to protect both human health and the environment. Unfortunately, the EPA's ecological risk-assessment paradigm has remained unchanged since its inception 30 years ago, despite repeated criticism by environmental scientists over the years.[22] And it appears that cleanup for these sites is a never-ending game of whack-a-mole, with new sites being added to the list faster than old sites can be cleaned up. The EPA has even set up an interactive Superfund search website where you can "search for sites near you" on a map and check their vicinity to your home, local school, and hospitals.[23] Not a fun thing to have to do!

Most Americans are not aware that nationally, military bases are among the most contaminated sites. Until recently, there were estimated to be about 140 contaminated military sites in the United States, but that number has grown dramatically due to findings that PFAS chemicals, a class of toxic fire-retardant chemicals, are pervasive throughout these sites, as well as at airports nationally. Approximately 1 in 10 Americans lives within 10 miles of a contaminated military site. The poisoning of soldiers and their families at Camp Lejeune in North Carolina for decades through drinking water wells contaminated with perchloroethylene (PCE or PERC), remains one of the greatest tragedies in US military history. Adding to this tragedy and enormous sickness and loss of life, the US government has not admitted fault for the pervasive contamination, paid reparations to stricken families, or addressed hundreds of other military bases that continue to expose military personnel and their families to toxic chemicals.[24-27]

Politics and Chemicals Safety

Today, an enormous number of the environmental mandates in laws passed by Congress are under political attack. It is astonishing that in the United States, having air, water, and food free of toxic chemicals has become a partisan political issue instead of a *basic right* for people. Many countries that do not have environmental regulatory agencies follow the behavior of US regulatory agencies as a guide for determining what is safe for *their own* citizens. Thus, the failures of US regulatory agencies have global implications.

Recently we have witnessed the bold moves by states, counties, and cities, to step in and pass legislation to regulate chemicals shown to be toxic. This is frequently countered by state or federal legislation mandating that only their legislatures can determine environmental policy, not local communities (this policy is referred to as "preemption"). However, states such as California continue to lead the way with progressive environmental policies and regulations, setting an example for other states to follow.

A Call to Arms: Environmental Activism

In 1962, Rachel Carson, a marine biologist and perhaps the finest nature writer of the 20th century, raised widespread public concern about the use of DDT and other pesticides with her book, *Silent Spring*. She detailed the reduction of bird species and numbers in areas sprayed with DDT, one of many pesticides that were used extensively beginning in the 1940s. She warned of the dangers to all natural systems from the misuse of chemical pesticides such as DDT, and questioned the scope and direction of modern science. Carson questioned the assumption by both government and private science that human domination of nature was the correct course for the future. She raised difficult questions, such as why humans had the right to control nature, to decide who lives or dies, to poison or to destroy non-human life. Although she was just one voice in a sea of naysayers, her voice and literary talent reverberated around the world, and she brought attention to the risks to healthy ecosystems posed by man-made chemicals as well as the potential effects on human health.

Other voices followed Carson: environmentalists, biologists, epidemiologists, and botanists. Zoologists, like Theo Colborn, and John Peterson Myers pioneers in the field of endocrine disruption. Colborn's research helped identify chemicals that interfere with hormones and other chemical messengers that control development in wildlife and humans. Colborn and Myers spoke up, and their 1996 book, *Our Stolen Future*, has been translated into dozens of languages.

In the 1970s physicians like Phillip Landrigan and Herbert Needleman raised awareness about the health effects of lead in children by asking mothers to send in their children's baby teeth for lead analysis. Their findings lead to the phasing out of lead in gasoline and paints in the late 1970s, culminating in an 88% drop in lead levels in American children by 2005.[28] They spoke up.

Students, community activists, tribal leaders—the list of voices that have fought against big pharma, corporate greed, and environmental pollution through the decades, is long. Standing on the shoulders of our predecessors, we can all speak up to raise awareness about environmental issues, and we can work together to take care of our planet and each other. Whether we are working in small academic laboratories, teaching elementary school, volunteering in the community, raising money to support communities in need, fighting for policy change on Capitol Hill, or just trying to raise our own healthy children, there is a role for all of us to clean up our planet and our bodies—NOW is the time!

> **Never doubt that a small group of thoughtful, committed citizens can change the world; indeed, it's the only thing that ever has.**
> —*Margaret Meade, American cultural anthropologist (1901–1978)*

Ways to Get Involved

- Get familiar with your environment: look up the air quality in your neighborhood (e.g., via the app AirNow from the EPA), monitor water reports for municipal water contamination, follow local environmental forums, become a member of local environmental boards, register to vote!
- Write to your senators and members of Congress about environmental issues that affect you and your family.
- Support vetted, reputable nonprofit organizations that work to improve local, state, and global environments.
- Stay informed about environmental issues on a daily basis through Environmental Health News (EHN.org) and their free Above the Fold, which delivers a daily news digest straight to your inbox, with links to top news worldwide on environmental health and climate (www.ehn.org/environmental-health-news-2507514432.html).
- Vote with your dollars: purchase non-toxic, ecofriendly, and sustainable products. Example: Mind the Store (https://saferchemicals.org/mind-the-store/), which is a nonprofit group that ranks retailers on toxic chemicals and creates a report card on retailer actions to eliminate toxic chemicals in their products published by the Mind the Store Campaign of the national nonprofit Safer Chemicals, Healthy Families (see Table 11.1).
- Contact manufacturers and let them know your opinion about their products.

- Learn about other communities that may be fighting for "environmental justice" over water contamination, air quality, disrupted ecosystems, and toxic waste disposal, and show your support!

Take-Home Message

Humans have evolved over millions of years and developed the mental capacity to create new materials and products to improve food storage, modernize transportation, and potentially reduce the use of natural resources. However, we have been shortsighted regarding downstream effects of many man-made inventions. Environmental chemicals are now pervasive and found in the bodies of all human beings who are examined throughout the world, and we are now discovering the health effects on humans, wildlife, and ecosystems. Since the regulatory system in the United States is not functioning as it should to protect the public from chemicals known to cause harm to human health, as well as pets and wildlife, it is *up to individuals* to learn how to reduce the number and amounts of toxic chemicals in your environment, and this book was written to guide you.

References

1. Eaton SB. The ancestral human diet: what was it and should it be a paradigm for contemporary nutrition? *Proc Nutr Soc.* 2006;65(1):1–6.
2. Thapa S, Short RV, Potts M. Breast feeding, birth spacing and their effects on child survival. *Nature.* 1988;335(6192):679–682.
3. Cordain L, Eaton SB, Sebastian A, et al. Origins and evolution of the Western diet: health implications for the 21st century. *Am J Clin Nutr.* 2005;81(2): 341–354.
4. Eaton SB, Eaton SB, 3rd. Paleolithic vs. modern diets—selected pathophysiological implications. *Eur J Nutr.* 2000;39(2):67–70.
5. Environmental Working Group (EWG). PCBs in farmed salmon: wild versus farmed, http://www.ewg.org/research/pcbs-farmed-salmon/wild-versus-farmed. Published 2003. Accessed May 16, 2016.
6. Jacobson JL, Jacobson SW. Intellectual impairment in children exposed to polychlorinated biphenyls in utero. *New Engl J Med.* 1996;335(11):783–789.
7. deFur PL, Kaszuba M. Implementing the precautionary principle. *Sci Total Environ.* 2002;288(1–2):155–165.

8. Hormann AM, vom Saal FS, Nagel SC, et al. Holding thermal receipt paper and eating food after using hand sanitizer results in high serum bioactive and urine total levels of bisphenol A (BPA). *PLoS One.* 2014;9(10):e110509.

9. Lorber M, Schecter A, Paepke O, Shropshire W, Christensen K, Birnbaum L. Exposure assessment of adult intake of bisphenol A (BPA) with emphasis on canned food dietary exposures. *Environ Int.* 2015;77:55–62.

10. Maffini MV, Neltner TG, Vogel S. We are what we eat: regulatory gaps in the United States that put our health at risk. *PLoS Biology.* 2017;15(12):e2003578.

11. Consumer Reports. GRAS: the hidden substances in your food. https://www.consumerreports.org/food-safety/gras-hidden-ingredients-in-your-food/. Published 2016. Accessed December 23, 2019.

12. Markowitz M. Lead poisoning. *Pedatr Rev/American Academy of Pediatrics.* 2000;21(10):327–335.

13. EPA's proposed "secret science" rule directly threatens children's health. https://theconversation.com/epas-proposed-secret-science-rule-directly-threatens-childrens-health-128769. Published 2020. Accessed January 10, 2020.

14. Markowitz G, Rosner D. *Deceit and Denial: Deadly Politics of Industrial Pollution.* 1st ed. Berkeley: University of California Press; 2002.

15. White House and Pentagon Bias National Academy Perchlorate Report. https://www.nrdc.org/resources/white-house-and-pentagon-bias-national-academy-perchlorate-report. Published 2005. Accessed January 1, 2020.

16. Ginsberg GL, Hattis DB, Zoeller RT, Rice DC. Evaluation of the U.S. EPA/OSWER preliminary remediation goal for perchlorate in groundwater: focus on exposure to nursing infants. *Environ Health Perspect.* 2007;115(3):361–369.

17. Herbicides & Trade Names. https://www.weedbusters.org.nz/weed-information/herbicides-trade-names/. Accessed January 10, 2020.

18. Mitro SD, Dodson RE, Singla V, et al. Consumer product chemicals in indoor dust: a quantitative meta-analysis of U.S. studies. *Environmental Science & Technology.* 2016.

19. Dishaw LV, Macaulay LJ, Roberts SC, Stapleton HM. Exposures, mechanisms, and impacts of endocrine-active flame retardants. *Curr Opin Pharmacol.* 2014;19:125–133.

20. Environmental Protection Agency (EPA). Superfund: National Priorities List (NPL). https://www.epa.gov/superfund/superfund-national-priorities-list-npl. Published 2019. Accessed December 9, 2019.

21. EPA. Superfund Site: Love Canal Niagara Falls, NY. https://cumulis.epa.gov/supercpad/SiteProfiles/index.cfm?fuseaction=second.Cleanup&id=0201290#bkground. Published 2019. Accessed December 15, 2019.

22. Tannenbaum LV. Commentary: an open appeal to the EPA for Superfund ERA reform. *Ennviron Pollut (Barking, Essex: 1987).* 2019:113308.

23. EPA. Search Superfund Site Information. https://cumulis.epa.gov/supercpad/cursites/srchsites.cfm. Accessed April 24, 2020.

24. Ruckart PZ, Bove FJ, Maslia M. Evaluation of exposure to contaminated drinking water and specific birth defects and childhood cancers at Marine Corps Base Camp Lejeune, North Carolina: a case-control study. *Environmental Health: A Global Access Science Source.* 2013;12:104.

25. Ruckart PZ, Bove FJ, Shanley E, 3rd, Maslia M. Evaluation of contaminated drinking water and male breast cancer at Marine Corps Base Camp Lejeune, North Carolina: a case control study. *Environmental Health: A Global Access Science Source.* 2015;14:74.

26. Morrison J. Perfluoinated chemicals linked to military bases, airports. https://cen.acs.org/articles/94/web/2016/08/Perfluorinated-chemicals-linked-military-bases.html. Published 2016. Accessed December 9, 2019.

27. Nazaryan A. Camp Lejeune and the U.S. military's polluted legacy. *Newsweek* July 16, 2014. https://www.newsweek.com/2014/07/25/us-military-supposed-protect-countrys-citizens-and-soldiers-not-poison-them-259103.html. Accessed April 24, 2020.

28. Benson SM, Talbott EO, Brink LL, Wu C, Sharma RK, Marsh GM. Environmental lead and childhood blood lead levels in US children: NHANES, 1999–2006. *Archives of Environmental & Occupational Health.* 2017;72(2):70–78.

29. Maffini MV, Neltner TG, Vogel S. We are what we eat: regulatory gaps in the United States that put our health at risk. *PLoS Biol* 2017;15;e2003578.

30. Vogel SA. *Is It Safe: BPA and the Struggle to Define the Safety of Chemicals.* Berkeley: University of California Press, 2013.

2

How the Human Endocrine and Immune Systems Are Disrupted by Chemical Exposures

I stand in awe of my body.

—Henry David Thoreau (1817–1862)

As described in chapter 1, in contrast to the initial millions of years of human evolution, modern humans have become increasingly inundated by a variety of exposures, particularly over the last few centuries. In addition to exposure to synthetic chemicals, other factors influence human health, including microwave radiation from cell phones, chronic emotional and physical stress, disruption of sleep wake cycles by synthetic light, and lack of adequate sleep.

This chapter presents the background information needed to understand how all of these *new* exposures and the modern lifestyle affect the human body and lead to poor health. The objective is to provide you with an understanding of the miraculous, intricate workings of the human body and a detailed look at how the endocrine and immune systems develop and are programmed to protect and defend us, particularly from man-made chemical "intruders" and other harmful environmental influences. We show that fetuses and infants are to a large degree defenseless while these defense systems are developing; in addition, the functioning of these systems throughout the remainder of life can be disrupted, contributing to many of chronic diseases that we face in modern society.

The Immune System 101: Our Defense Systems against Toxins

Our first line of defense against invaders consists of physical barriers such as skin. Skin is the largest organ of the human body, covering roughly 2 square meters in a fully grown adult. Skin is pretty tough, because it has several layers of cells; these cells keep it mostly waterproof, allow it to protect and cushion interior organs, and help manage body temperature. But skin is also very absorbent, as we know from using skin-softening lotions and topical medications (used for conditions such as arthritis, nausea, and menopause symptoms), which are specifically designed to get into the blood stream through the skin. Harnessing this absorptive property for medications has been an advancement in the treatment of many health conditions, as we will see in chapter 6 ("Medications Are Chemicals Too"), but we now know that human skin cannot always differentiate between what is *healthy* for the body and what it *harmful* to it. Skin-penetrating chemicals that are used in medications are *also* added to personal care products to allow other chemicals to be absorbed rapidly into the blood stream, perhaps to one's own detriment! On average, women use more products with skin-penetrating chemicals than men, whose skin is thicker and therefore more protective than women's skin.

The human immune system is basically composed of two systems or "teams," which are each made up of many "players." The teams are the "innate" and the "adaptive immune system," and each system has within its ranks numerous molecules that all work together to fight off invaders (see Figure 2.1.)

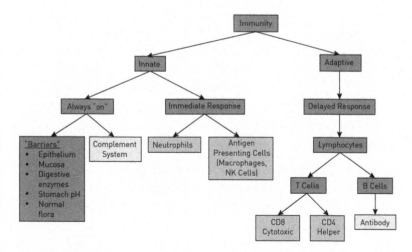

Figure 2.1 The human immune system.

The innate immune system is a "hard-wired" defense that has evolved over millions of years to recognize pathogens (bad guys) that have commonly infected humans. Essentially, the innate immune system acts as a powerful, rapid alert system to respond to common, everyday invaders. It is composed of a many foot soldiers: complement, macrophages, phagocytes, neutrophils and natural killer (NK) cells.

The adaptive immune system, on the other hand, changes throughout our entire lifespan to protect us against invaders that we have never encountered before. For example, doctors take advantage of the adaptive immune system by using vaccines to intentionally prime the body to protect it from likely invaders, such as the flu; measles, mumps, and rubella infections; common pneumonias; and the herpes virus that can cause shingles.

B-Cells and T-Cells

The "foot soldiers" in the adaptive immune system, called B-cells, make antibodies ("resistance fighters") specifically directed to attack something infectious, such as a virus or bacteria. Antibodies fan out throughout the body to attack the invader. The four main classes of antibodies—IgG, IgM, IgA, and IgE—have a unique structure in order to pair up with a specific "invader." Antibodies will "remember" that invader for the rest of the life of that human, and if it should ever strike again, the response will be faster and more directed, thanks to the "memory" of those B-cells.

T-cells, of which there are several types, are another weapon of the adaptive immune system. T-cells only recognize invaders that are "properly presented" by specialized antigen-presenting cells (APCs). Before T-cells can spring into action they must be activated, which helps ensure that only useful weapons will be mobilized. Once T-cells are activated, helper-T cells orchestrate the immune response, and killer T-cells destroy infected cells. Essentially, weapons in the adaptive immune system are made on demand so as not to waste energy and resources!

So, why is all of this important? First, because it illustrates the vast intricacies of the human immune system, and second, it shows that the slightest provocation or irritant, be it intentional (e.g., medication or personal care exposure) or by chance (e.g., pollen) can set off a whole host of events; thus doing its job to surveil and respond. However, an error in the normal workings of the immune system may even direct its weapons toward its own body—also known as an autoimmune response. Throughout our lifetime, the healthy immune system tolerates itself, but when self-tolerance is disturbed, the immune system becomes dysregulated, resulting in the emergence of an autoimmune disease. Autoimmune diseases, such as rheumatoid arthritis, lupus, multiple sclerosis, and Crohn's disease, are diseases in which the human body has essentially turned on itself, mistaking friend (your body) for foe (foreign invaders), and unleashing an erroneous attack. The ability to recognize the difference between your cells and invading cells begins in early embryonic life, and this ability continues to gradually develop. During "critical windows" in development, such as embryonic life, chemical exposures may affect different components of the immune system.[1]

So, can exposure to a specific chemical *cause* autoimmune disease? It's never an easy task to establish a true cause-and-effect relationship in the human body, given each individual's genetics as well as the host of outside influences or confounders that may contribute (such as lifestyle, diet, stress, medications, history of infection, and other environmental exposures). However, we can learn a lot from occupational exposures, where several workers may experience similar health problems due to being exposed to a specific chemical. For example, several studies looked at workers who were exposed to vinyl chloride in plastic factories and developed autoimmune liver disease.[2] Workers exposed to silica dust, industrial solvents, and heavy metals develop scleroderma, an autoimmune disease involving the skin, lungs, and heart, at higher rates than the general population.[3]

But it's not just factory workers exposed to high levels of a specific chemical that scientists are looking at, it's also the general public, the everyday consumer. Researchers have discovered that many chemicals in products that we use *every day* have the ability to affect our highly sensitive immune systems. Take BPA, which we described earlier as a pervasive plastic chemical found in canned foods and drinks, on cash register receipts, in plastic food storage containers, and in plastic toys. Although much attention has been focused on BPA for its ability to disrupt endocrine hormone function, it also has the ability to activate many immune pathways involved in autoimmunity. It is believed that BPA has the potential to amplify and disrupt signaling between the foot soldiers of both the innate and adaptive immune system, increase fighting-cell activity, disrupt liver enzymes that are supposed to alter BPA to facilitate removal by the kidney, and reduce cells that keep the immune system "quiet" and inactive[4] (see Figure 2.2).

Lab tests have shown that chemicals in processed foods (e.g., sodium) increase immune system activity.[5] One study showed that sugar-sweetened soda increased the development of rheumatoid arthritis![6] Other risks for developing an autoimmune reaction include other "chemicals," such as heavy antibiotic use as a child, first- and second-hand tobacco smoke exposure, pesticide exposure, and not having been breast-feed. Exposure to some infections, vitamin D deficiency, and even childhood trauma have also been shown to increase risk for some autoimmune diseases.[7-14] It is estimated that almost 5% of the world's population will eventually develop an autoimmune disease,

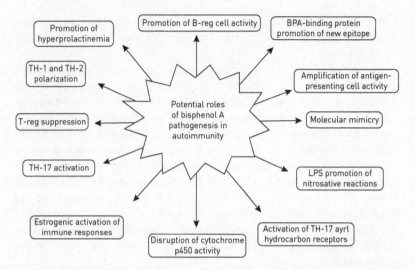

Figure 2.2 This diagram illustrates the potential mechanisms of bisphenol A's promotion of autoimmunity. BPA: bisphenol A; B-reg cell: regulatory B cell; LPS: lipopolysaccharide; TH: T-helper; T-reg: regulatory T cell.[3-5]

and that number continues to grow.[15,16] Whether this growth is due to better detection and reporting by doctors, or because of an actual increase in environmental exposure, is unclear.

So should we all stop eating, drinking, and taking our medications? No, of course not. It's about making smart choices when it comes to our lifestyle, including food quality and preparation method, drinking water, exercise, sleep, stress management, and thoughtful and judicious medication use.

The Endocrine System 101

For most of us, hormones are about all we know of the human endocrine system. Hormones are created by many different glands in the body, in order to signal or communicate between organs (see Figure 2.3). For instance, the female ovaries produce the hormone estrogen to regulate the development of an egg in order to make a baby, but estrogen is essential for the functioning of the testes in males.[17] Testosterone, which is critical for male reproductive function by signaling the formation of sperm in the testes, also influences libido in women. Thyroid hormone, produced by the thyroid gland, tells different parts of the human body what level of energy to use, coordinates heart rate and metabolism, controls digestive function, and is critical for normal brain development (during the initial period of fetal development, the fetus is entirely dependent on thyroid hormone produced by the mother, and even a small decrease in maternal thyroid levels can lead to a permanent decrease in the child's IQ).[18]

Endocrine-Disrupting Chemicals: How the Endocrine System Can Get Fooled

One class of environmental chemicals is the endocrine-disrupting chemicals (EDCs), so named because they can disrupt the normal workings of the endocrine system. They may look and act like a hormone (estrogen, for example), but continuous exposure to extra estrogenic chemicals can cause a whole host of unwanted changes, such as breast tumor development; conversely, they may act as a hormone antagonist (e.g., the drug tamoxifen, which blocks estrogen action and is used to treat breast cancer). A chemical with either antiestrogen or antitestosterone activity would impair fertility. Other chemicals may cause hypothyroidism, interfering with the thyroid gland's ability to produce sufficient thyroid hormone; effects include weight gain, fatigue, joint pain, and hair loss. If this occurs while a women is pregnant, permanent damage to fetal brain development (leading to lower IQ of the child) will be the result. (See figure 2.5.)

The science of medicine has come a long way from the time of blood-letting and amputations in order to cure simple infections, and new discoveries about the human body and its inner workings continue to emerge. In the early 1980s, researchers discovered the vast interplay of the stomach bacteria *Helicobacter pylori* that had the odd ability to create ulcers in the stomach lining; this discovery was initially ridiculed by the scientific community. In the early 1990s, there was a similar skeptical response to the prediction that EDCs could be the cause of both infertility in wildlife and a dramatic increase in noncommunicable disease in the US population and elsewhere.[19]

In April 2018, a new human organ called the mesentery was discovered. The mesentery is a network of tissues found throughout the body, wrapping around the entire digestive tract, the lungs, and every artery and vein. It was originally thought to be a fragmented structure, made up of several parts, but new evidence shows that the mesentery is one continuous organ, defined as being made up of cells adapted to perform a specific function. It now holds the distinct honor of being the 79th organ in the human body, reclassified a mere 100 years after its original discovery as merely an anatomical finding.[20]

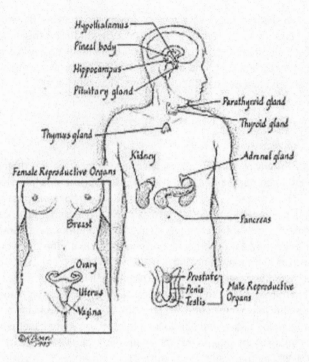

Figure 2.3 The human endocrine system and glands.

Similar to these new discoveries and the bounty of information that followed, there are now tens of thousands of peer-reviewed studies in the scientific literature regarding endocrine disrupters. This new class of chemicals has shaken the foundations of the field of toxicology. Back in the 1500s Paracelsus, the physician known as the forefather of toxicology, famously described an increase in health risk with an increase in dose as the core assumption in toxicology; toxicologists today have shortened this to "the dose makes the poison." His theory was that dose and effect move together in a predictable direction, never changing direction of the response as the dose increases, such as first stimulating and then inhibiting a response. In other words, lower exposures to hazardous compounds were predicted to always generate lower risks. This core assumption has defined our actions in medicine, chemical safety testing, and in everyday life. This asssumption seemed reasonable: the greater the amount of ice cream you eat, the more likely you are to get a stomach ache.

However, the ice cream analogy is completely irrelevant with regard to understanding the risks posed by very low doses of EDCs, because hormones act through specialized receptors at minute doses. Jumping forward to the 1990s, centuries after Paracelsus proposed his foundation assumption, scientists discovered that many environmental chemicals don't follow that playbook—and in fact they can cause harm at very, very small dosages, and the type of harm can differ between very low and higher exposures! Instead of a linear or monotonic response, EDCs often show a nonmonotonic response that when graphed looks like a "U" or an "inverted U" (see Figure 2.4). There are over 1000 known EDCs, and many have been shown to exhibit a nonmonotonic dose-response relationship. This includes the chemical BPA, the widely used pesticide atrazine, phthalates used in plastics and fragrances, as well as flame-retardant chemicals, several vitamins, essential nutrients, and pharmaceuticals. One example that is acknowledged by physicians is the estrogenic drug tamoxifen, which is prescribed to women with estrogen-responsive breast cancer to inhibit tumor progression. At high doses tamoxifen blocks the ability of estrogen to stimulate breast cancer cells, but it has been known for over 40 years that at low doses tamoxifen stimulates breast cancer (known as "tamoxifen flare"), showing that low doses of this drug can result in an effect opposite to that seen at high doses.[21,22] The fact that natural hormones, hormonal drugs, and EDCs all commonly show nonmonotonic dose-response relationships demonstrates that the core assumption of toxicology, that only very high doses of chemicals need to be studied to understand their risks to the public at much lower exposures, is false. Yet, as of 2020, the FDA, EPA, and other federal agencies still refuse to abandon the 16th-century dogma that testing only high doses of a chemical is sufficient to predict what EDCs will do at the low doses commonly encountered by people.

Even over-the-counter medications, such as Tylenol and ibuprofen, which we use every day, including during pregnancy, have been shown to behave as endocrine disruptors. Mixtures of many endocrine-disrupting chemicals (typical of human exposures) can also lead to additive effects, not seen if only individual endocrine-disrupting chemicals are studied, which is how regulatory agencies assess chemical risks.[23]

Endocrine-disrupting chemicals are the subject of worldwide concern. A report published in February 2013 by the United Nations Environment Programme (UNEP) and WHO, titled "State of the Science of Endocrine-Disrupting Chemicals—2012," stated that EDCs are "a global threat that should be addressed."[24] European and US medical and scientific societies have come out with statement policies on the health effects of EDCs:[25]

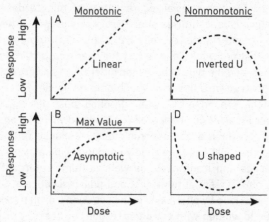

Nonmonotonic Dose-Response Relationships are Common for Endocrine-Disrupting Chemicals

FIGURE 2.4 Dose-response (D-R) curves in toxicological experiments showing D-R-relationships that are monotonic (Panel A and B), where the direction of the response does not change as dose increases) and nonmonotonic (Panel C and D), where the direction of the response changes as dose increases. The central assumption governing evaluation of safety of environmental chemicals by regulatory agency toxicologists is that D-R relationships are always monotonic, based on the proposition from the early 1500s that "the dose makes the poison" (i.e., the higher the dose the greater the effect). However, this assumption is false for hormones, hormonal drugs and endocrine-disrupting chemicals (EDCs). EDCs stimulate an increase in response at low (parts-per-trillion to parts-per-billion) doses via activating specific receptors in target tissues, but inhibit the same responses via inhibiting those receptors while eliciting other unexpected responses at high doses (via "cross-talk" with different receptors for other hormones), resulting in inverted U D-R curves (Panel C). Monotonic D-R curves can be linear (Panel A) or reach a maximum value (the asymptote) and then level off (Panel B). Nonmonotonic D-R curves can start to increase at low doses (Panel C) and then decrease (change direction) as dose continues to increase forming an inverted U D-R curve. For a response that is naturally high to begin with (Panel D), as dose begins to increase the response decreases, but then as dose further increases the response changes direction and begins to increase, forming a U-shaped response.

the American Academy of Pediatrics Council on Environmental Health expressed their concern in 2011;[26] the American Academy of Obstetrics and Gynecology and the American Society for Reproductive Medicine responded in 2013;[27] and the International Federation of Gynecology and Obstetrics made their statement in 2015.[28,29] The Endocrine Society has published many policy statements regarding EDC health risks.[30-32] But risk to human health is not the only alarming issue. The economic impact on society of EDCs and other toxic chemicals is growing; the cost to the US economy alone due to disease management and lost wages is estimated to be $340 billion annually.[33,34]

Body Burden: Measuring Chemicals in Humans

So how do we know if humans are truly exposed to harmful environmental chemicals? Many biomonitoring studies in the United States and around the world look at human bodily fluids and tissue to assess exposure levels to a variety of chemicals. Body fluids such as blood, urine, sweat, semen, breast milk, as well as human tissues such as fat, bone, and organ samples, are analyzed to estimate exposures to an array of worldwide industrial, food, and agricultural chemicals.

In 1956 Congress mandated that the CDC set up ongoing assessments of diseases in adults all across the US population. Over time, nutrition and environmental chemicals were added to this ongoing study. An environmental chemical refers to a chemical compound or chemical element present in air, water, food, soil, dust, or other environmental media (e.g., consumer products). The CDC National Health and Nutrition Examination Survey (NHANES) involves a set of mobile trucks that travel to selected parts of the country to set up shop. Researchers and clinicians examine a total of approximately 2,500 US residents during each 2-year exam period, asking them questions about their medical conditions, medication use, diet and lifestyle, and psychiatric status. Volunteer residents undergo extensive physical exams and diagnostic tests, and researchers collect blood and urine samples. This ongoing study collects enormous amounts of data that are posted online (https://www.cdc.gov/nchs/nhanes/index.htm) and are thus available for use by researchers to learn about a variety of medical conditions and human habits. With the advent in the early 21st century of testing for environmental chemicals, researchers have been able to relate diseases, and many other outcomes that are recorded, to chemical exposures and other aspects of the volunteer's lifestyle. Each year more questions are added and more chemicals are measured. The most recent report, which came out in 2019, contains information on 75 previously untested compounds, for a total of 212 compounds measured; for the first time, it included levels of 30 previously unlisted solvents. Called the CDC Fourth National Report on Human Exposure to Environmental Chemicals or "the fourth report," the CDC looked at US residents from 1999 through 2016. It showed that the majority of individuals tested were exposed to a vast array of chemicals; acrylamides, cotinine (found in smokers), trihalomethanes, bisphenol A, phthalates, chlorinated pesticides, triclosan, organophosphate pesticides, pyrethroids, heavy metals, aromatic hydrocarbons, polybrominated diphenyl ethers, benzophenone from sunblock, perfluorocarbons from nonstick coatings and flame retardants, and a host of polychlorinated biphenyls and solvents in their blood and urine samples.

Using NHANES data, folate use among pregnant women was studied, leading to a recommendation for changes to pre-pregnancy and pregnancy nutrition policy in order to help prevent neural tube defects, like spina bifida, from low folic acid intake, which is common in the United States. The obesity epidemic is followed through the data gleaned from NHANES. Researchers and doctors continue to use these results to adjust nutrition standards, the number and classes of chemicals tested, epidemiological trends, and to identify exposures of various populations. NHANES data have revealed the importance of socioeconomic background and different subcultures, zip codes (identifying cancer and other disease clusters), and age groups, which can be compared with national averages.[35] A disturbing recent development is that because of a lack of adequate funding, the CDC's assay methods rely on indirect methods to estimate (using models that are not appropriate) the total amount of many of these chemicals that people in the United States are exposed to. These findings raise the possibility that the actual amount of exposure to many of these chemicals may be significantly underestimated by the assay methods used by the CDC.[36]

The underestimation of exposure to various chemicals is a serious problem. For example, the FDA has considered BPA, for example, to be safe even though both animal and human research shows otherwise, and the NHANES data since 2003–2004 has shown that virtually all Americans have measurable BPA exposure. However, the indirect assay used to measure BPA could be underestimating actual exposure to BPA by as much as 170-fold, which dramatically changes the risk calculation for this, and likely numerous other chemicals. Clearly, adequate funding for the CDC to have the best assay tools available to conduct this critical survey of the health and exposures of Americans should be a national priority.

How Chemical Exposures Can Affect Multiple Generations at Once

As if risk posed by EDCs and other types of toxic chemicals (e.g., heavy metals) to fetuses while growing in the uterus is not scary enough, environmental exposures can actually create changes beyond the future lifespan of the fetus that may affect subsequent generations, even if they are not directly exposed to the chemical. How does this work? When a pregnant woman experiences an environmental exposure of any kind (e.g., chemical, behavioral such as severe stress, nutritional), *she is affected, her fetus is affected throughout life, and the offspring produced by her fetus* are also actually exposed to that chemical because the fetus has already created their very own sperm stem cells (males) or eggs (females) that will be used to produce offspring (the grandchildren of the exposed mother). During human pregnancy, a female fetus will develop her entire set of eggs. These

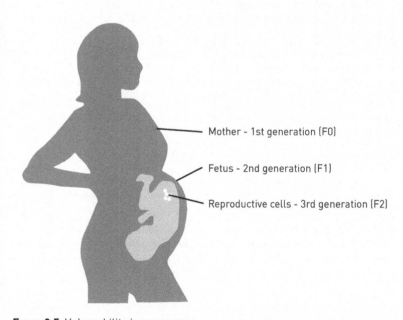

Mother - 1st generation (F0)

Fetus - 2nd generation (F1)

Reproductive cells - 3rd generation (F2)

FIGURE 2.5 Vulnerability in pregnancy.
When a pregnant woman is exposed to an environmental toxin, three generations are exposed at the same time (multigenerational exposure), the pregnant woman (F0), the fetus (F1), and the reproductive cells of the fetus (F2), which are the sperm or egg cells that produce a child when the fetus grow to adulthood and reproduces.

eggs are stored in her two ovaries for later use; they will be released monthly when menstrual cycles begins after puberty, until they are used up leading to menopause. A male fetus develops testes containing the sperm stem cells that will go on after puberty to create sperm throughout their lifespan. The sperm stem cells are never used up, and all sperm created by that male will reflect any damage that has occurred to the sperm stem cells during fetal life. Therefore, any exposure by a pregnant mom can have bad consequences to *three generations*: the mother, her children, and her grandchildren! (see Figure 2.5) This is called a *multigenerational effect*.[37]

Many environmental exposures (with the exception of some forms of radiation) may not actually affect our DNA directly by altering the genetic code. Rather they affect the proteins that control gene expression as well as other mechanisms involved in controlling gene function—that is, whether or not the gene stays quiet or is actually expressed and becomes active as well as the level of activity of the gene. The effects of such an exposure during prenatal and/or childhood development are permanent, and there is now clear evidence that they can persist for multiple generations, even beyond the exposed mother's grandchildren.[38] When the effects extend beyond the directly exposed generations—the pregnant mother, her baby, and her future grandchildren—this is called transgenerational effects of exposure, due to changes in the control of genes through multiple mechanisms. These effects are referred to as epigenetic effects, meaning that they are different than the gene-mutation effects that have been the focus of genetics for the past hundred years.[39,40]

Transgenerational Effects

Transgenerational changes occur when epigenetic changes are passed on to later generations that were not directly exposed—that is, the generations beyond one's grandchildren. For over a century, biologists dismissed the idea that the environment could modify the epigenome. The dogma was that these "modifications" could not be transmitted to future generations, only changes in the genetic code could do that—the idea of inheritance of environmentally induced changes in traits was known as Lamarkian Inheritance. However, many industrial chemicals have now been tested in animal studies and have been shown to cause epigenetic changes that are passed down to successive generations of offspring. This research has uncovered plausible molecular mechanisms thought to provide the basis for transgenerational inheritance of traits induced by environmental exposures.

In humans, researchers now know that childhood trauma, major infections, malnourishment, and smoking and other environmental pollutants have the capability to change our epigenomes in ways that carry out to generations beyond the original exposure. As with the Dutch Hunger Winter that will be discussed in chapter 3, the nutritional and social stress from starvation experienced by pregnant women in the Netherlands during World War II affected their children and grandchildren who have shown increased risk for obesity and heart disease as adults. These multigenerational changes in these diseases have not been found to be consistent with classical mutations in the genetic code and cannot be explained by random genetic changes alone. They are due to environmental exposures.

Diet and Epigenetic Changes

Epigenetics represents the way by which our environment is able to affect and modulate the way our genes function. Epigenetic changes refer to chemical modifications of DNA and the proteins they are attached to that together make up chromosomes. The DNA material we inherit from our parents is still there, but may not function normally due to environmental exposures. These epigenetic modifications refer to any chemical change in the chromosomes and DNA other than changes to the genetic code—the "genetic letters" that together make up the genetic code of each species. Disruption of the epigenome (the control systems that regulate gene function) can disrupt the normal activity of critical genes, particularly when the disruption occurs at the point of fetal development when organs are differentiating from the original single ovarian oocyte that was fertilized by a sperm. It is important to know that every cell in a person's body contains the same genes, but that specific genes controlling, for example, nerve cell function, are not active in other tissues such as bone or skin cells; this is because during development of different organs, epigenetic changes in genes shut down expression of genes that are not appropriate for that type of cell in that organ.

But not all exposures cause *harmful* epigenetic changes. Eating foods with healthy nutrients, for example, can affect our epigenome *positively* by helping to reduce a variety of chronic illnesses. In addition, certain nutrients (such as some vitamins) actually *protect the epigenome* from the harmful effects of exposures to toxic chemicals.

The following are some examples of substances that create positive epigenetic effects or that can counter negative epigenetic effects of toxic chemicals on gene function:

- **Folic acid**, a water-soluble B vitamin, also known as folate or B9, is commonly found in green leafy vegetables and has been shown to offset the damaging effects of BPA in mice that were exposed to BPA in their mother's womb.[41]
- **Omega-3 fatty acids**, which are found in fish, eggs, nuts, oils, chia and flax seeds, and leafy greens, have been shown to offset the toxic effects of BPA, lead, mercury, and dioxin (found in air pollution from trash incinerators), in both animal and human studies.[42]
- **Iodine** intake (in appropriate amounts) during pregnancy and while nursing can offset the effects of various environmental pollutants, such as nitrates, thiocyanate, and perchlorate (found in rocket fuel and industrial-level produce washes), which can disrupt normal thyroid function and negatively affect fetal brain development.[43]
- **Quercitin**, an antioxidant nutrient also known as a "flavonoid," found under the skin of apples and onions, has been shown to be protective against polychlorinated biphenyls (PCBs), BPA, and methylmercury exposure in animal studies.[44]
- **Iron, calcium, and vitamin C** intake, resulting in sufficient blood levels, have been shown to be protective in children exposed to lead, resulting in less lead absorption.[45]
- **Iron** intake, ensuring adequate levels in the blood, helps to reduce absorption in children of cadmium, a metal that is toxic to the brain.[46]
- **Cruciferous vegetables** (discussed in chapter 13), have a variety of vitamins, antioxidants, and sulfur-containing compounds that help detoxify the body, assisting in the breakdown of many environmental chemicals into less-harmful compounds.[47,48]

Bottom line

Eating certain nutrient-rich, pesticide-free foods can offset the epigenetic effects from our chemical environment, thereby reducing harm to our bodies, and for those who plan to have children (this applies to men and women), also reducing the risk for harmful epigenetic changes for future generations to come.

Humans are absorbing their environment and filling up on many of the industrial chemicals that have been created, many of which were originally thought to improve the quality of our lives and make us healthier. Despite the fact that humans have evolved over millions of years, the 90,000+ industrial, food, agricultural, and personal care chemicals have been in existence for only 200 years, with the greatest increase in production occurring after WWII. Now that many of these chemicals are making their way into our bodies, it is no wonder that the consequence for humans is an increase in chronic diseases. There hasn't been enough time for the human body to adapt to this chemical onslaught! The dramatic increase in man-made chemicals since WWII has been accompanied by dramatic increases in chronic diseases, such as disorders of metabolism (obesity, diabetes, heart and liver disease) and the immune system (allergy, asthma, and autoimmunity). The increases are occurring too rapidly to be due to genetic mutations alone, but sadly, most federal research money is directed at finding gene mutations associated with these diseases rather than looking for environmental factors that surround us every day.

Now that we know so many harmful chemicals are capable of getting into our bodies, and that federal agencies have not set up needed protections to keep us safe, it is up to each and every one of us to make smarter choices moving forward.

References

1. Landreth KS. Critical windows in development of the rodent immune system. *Human & Experimental Toxicology.* 2002;21(9–10):493–498.
2. Mundt KA, Dell LD, Crawford L, Gallagher AE. Quantitative estimated exposure to vinyl chloride and risk of angiosarcoma of the liver and hepatocellular cancer in the US industry-wide vinyl chloride cohort: mortality update through 2013. *Occupational and Environmental Medicine.* 2017;74(10):709–716.
3. Rubio-Rivas M, Moreno R, Corbella X. Occupational and environmental scleroderma. Systematic review and meta-analysis. *Clinical Rheumatology.* 2017;36(3):569–582.
4. Kharrazian D. The potential roles of bisphenol A (BPA) pathogenesis in autoimmunity. *Autoimmune Diseases.* 2014;2014:743616.
5. Manzel A, Muller DN, Hafler DA, Erdman SE, Linker RA, Kleinewietfeld M. Role of "Western diet" in inflammatory autoimmune diseases. *Current Allergy and Asthma Reports.* 2014;14(1):404.

6. Hu Y, Costenbader KH, Gao X, et al. Sugar-sweetened soda consumption and risk of developing rheumatoid arthritis in women. *Am J Clin Nutr.* 2014;100(3):959–967.

7. Parks CG, Walitt BT, Pettinger M, et al. Insecticide use and risk of rheumatoid arthritis and systemic lupus erythematosus in the Women's Health Initiative Observational Study. *Arthritis care & research.* 2011;63(2):184–194.

8. Cohen A. Rheumatology and the environment: an integrative view. *Alternative and Complimentary Therapies (CAM).* 2017;23(1).

9. Miller FW, Alfredsson L, Costenbader KH, et al. Epidemiology of environmental exposures and human autoimmune diseases: findings from a National Institute of Environmental Health Sciences Expert Panel Workshop. *Journal of Autoimmunity.* 2012;39(4):259–271.

10. Huan Song M, PhD; Fang Fang, MD, PhD; Gunnar Tomasson, MD, PhD; Filip K. Arnberg, PhD; David Mataix-Cols, et al. Association of Stress-Related Disorders With Subsequent Autoimmune Disease. *Journal of the American Medical Association.* 2018;319:2388–2400.

11. Sharif K, Watad A, Coplan L, et al. The role of stress in the mosaic of autoimmunity: An overlooked association. *Autoimmunity Reviews.* 2018;17(10):967–983.

12. Sharif K, Sharif Y, Watad A, et al. Vitamin D, autoimmunity and recurrent pregnancy loss: More than an association. *American Journal of Reproductive Immunology (New York, NY: 1989).* 2018;80(3):e12991.

13. Vieira Borba V, Sharif K, Shoenfeld Y. Breastfeeding and autoimmunity: Programing health from the beginning. *American Journal of Reproductive Immunology.* 2018;79(1).

14. Gomes JP, Watad A, Shoenfeld Y. Nicotine and autoimmunity: the lotus' flower in tobacco. *Pharmacol Res.* 2018;128:101–109.

15. Anaya JM, Shoenfeld Y, Rojas-Villarraga A, Levy RA, Cervera R, eds.. *Autoimmunity from Bench to Bedside.* El Rosario University Press; 2013.

16. Agmon-Levin N, Lian Z, Shoenfeld Y. Explosion of autoimmune diseases and the mosaic of old and novel factors. *Cell Mol Immunol.* 2011;8(3):189–192.

17. Hess RA. Oestrogen in fluid transport in efferent ducts of the male reproductive tract. *Rev Reprod.* 2000;5(2):84–92.

18. Haddow JE, Palomaki GE, Allan WC, et al. Maternal thyroid deficiency during pregnancy and subsequent neuropsychological development of the child. *The New England Journal of Medicine.* 1999;341(8):549–555.

19. Colborn T, vom Saal FS, Soto AM. Developmental effects of endocrine-disrupting chemicals in wildlife and humans. *Environ Health Perspect.* 1993;101(5):378–384.

20. Coffey JC, O'Leary DP. The mesentery: structure, function, and role in disease. *The Lancet Gastroenterology & Hepatology.* 2016;1(3):238–247.

21. Arnold DJ, Markham MJ, Hacker S. Tamoxifen flare. *JAMA*. 1979;241(23):2506.

22. Plotkin D, Lechner JJ, Jung WE, Rosen PJ. Tamoxifen flare in advanced breast cancer. *JAMA*. 1978;240(24):2644–2646.

23. Drakvik E, Altenburger R, Aoki Y, et al. Statement on advancing the assessment of chemical mixtures and their risks for human health and the environment. *Environ Int*. 2019;134:105267.

24. World Health Organization and United Nations Environment Programme. State of the Science of Endocrine Disrupting Chemicals-2012. https://www.who.int/ceh/publications/endocrine/en/. Accessed April 23, 2020.

25. Kortenkamp A, Martin O, Faust M, et al. State of the art assessment of endocrine disruptors: final report. *Brussels: European Commission*. 2011:442.

26. Council on Environmental Health. Chemical-management policy: prioritizing children's health. *Pediatrics*. 2011;127(5):983–990.

27. American College of Obstetricians and Gynecologists. Exposure to toxic environmental agents. *Fertility and Sterility*. 2013;100(4):931–934.

28. The American Academy of Obstetricians and Gynecologists. Committee Opinion; Exposure to Toxic Environmental Agents. 2013(575).

29. Di Renzo GC, Conry JA, Blake J, et al. International Federation of Gynecology and Obstetrics opinion on reproductive health impacts of exposure to toxic environmental chemicals. *International Journal of Gynaecology and Obstetrics: The Official Organ of the International Federation of Gynaecology and Obstetrics*. 2015;131(3):219–225.

30. Diamanti-Kandarakis E, Bourguignon JP, Giudice LC, et al. Endocrine-disrupting chemicals: an Endocrine Society scientific statement. *Endocrine Reviews*. 2009;30(4):293–342.

31. Zoeller RT, Brown TR, Doan LL, et al. Endocrine-disrupting chemicals and public health protection: a statement of principles from the Endocrine Society. *Endocrinology*. 2012;153(9):4097–4110.

32. Gore AC, Chappell VA, Fenton SE, et al. EDC-2: the Endocrine Society's Second Scientific Statement on Endocrine-Disrupting Chemicals. *Endocrine reviews*. 2015;36(6):E1-e150.

33. Trasande L, Landrigan PJ, Schechter C. Public health and economic consequences of methyl mercury toxicity to the developing brain. *Environ Health Perspect*. 2005;113(5):590–596.

34. Attina TM, Hauser R, Sathyanarayana S, et al. Exposure to endocrine-disrupting chemicals in the USA: a population-based disease burden and cost analysis. *Lancet Diabetes Endocrinol*. 2016;4:996–1003.

35. US Centers for Disease Control and Prevention. CDC National Biomonitoring Program. https://www.cdc.gov/biomonitoring/. Published 2019. Accessed April 14, 2019.

36. Gerona R, Vom Saal FS, Hunt PA. BPA: have flawed analytical techniques compromised risk assessments? *The Lancet Diabetes & Endocrinology.* 2019.

37. Vrooman LA, Oatley JM, Griswold JE, Hassold TJ, Hunt PA. Estrogenic exposure alters the spermatogonial stem cells in the developing testis, permanently reducing crossover levels in the adult. *PLoS Genet.* 2015;11(1):e1004949.

38. Viluksela, M. Pohjanvirta, R., Multigenerational and transgenerational effects of dioxins. *Int J Mol Sci* 2019, *20* (12). DOI: 10.3390/ijms20122947.

39. Casati L, Sendra R, Sibilia V, Celotti F. Endocrine disrupters: the new players able to affect the epigenome. *Frontiers in Cell and Developmental Biology.* 2015;3:37.

40. Crews D, Gillette R, Miller-Crews I, Gore AC, Skinner MK. Nature, nurture and epigenetics. *Molecular and Cellular Endocrinology.* 2014;398(1–2):42–52.

41. Dolinoy DC, Huang D, Jirtle RL. Maternal nutrient supplementation counteracts bisphenol A-induced DNA hypomethylation in early development. *Proceedings of the National Academy of Sciences of the United States of America.* 2007;104(32):13056–13061.

42. Rice DC. Overview of modifiers of methylmercury neurotoxicity: chemicals, nutrients, and the social environment. *Neurotoxicology.* 2008;29(5):761–766.

43. Rogan WJ, Paulson JA, Baum C, et al. Iodine deficiency, pollutant chemicals, and the thyroid: new information on an old problem. *Pediatrics.* 2014;133(6):1163–1166.

44. Barcelos GR, Grotto D, Serpeloni JM, et al. Protective properties of quercetin against DNA damage and oxidative stress induced by methylmercury in rats. *Arch Toxicol.* 2011;85(9):1151–1157.

45. Jiao J, Lu G, Liu X, Zhu H, Zhang Y. Reduction of blood lead levels in lead-exposed mice by dietary supplements and natural antioxidants. *J Sci Food Agric.* 2011;91(3):485–491.

46. Silver MK, Lozoff B, Meeker JD. Blood cadmium is elevated in iron deficient US children: a cross-sectional study. *Environmental Health: A Global Access Science Source.* 2013;12:117.

47. Atwell LL, Beaver LM, Shannon J, Williams DE, Dashwood RH, Ho E. Epigenetic Regulation by Sulforaphane: Opportunities for Breast and Prostate Cancer Chemoprevention. *Current Pharmacology Reports.* 2015;1(2):102–111.

48. Kapusta-Duch J, Kopec A, Piatkowska E, Borczak B, Leszczynska T. The beneficial effects of Brassica vegetables on human health. *Rocz Panstw Zakl Hig.* 2012;63(4):389–395.

3

Chemicals and Kids
What Parents and Parents-to-Be Need to Know!

Neurons are being formed at a rate of 250,000 per minute on average over the course of a pregnancy—and that's a lot of opportunity for things to go awry.
> —Irva Hertz-Picciotto, Ph.D, University of California-Davis
> Environmental Health Sciences Center

Fertility

The ability to become pregnant is complex, and many factors such as age of the parents, nutritional status, stress levels, and medication use, all play a role. But, if the couple is unable to become pregnant despite frequent, carefully timed, unprotected sex for 1 year, environmental chemical exposures should be explored. Here's why: fertility is dependent on the fine balance of hormones in men and women to work efficiently, and endocrine-disrupting chemicals, from products we use every day, can disrupt this balance and make conception more difficult. Prior to trying to have a child, both men and women should be counseled on avoiding synthetic chemicals in the air that they breathe, reducing and vetting personal care products, and consuming food and drinks that are unprocessed and contain low/no pesticides. In addition, fragile sperm and eggs take months to develop in men and women and their quantity *and* quality may be affected by chemicals or low-level radiation exposure through the placement and everyday use of modern technology such as laptop and cell phones. Laptops placed on the lap and active cell phones (i.e., *not* on airplane mode) carried in front pants pocket of males, have been shown to decrease both sperm quantity and quality![1,2]

Pregnancy

The human body is quite miraculous in that it is able to manage nutrients, detoxify, and eliminate many foreign substances as protection for its own existence. BUT, when it comes to protecting a fetus in the mother's womb (Figure 3.1), we now know, from both animal *and* human studies, that the placenta, once believed to be highly protective for a growing fetus, in fact

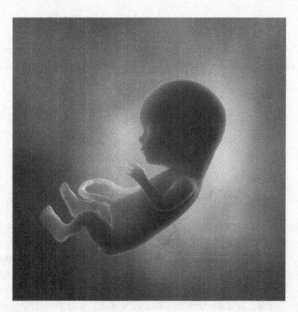

FIGURE 3.1 Human fetus in the womb photo.

does *not act as a barrier* against many harmful chemicals. In 2004, the Environmental Working Group (EWG), a nonprofit consumer advocacy group, analyzed the umbilical cord blood of 10 random newborns. They found an average of 200 industrial chemicals in each newborn, along with persistent pesticide-breakdown products that had been banned 30 years prior to the study.[3] Many other studies confirm that chemicals from everyday products not only get into our bodies, they also get into the bodies of vulnerable fetuses through the blood-stream of pregnant mothers. Chemical exposures include PCBs and mercury from fish intake, phthalates from personal care products applied to skin, flame retardants from couches, secondhand smoke, pesticides from produce, and many other common chemicals. So it makes sense for a woman and her partner to reduce exposures to harmful chemicals and microwave radiation (from cell phones, tablets etc.) as much as possible, *before considering having a baby*, in order for the fetus to have the best opportunity for healthy brain and body development. Of course, during pregnancy deliberate exposure to toxic chemicals from tobacco, alcoholic drinks, radiation, and other sources should be eliminated, and the use of any drug (prescription or over-the-counter) should be considered a potential hazard—acetaminophen, for example, which is used by pregnant women, interacts with phthalates to interfere with masculinization in male fetuses. Nonmedicinal pain management methods are discussed in chapter 6.

NOTE: Talk with your healthcare provider before stopping any prescription medications, but recognize that many healthcare providers have little knowledge of the impact that toxic chemicals have on your health. Also, for many drugs, the effects on fetuses are not known.

Critical Periods of Risk from Chemical Exposures

As mentioned throughout this book, the *timing of exposure* can be just as critical as the *type of exposure,* whether the exposure is a neurotoxin, an endocrine disruptor, or both. Critical periods include pregnancy, newborn and toddler years, adolescents through late teens, and even menopause; these are all periods characterized by surges in hormone levels resulting in physiologic changes (see Figure 3.2). During menopause, for instance, a loss of hormone activity (estrogen) may result in hot flashes, joint pain, and loss of libido. The primary focus of research on endocrine-disrupting chemicals has been on the effects of exposure during fetal, infant, and childhood exposure. Some

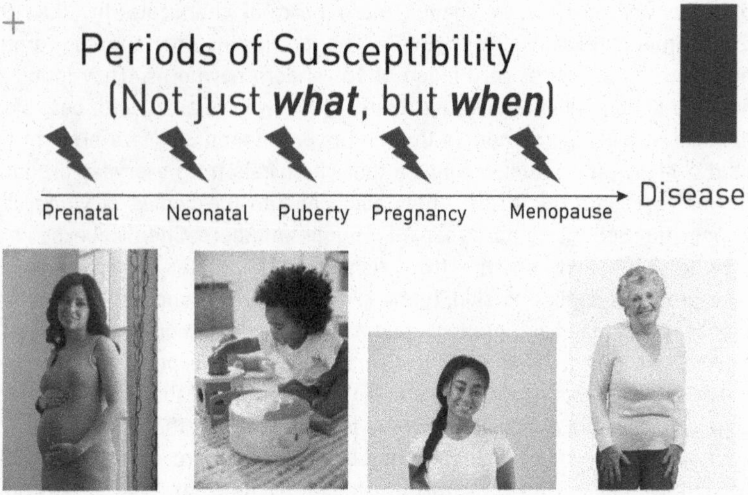

Periods of Susceptibility
(Not just *what*, but *when*)

Prenatal   Neonatal   Puberty   Pregnancy   Menopause → Disease

FIGURE 3.2 Vulnerable periods of human development due to rapid changes in hormone activity.

chemical compounds, even some medications, may cause specific harmful effects, such as birth defects in a fetus if a pregnant mother is exposed to them. However, these same compounds may have *no* harmful effect when a person is exposed to them during adulthood (see Figure 6.1 fetal development chart). A classic example of this is the medication thalidomide, which was prescribed in the 1960s as a sedative to treat anxiety and sleeplessness. By 1960, thalidomide was marketed in 46 countries, and within a few years, one in seven Americans took thalidomide, including thousands of pregnant women. Many of the children exposed to this medication in utero were born with severely shortened arms and legs (a birth defect known as phocomelia) as well as other neurologic problems. However, it was also discovered by researchers that thalidomide could be used safely to treat many diseases when prescribed to adults who were *not* pregnant. Its success in treating multiple myeloma, leprosy, sarcoidosis, Crohn's, Behcet's, lupus, and other diseases has brought thalidomide back to the market, though amid considerable controversy.[4]

What about industrial chemicals such as phthalates? This group of chemicals is used in fragrances (to make the smell last longer), plastic toys, vinyl flooring, shower curtains, nail polish, and IV tubing. Phthalates are particularly harmful when a fetus is exposed during the first and second trimesters of fetal growth, because of the sensitivity to hormone-disrupting effects during the stage of fetal growth when the reproductive organs are developing under the influence of sex hormones.[5,6] *Time* magazine even wrote about this phenomenon in their October 2010 issue highlighting fetal vulnerability during pregnancy in ways most of us would never expect.

One tragic example of multigenerational effects seen in humans occurred after a medication, a synthetic form of estrogen called diethylstilbestrol (DES), was given to millions of women in the United States. DES was prescribed from 1938 to 1971 to prevent spontaneous abortion and preterm delivery in pregnant women. Although the mothers themselves were relatively unharmed by the medication (there is some evidence that they had a moderately increased risk for developing breast cancer), their daughters (known as DES daughters), exposed in utero had much more severe health outcomes, including malformations of the female reproductive tract, infertility, increased incidence of a rare vaginal cancer (clear cell adenocarcinoma), altered timing of menopause, and increased risk of breast cancer in middle age, 40+ years after exposure in utero. These health effects did not become apparent until the DES daughters reached puberty, attempted to become pregnant, or reached middle age and menopause. There were no externally obvious physical changes on examination at birth, which is

---

Box 3.1 Ways in which Children Are Vulnerable to Chemicals in Their Environment.

+ Children...uniquely vulnerable
  - Pound-for-pound, greater exposure
  - Close to the ground
  - Hand-to-mouth behavior
  - Lack of variety in diet
  - Immature metabolism
  - Greater absorption through skin
  - Continuously developing
    - Reproductive system
    - Nervous system
  - More years of future life

the only outcome used by physicians of that era as well as in standard toxicologic testing for risk assessment, showing that exposures can often take months to manifest in exposed laboratory animals and decades to manifest in exposed humans.[7]

Toddler Exposures

Toddlers are uniquely vulnerable to chemicals in their environment (see Box 3.1). Pound for pound, they have greater exposure than adults, they are often close to or on the ground where harmful dust lurks, and coupled with hand-to-mouth behavior, they are at increased risk of ingestion of chemicals from dust and chemicals in carpets and vinyl flooring. Toddlers tend to lack variety in their diet, so they do not typically consume many healthful and protective nutrients. Because they are still developing, toddlers have immature "detoxification" systems with reduced liver enzyme activity, which decreases their ability to breakdown chemicals. Their reproductive and nervous systems are still actively growing and therefore more vulnerable to environmental factors than those of fully grown adults. Additionally, when children are exposed to chemicals starting from a young age, they have many more years of exposure ahead of them, increasing their risks from cumulative exposures.

Exposures Outside the Home: Focus on Daycares

Infants, toddlers, children, and teens spend an enormous amount of time outside of the house, in places such as daycares, schools, cars and buses, recreational facilities (e.g., swimming pools, soccer turf), and jobs. Daycares that are owned by large corporations, often follow the same cleaning protocols, buy the same furnishings (e.g., play area rugs, desks, toys), and employ similar outdoor landscaping routines. If you notice lawn signs that warn of pesticide spraying, automated air fresheners in every classroom, plastic toys that look worn and overused, it would be warranted to contact the director of the facility to share your concerns about exposure to environmental toxins.

Teen Exposures: Another Critical Period of Exposure

Sex hormones are active at different stages of human development (see Figure 3.2). During fetal life sex hormones are responsible for sexual differentiation (boy vs. girl), brain development, hormone glands development, and a host of other critical activities and signaling. The next major phase of sex hormone activity begins at puberty; a person in this age group is referred to as a "tween," between being a child and a teenager.

The adolescent years represent the time of human (and animal) development where hormone activity is at its highest level. "Raging hormones" is often used to describe puberty, when sex hormones such as testosterone and estrogen surge and create physical changes seemingly overnight. A new spurt in growth, as well as body hair growth, breast development in girls and penile development in boys, acne, emotional variability, and voice changes are all part of the normal changes of puberty, essentially readying the body to be able to reproduce.

Given the enormous hormonal activity during puberty, it is prudent to consider the effects that environmental chemicals, particularly EDCs, may have on the normal balance and activity of these hormones. Researchers have found that several hormones may be disrupted in teens exposed to elevated levels of known endocrine disruptors such as phthalates, BPA, pesticides, and flame-retardant chemicals. Researchers have also found increased rates of obesity, thyroid dysfunction, elevated blood pressure, earlier onset of puberty, and higher rates of blood sugar levels (i.e., insulin resistance) associated with elevated levels of EDCs in tests of children, tweens and young teenager's blood and urine samples.[8-14] There is also evidence that African American girls, more so than Caucasian girls the same age, have earlier onset of puberty than prior generations. Menstruation among these young girls is occurring as early as ages seven and eight, which increases their lifetime exposure to estrogen, putting them at greater risk for developing breast cancer than girls exposed to estrogen for fewer overall years of life. Researchers believe that increased marketing and use of personal care products at young ages, especially synthetic estrogenic hair products, may be to blame.[15-18] Clearly, the enormous body of evidence now showing increased risk of chronic health issues in young people, plus the ever-growing cost of healthcare in the United States should be a wake-up call that teens, parents, doctors, high school educators, and politicians cannot ignore.[19-23]

Adolescent and Teen Health Education

Teens are a unique audience for learning environmental health information, and based on the author's (AC) work with high schools, teens are a critical demographic for several reasons.

First, adolescents and teens are extremely self-conscious of their changing bodies, and they face an enormous amount of social pressure to look and smell good every day. It's no surprise that teenagers use more personal care products daily than any other demographic, which exposes them to more synthetic chemicals on a regular basis than adults. Adolescents and teens are "body aware," curious, and receptive to vetted information about their bodies.

Second, teens are continuing to form the habits that they'll maintain throughout their lifetime. If we can put them on the right track now, they'll lead healthier lives as adults. They are also at a time in their lives when they must learn to make better decisions for their health, whether it concerns preventing date rape, saying "no" to drugs and alcohol, dealing with bullying, seeking help for depression, or discussing sexuality and contraceptive options. Chemical and radiation information is an added layer of health and well-being that is relevant for our time; it is a growing topic of concern, and there is increasing awareness among teens. Thus, with teens, it is an opportunity to make a real difference at a young age, a difference that will affect their health for the rest of their lives.

Third, adolescents and teens may one day have kids of their own, which means that educating them now about harmful chemicals will help lower their exposure to chemicals before and during pregnancy. They will likely disseminate this information to their parents and siblings, and they will also set a healthy example for their *own* children's behaviors.

Fourth, teens not yet 18 will soon be able to vote and make changes to the political landscape, demanding better policy and stricter regulations. They will likely move the consumer product market in a safer direction just through purchasing power, and they will be able to understand the chemical exposures on a global level and help fight for environmental justice for communities in need.

Here are a few points about teens and chemicals and WHY environmental health information needs to get to THIS demographic:

- Teens use the most personal care products per day (15 each) of any segment of the US population, followed by adult women (12 each) and adult men (6 each).
- A study from 2014 showed that half of 12- to 14-year-old girls wear makeup most days and 17% refuse to leave the house without make-up; 63% of those who wear makeup go to bed with their makeup on at least once per week.
- There is no federal regulatory oversight in the United States for personal care products, and the vast majority of chemical ingredients have *not*

been tested for safety or toxicity, especially in children, teens, and pregnant women—times when humans are most vulnerable to health effects.

- Research shows that when teenage girls are given safer, less toxic personal care products to use, the levels of many harmful chemicals (e.g., parabens, phthalates, triclosan, oxybenzone) in their urine drop dramatically.
- Issues critical to teen wellness include: turf on sports fields containing PFAS chemicals, radiation exposure due to cell phone/tablet/computer use, air pollution and asthma risk, smoking and vaping, toxic food additives in processed foods, chemicals in feminine care products, environmental changes to improve mental health, clean drinking water and use of sports bottles, unregulated chemicals in food packaging and cookware.

> **Give a man a fish and you feed him for a day.**
> **Teach a man to fish and you feed him for a lifetime.**
>
> — Chinese proverb

Plastics in the Mouth: Baby Bottles and Sports Mouth Guards

Which plastics are safe for kids? After the prohibition of BPA-containing polycarbonate baby bottles in the European Union (EU) and United States, alternative materials such as polypropylene, polyethersulphone, Tritan, and copolyester, have appeared on the market. According to one study, repeated use of baby bottles made from these materials under "real-life" conditions (including placing them in a microwave or dishwasher) did not result in detection of most, but not all, chemicals above government regulatory limits—regulatory limits that are far higher than levels shown to cause adverse effects for many chemicals.[24] At this time, silicone appears to be safe for teething infants and baby bottle nipples,[25] and we recommend using glass bottles with silicone nipples and washing the nipples well with soap, by hand, as opposed to heating them to a high temperature in a sanitizing dish washer (buy glass bottles with a silicone or fabric sleeve in case they are dropped).

For parents whose children participate in sports, a mouth guard is encouraged and often required to avoid injuries to the mouth and teeth.

Mouth guards come in a variety of plastics and often are made in countries that do not require the ingredients to be listed on the packaging. Because there are no studies available investigating the various types of plastic used for mouth guards and their safety, we suggest the folloiwng:

- Look for clear silicone products.
- After molding the mouth guard in hot water, as many of them require, rinse the mouth guard well with cold water.
- After use, clean with soap and cold water and avoid exposure to high temperatures in hot water or by leaving in hot cars and storage closets, since high heat facilitates leaching of chemicals and a gradual break-down of the products.

Synthetic Sports Turf

Synthetic sports turf, has grown wildly popular, replacing the traditional mowed grass typically found in indoor sports centers, schools, playgrounds, and doggy daycares. But despite its benefits of being weatherproof, easy to maintain, and able to move a ball down the field faster, synthetic turf raises many health concerns. It was originally argued that synthetic turf helped reduce knee injuries for athletes, but several studies have debunked that claim, including a 2019 study published in the the *American Journal of Sports Medicine* that looked at knee injuries during NCAA (National Collegiate Athletic Association) football events on natural grass and artificial turf playing surfaces. The study showed that, among NCAA Division I college football players who played from 2004 to 2014, there was an increased number of ligament and meniscal knee injuries or rotational injuries to the knees. Posterior cruciate ligament (PCL) tears significantly increased during competitions played on artificial turf as compared with those played on natural grass. Players in NCAA Divisions II and III also experienced higher rates of anterior cruciate ligament (ACL) injuries during competitions on artificial turf versus natural grass.[26,27] These same issues apply to other sports, such as soccer, field hockey, lacrosse, etc. The lifespan of artificial turf is shorter than initially predicted, and there are no good recycling options for the tons of artificial turf that are being replaced at 5- to 10-year intervals, with the old turf being dumped in landfills. The toxic PFAS chemicals and lead found in turf are neurotoxins and persistent (they do not break down in our environment over time), resulting in them being referred to as "forever chemicals."

In addition to physical injuries, chemical exposure to synthetic turf chemicals is now an issue of growing concern. First, manufacturers of turf are not required by US law to reveal any of the materials used in its production or to test the materials for chemicals that might be harmful to human health. The blades of this fake grass have been shown to contain lead, which is not considered safe at any level, particularly in growing children who are often the biggest users of synthetic turf. Under extreme heat and continued wear-and-tear, the synthetic grass can release lead into its surroundings. As mentioned previously, lead was removed from gasoline and paints in the mid-1970s because it is a neurotoxin that affects brain development and leads to learning disabilities and lower IQ.[28,29] The tiny black pieces often found on turf are called "tire crumb" and are made from old tires (see Figure 3.3). These pellets contain an array

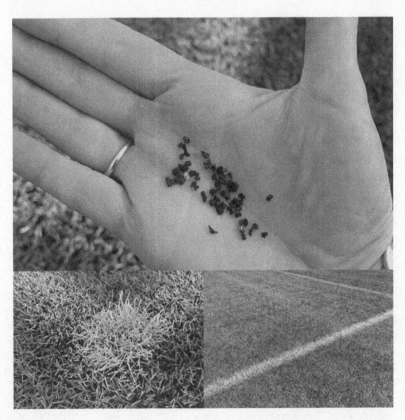

Figure 3.3 Synthetic soccer turf with "tire crumb," taken by author AC at her son's soccer game.

of petroleum-based chemicals, such as benzene, neurotoxic fluorinated compounds or PFAS, and formaldehyde, which is a known carcinogens and contributes to a host of health risks.[30]

So what is a parent to do? Especially if their child loves to play soccer and other sports played on turf?

Synthetic Turf Recommendations

- Wash well with lots of soap immediately after playing on synthetic turf. Petroleum-based chemicals are made from oil, so they need soap as a detergent to remove them.
- Skin abrasions on knees and elbows allow for easier entry of turf chemicals, so clean and cover wounds promptly.
- After time spent on turf, check and remove all tire crumb from ears, hair, between toes, and even underwear. This stuff gets everywhere!
- Keep sneakers and cleats outside in a plastic bucket so toxic chemicals can be safely washed away outside and aren't brought inside.
- Wash your pet's paws after spending time on synthetic turf.
- Lobby your school, daycare, and doggy daycare to change to a grass field and also offer ideas to avoid pesticide spraying.

Top 12 Tips for Parents and Parents-to-Be

- **Create a healthy water "system":** Whether you use well water or municipal tap water, always filter drinking and cooking water at the point of use, that is, your faucet (see chapter 5). Choose a filtering system that is affordable and change out the filter portion regularly. Carry water in glass and stainless steel containers. Avoid BPA-containing as well as "BPA-Free" plastics.
- **Eat clean foods:** Reduce consumption of foods with pesticides, coloring, preservatives, artificial flavoring, or genetically modified ingredients (GMO) that are designed to tolerate dangerously high levels of pesticides. Look for labels that read "USDA Organic" and "Non-GMO Project Verified," which indicate foods with fewer pesticides residues.
- **Reduce consumption of canned food and drinks:** This will help to reduce exposure to BPA that is used to coat the inside of most cans. Switch to frozen organic produce where available, and transfer frozen foods to glassware when you heat and reheat. Buy organic produce in-season when it is cheapest; alternatively, look up the Dirty Dozen and Clean Fifteen lists from EWG.org, to choose conventional (non-organic produce) with fewer pesticides residues, as discussed in chapter 4.

- **Beware of some toys:** Toys, which are not generally labeled with date of manufacture and may contain harmful phthalates if manufactured in the United States prior to 2006. Avoid old plastic toys, hand-me-downs, and toys made in China or overseas, which are not tested or regulated for phthalates, BPA and other harmful chemicals.
- **Change out cookware:** Replace "nonstick" pans with stainless steel and replace plastic storage containers and utensils with stainless steel, bamboo, and glass. Avoid eating soup and other hot foods in plastic, and never heat food or drinks in any type of plastic container.
- **Clean often:** Dust, mop, and/or vacuum 1–2 times per week to reduce dust that sticks to many harmful chemicals, such as from smoke, cleaning products, flame retardants, and chemical fragrances.
- **Reduce and check personal care products**: Pregnant moms and children should avoid any chemicals on skin or hair that are unnecessary; check the products on the EWG.org/Skindeep website or phone app (Healthy Living) for safety, and if possible, choose safer options. Hair products used by African American women are particularly toxic (see chapter 8).
- **Reduce and check cleaning products:** Avoid any unnecessary cleaning products, such as carpet powders, fabric softeners, stain-guard products, and surface cleaners; check EWG.org to choose safer cleaning products. Make your own cleaning products with simple ingredients, such as white vinegar, sea salt, lemon juice, and organic essential oils (see chapter 9).
- **Keep the indoor air clean:** Avoid plug-in, spray, incense, and candle air-fresheners which often contain phthalates and other synthetic chemicals. Open windows often to recirculate fresh air if the outside air is not polluted. Use indoor air purifiers to keep indoor air clean (see chapter 7).
- **Limit radiation exposure**: Avoid lowering sperm count by not placing laptop computers on your lap and carrying cell phones in front pants pockets. Do not rest cell phones or laptops on a pregnant belly. Children should not hold cell phones up to their heads or sleep near cellular devices, including baby monitors, tablets, cell phones, and WIFI linked stuffed animals. Pay attention to the location of the WIFI router in your house in terms of proximity to where children play and sleep. There are radiation (EMF) protection devices that can be purchased (see chapter 12).
- **Survey all areas where your children spend time:** Children spend a great deal of time in daycares, schools, on playgrounds, lawns, turf, and in automobiles, so check these spaces for ways to reduce exposure to chemicals and EMF radiation.

- **Fire and carbon monoxide protection**: Make sure your home has appropriate fire and carbon monoxide detectors/alarms installed, and that the batteries and function are checked every 6 months.

Bottom Line

What we do today can have lasting effects on ourselves, our children, and even our grandchildren. Educating young people on ways to reduce exposures is vital to prepare them for choices that they may make throughout life. Parents and parents-to-be can make a real difference in the health of their children's lives by planning ahead before conception to make lifestyle and environmental changes and by helping their children reduce exposures throughout their entire lifespan.

References

1. Avendano C, Mata A, Sanchez Sarmiento CA, Doncel GF. Use of laptop computers connected to internet through Wi-Fi decreases human sperm motility and increases sperm DNA fragmentation. *Fertility and Sterility.* 2012;97(1):39–45.e32.
2. Adams JA, Galloway TS, Mondal D, Esteves SC, Mathews F. Effect of mobile telephones on sperm quality: a systematic review and meta-analysis. *Environ Int.* 2014;70:106–112.
3. Environmental Working Group. Body burden—the pollution in newborns: a benchmark investigation of industrial chemicals, pollutants and pesticides in umbilical cord blood. 2005.
4. Chen M, Doherty SD, Hsu S. Innovative uses of thalidomide. *Dermatologic Clinics.* 2010;28(3):577–586.
5. Swan SH, Sathyanarayana S, Barrett ES, et al. First trimester phthalate exposure and anogenital distance in newborns. *Human Reproduction.* 2015;30(4):963–972.
6. Watkins DJ, Sanchez, BN, Téllez-Rojo MM, et al. Impact of phthalate and BPA exposure during in utero windows of susceptibility on reproductive hormones and sexual maturation in peripubertal males. *Environmental Health.* 2017;16(69).
7. Hoover RN, Hyer M, Pfeiffer RM, et al. Adverse health outcomes in women exposed in utero to diethylstilbestrol. *The New England Journal of Medicine.* 2011;365(14):1304–1314.

8. Trasande L, Sathyanarayana S, Trachtman H. Dietary phthalates and low-grade albuminuria in US children and adolescents. *CJASN*. 2014;9(1):100–109.

9. Trasande L, Attina TM, Blustein J. Association between urinary bisphenol A concentration and obesity prevalence in children and adolescents. *JAMA*. 2012;308(11):1113–1121.

10. Trasande L, Attina TM. Association of exposure to di-2-ethylhexylphthalate replacements with increased blood pressure in children and adolescents. *Hypertension*. 2015;66(2):301–308.

11. Suhartono S, Kartini A, Subagio HW, et al. Pesticide exposure and thyroid function in elementary school children living in an agricultural area, Brebes District, Indonesia. *The International Journal of Occupational and Environmental Medicine*. 2018;9(3):137–144.

12. Trasande L, Spanier AJ, Sathyanarayana S, Attina TM, Blustein J. Urinary phthalates and increased insulin resistance in adolescents. *Pediatrics*. 2013;132(3):e646–655.

13. Harley KG, Berger KP, Kogut K, et al. Association of phthalates, parabens and phenols found in personal care products with pubertal timing in girls and boys. *Human Reproduction (Oxford, England)*. 2019;34(1):109–117.

14. McMullen AG, Kohn B, Trasande L. Identifying subpopulations vulnerable to the thyroid-blocking effects of perchlorate and thiocyanate. *The Journal of Clinical Endocrinology & Metabolism*. 2017.

15. James-Todd T, Terry, MB, et. al. Childhood hair product use and earlier age at menarche in a racially diverse study population: a pilot study. *Annals of Epidemiology*. 2011;21(6):461–465.

16. American S. Hair products popular with black women may contain harmful chemicals. https://www.scientificamerican.com/article/hair-products-popular-with-black-women-may-contain-harmful-chemicals/. Published 2018. Updated May 11, 2018. Accessed March 4, 2019.

17. Helm J, Nishioka, M et. al. Measurement of endocrine disrupting and asthma-associated chemicals in hair products used by Black women. *Environ Res*. 2018(165):448–458.

18. Stiel L, Adkins-Jackson PB, Clark P, Mitchell E, Montgomery S. A review of hair product use on breast cancer risk in African American women. *Cancer Medicine*. 2016;5(3):597–604.

19. Attina TM, Hauser R, Sathyanarayana S, et al. Exposure to endocrine-disrupting chemicals in the USA: a population-based disease burden and cost analysis. *Lancet Diabetes Endocrinol*. 2016;4:996–1003.

20. Legler J, Fletcher T, Govarts E, et al. Obesity, diabetes, and associated costs of exposure to endocrine-disrupting chemicals in the European Union. *J Clin Endocrinol Metab*. 2015;100(4):1278–1288.

21. Trasande L, Chatterjee S. The impact of obesity on health service utilization and costs in childhood. *Obesity.* 2009;17(9):1749–1754.
22. Attina TM, Hauser R, Sathyanarayana S, et al. Exposure to endocrine-disrupting chemicals in the USA: a population-based disease burden and cost analysis. *The Lancet Diabetes & Endocrinology.* 2016.
23. Trasande L, Liu Y. Reducing the staggering costs of environmental disease in children, estimated at $76.6 billion in 2008. *Health Affairs (Project Hope).* 2011;30(5):863–870.
24. Onghena M, Van Hoeck E, Negreira N, Quirynen L, Van Loco J, Covaci A. Evaluation of the migration of chemicals from baby bottles under standardised and duration testing conditions. *Food Addit Contam Part A Chem Anal Control Expo Risk Assess.* 2016;33(5):893–904.
25. Zhang K, Wong JW, Begley TH, Hayward DG, Limm W. Determination of siloxanes in silicone products and potential migration to milk, formula and liquid simulants. *Food Addit Contam Part A Chem Anal Control Expo Risk Assess.* 2012;29(8):1311–1321.
26. Wannop JW, Foreman T, Madden R, Stefanyshyn D. Influence of the composition of artificial turf on rotational traction and athlete biomechanics. *Journal of Sports Sciences.* 2019:1–8.
27. Loughran GJ, Vulpis CT, Murphy JP, et al. Incidence of knee injuries on artificial turf versus natural grass in National Collegiate Athletic Association American football: 2004–2005 through 2013–2014 seasons. *The American Journal of Sports Medicine.* 2019;47(6):1294–1301.
28. Bleyer A. Synthetic turf fields, crumb rubber, and alleged cancer risk. *Sports medicine.* 2017;47(12):2437–2441.
29. Almansour KS, Arisco NJ, Woo MK, Young AS, Adamkiewicz G, Hart JE. Playground lead levels in rubber, soil, sand, and mulch surfaces in Boston. *PLoS One.* 2019;14(4):e0216156.
30. Lerner S. Toxic PFAS chemicals found in artificial turf. *The Intercept.* https://theintercept.com/2019/10/08/pfas-chemicals-artificial-turf-soccer/. Published 2019. Accessed October 21, 2019.

4

We Are What We Eat
Chemicals in Our Food

Let food be thy medicine and medicine be thy food.
—Hippocrates, ancient Greek physician, "Father of Medicine"
(c. 460–c. 370 BC)

We've been hearing for years that processed foods contribute to the "body burden" (total amount of chemicals present) of toxic chemicals and a long list of illnesses. Nitrates in our hot dogs, pesticides on our produce, "smoothing" chemicals (i.e., emulsifiers) in our dairy products, antibiotics in our chicken, food coloring in our cereal—the list is enormous and daunting.

Scientists have discovered that ingredients such as sodium, high fructose corn syrup, and *trans* fats, as well as synthetic food additives and preservatives, increase the risk of obesity, diabetes, hypertension, stroke, heart and liver disease (collectively referred to as metabolic syndrome) and immune system disease in both adults and children.[1-3] Other chemicals in food and food packaging can contribute to endocrine disorders, infertility, neural tube defects, reduced anogenital distance in male offspring (a biomarker of reduced fetal masculinization), decreased sperm count and quality, developmental delay, and attention deficit hyperactivity disorder (ADHD); this has been recognized by the World Health Organization, the Endocrine Society, the American Academy of Pediatrics, and the American Academy of Obstetricians and Gynecologists.[4-9]

Processed foods remain one of the biggest threats to our health because they contain a vast array of chemicals to improve taste, smell, color, "mouth feel" (such as crunch or the melt-in-your-mouth sensation), consistency, nutritional content, and shelf-life. And it's not just food itself that we have to watch out for, but the containers food is stored in, which can leach toxic chemicals such as styrene, vinyl chloride, and BPA into our food. Not only do these chemicals sound unappetizing, they're actually really bad for you! Given that we all must eat to survive, it would seem that the most important exposure that we can try to control is related to our food.

Major Shortcomings with Our Food Regulations

One of the first food regulation policies put into place in the United States was the Federal Food, Drug, and Cosmetics Act of 1938, although this law did not require any safety testing of chemicals used in personal care or food items. However, in 1958, the Food Additive Amendment was passed, which was intended to fundamentally change the rules regarding chemicals used in food production by requiring food additive manufacturers to test any potentially unsafe substances before being added to food at levels deemed "safe." Sadly, the requirements in this law have not been enforced by the food safety division of the FDA.

What *is* a food additive? Food additives are coloring, flavoring, sweeteners, preservatives, emulsifiers, and other chemicals *deliberately* added to food during processing. These are also called *direct food additives*. Food additives may also be unintentional or *indirect additives* that come from the production (preparation and transport) of foods and drinks, and they include chemicals from manufacturing equipment, dyes, coatings, adhesives, paper, and plastic. Also included as indirect additives are chemicals that leach from the packaging into food and beverages. These indirect additives include many chemicals now known to be harmful to human health, such as BPA, perchlorate, phthalates, parabens, trans fats, and even microscopic pieces of plastic known as microplastics. As if all of the intentionally added food chemicals weren't enough to be worried and angry about, microplastics are being detected at an alarming rate in packaged foods, fish and shellfish, honey, salt, beer, and even bottled water.

In the United States, more than 10,000 chemicals are currently allowed to be added to food and drinks as well as to their packaging. An estimated 1000 additional chemicals are allowed to be added to foods and drinks, but these chemicals are "outside" of the FDA approval process, and subsequently designated by the FDA and US Food and Agricultural Department as "generally regarded as safe" (GRAS). GRAS designation for a chemical allows food manufacturers to state that the chemical is safe with limited or no safety information about the chemical.[9,10]

The Food Additives Amendment of 1958, which is the last time food additives were defined, states that a food additive is "any substance the intended use of which results or may reasonably be expected to result, directly or indirectly, in its becoming a component or otherwise affecting the characteristics of any food." This amendment is the foundation for the US food additive regulatory program, which oversees most substances added to food, but we now know there are many shortcomings to this amendment. To begin with, out of the thousands of food chemicals allowable today in food production, many were grandfathered in prior to the 1958 amendment without adequate testing for safety or toxicity. In addition, science has advanced since 1958 to show that many food additives can affect brain function and behavior as well as disrupt the human endocrine system, which is critical to a multitude of biologic processes in the human body—especially for a growing fetus and developing child. Endocrine-disrupting chemical effects occur at *low* levels, below EPA "safe" exposure levels; these safe-exposure levels provide the incorrect assumption that they are "safe" if exposure is below that level, but the levels were not established taking endocrine disruption into account. The 1958 law also does not address this.

What about reevaluating existing additives for safety? The FDA does not have the authority to obtain data on or to reassess the safety of chemicals already on the market, even those chemicals approved in the 1960s without any testing for toxicity that are now in hundreds of other foods, drinks, and packaging. Consider this: the FDA recommends that manufacturers perform a month-long feeding study in laboratory animals for preservatives, sweeteners, and flavors purposely added to food; yet less than 22% of approximately 4000 chemicals in question have sufficient data to even estimate how much of the additive is safe to eat, and less than 7% of the 4000 chemicals in question were tested for developmental or reproductive effects.[11,12] With outdated safety standards, limited funding, powerful food lobbyists impacting FDA decisions, and legislators dragging their feet, the challenges to improving food safety no doubt seem daunting. We hope the following recommendations will help you feel more empowered to navigate our complicated food system and make healthier choices for you and your families.

Organic versus Conventional Foods

Spraying pesticides on produce is a worldwide phenomenon, occurring in the United States for decades, particularly after WWII, when the manufacturing of pesticides began to explode. Recent data from the FDA Pesticide Residue Monitoring Program show that approximately 47% of domestic foods and 49% of imported foods sampled had detectable levels of pesticide residue. For example, apples tested positive for 47 different pesticide residues—6 of which are known or probable carcinogens, 16 are suspected endocrine disruptors, 5 are neurotoxic, and 6 show evidence of developmental or reproductive toxicity.[13]

While there are more than 900 synthetic pesticides registered by the EPA for use in conventional farming in the United States, under US law organic farming is allowed only *25* synthetic pest control products for use. In addition, the organic farmer must first use "mechanical, cultural, biological and natural materials" to eradicate pests before utilizing any of the 25 synthetic pesticides. Included in the 25 allowable synthetic pesticides are hydrogen peroxide, calcium hypochlorite, boric acid, and soaps.[14]

While the dispute over whether or not organic produce has more nutrients than non-organic food continues, what *cannot* be disputed is the vast reduction (but not elimination) in pesticides that one is exposed to when eating an organic diet. Monitoring data of residue from the use of numerous pesticides have shown that organically grown foods have lower levels of pesticide residue compared with conventionally grown foods.

These pesticides are getting into our bodies. When the diets of a large population of preschoolers in Seattle, Washington, were compared, children eating organic diets had far lower levels of pesticides in their urine than children who did not eat organic diets.[15] Many studies have shown that when conventional foods are swapped out for organic substitutes, toxic pesticide levels in the participants drop dramatically.[16,17]

All of these exposures add up. Given the sheer amount and variety of foods people consume, it should not be surprising that we are exposed to a cocktail of harmful pesticides, each of which may fall below the legal limits designated by the EPA. However, when added together, these amounts can reach unsafe levels and cause real harm, especially to a growing brain. One study showed that, due to the wide assortment of foods containing organophosphate pesticides, 40% of US children may be exposed to these pesticides at greater levels than are known to cause neurological harm. And synergistic effects of multiple types of pesticides on food are also likely to add health risks.[18,19] There are two types of ways that chemicals in mixtures can interact: chemicals that act through the same mechanism (for example through activation of estrogen receptors) can have *additive* effects (1+1=2), or chemicals in a mixture that operate through different mechanisms have the potential for *synergistic* interactions (1+1=100). Synergy is a common finding for hormonal interactions (e.g., estrogen and progesterone) but is not as well studied as additive effects for chemical mixtures.

According to Philip Landrigan, MD, former dean of Global Health and director of the Children's Environmental Health Center at Mount Sinai in New York, "Even low levels of pesticide exposure can be harmful to infants, babies, and young children, so when possible, parents and caregivers should take steps to lower children's exposures to pesticides while still feeding them diets rich in healthy fruits and vegetables."[20,21]

GMO

Genetically modified organisms (GMOs) are living organisms whose genetic material (or DNA) has been artificially manipulated in a laboratory through the use of specialized engineering. Splicing out segments of DNA from one species and adding them into the DNA of another can create combinations of animal, plant, bacterial, and viral genes that do not occur naturally or are not created through traditional crossbreeding methods. Most GMOs were created to withstand pesticide applications so that surrounding weeds and pests would be affected by spraying but the plant itself would not. However, the pesticide-resistant plant can survive when exposed to higher levels of pesticides than are healthy to consume. Other examples of genetic engineering in farming include the insertion or deletion of genetic material into apple seeds to keep the apples from browning, into strawberries so they survive freezing temperatures, and into potatoes to keep them from bruising.

GMOs and genetic engineering in agriculture are perhaps the most disputed fields of modern biotechnology. GMO crops were first approved for commercial use and introduced into US farming in 1996. Since then, their

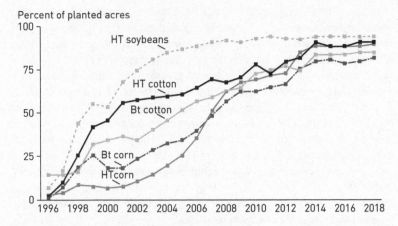

Figure 4.1 USDA. Adoption of genetically engineered crops in the United States, 1996–2018. Note: HT indicates herbicide-tolerant varieties; Bt indicates insect-resistant varieties (containing genes from the soil bacterium Bacillus thringiensis). Datafor each crop catetgory include varieties with both HT and Bt (stacked) traits.

use has increased rapidly (see Figures 4.1 and 4.2). More than 90% of all soybean, cotton, and corn farmland in the United States is currently used to grow genetically engineered (GE) crops designed to withstand exposure to high levels of pesticides such as Roundup.

Much of the argument in favor of GMO foods surrounds global famine initiatives, with the idea that GMO crops will produce greater yield through the introduction of pesticide-resistant seeds. However, the impact of GMO technology to increase crop yield has become a highly politicized issue, with industry-supported studies identifying significant increases and other independent studies not supporting an increase in yield related to GMO. However, even if it were accepted that yield is increased for at least some GMO crops, this has to be viewed in relation to the potential health problems associated with eating crops with high levels of pesticide residues. There is genetic resistance that allows the crop to survive when exposed to much higher levels of pesticides than were initially intended to be used on crops. Thus, despite the argument from industry that GMO farming is necessary and appropriate for the production of adequate food supplies worldwide, it is not clear that GMOs currently on the market increase yield, improve tolerance to drought conditions, enhance nutrition,

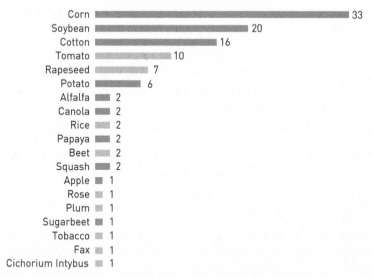

USDA Approved Genetically Modified Crops
Produced in US   Not currently produced

Crop	Value
Corn	33
Soybean	20
Cotton	16
Tomato	10
Rapeseed	7
Potato	6
Alfalfa	2
Canola	2
Rice	2
Papaya	2
Beet	2
Squash	2
Apple	1
Rose	1
Plum	1
Sugarbeet	1
Tobacco	1
Fax	1
Cichorium Intybus	1

Figure 4.2 This bar chart shows all deregulated crops, sized by the number of genetic varieties approved for each. The darkly shaded ten crops are currently produced in the United States.

or provide any other consumer benefit. Studies have shown that weeds and other pests designed to be "killed off" by spraying of GMO seeds have instead become increasingly resistant to the pesticides, requiring multiple rounds of spraying, leading to greater amounts of pesticide residues being found on GMO crops (see EWG's Annual Shopper's Guide to Pesticides in Produce for lists of the "Dirty Dozen" and "Clean Fifteen" produce; see Table 4.2 for 2020 EWG lists).

The most famous example of GMO food used to reduce or solve a public health problem is "golden rice," which was bioengineered or "biofortified" to contain betacarotene as a source of vitamin A. Vitamin A deficiency often leads to blindness in children if adequate amounts are not consumed; it is a worldwide problem. Unfortunately, the use of golden rice was found to have limited impact on the populations it was designed to help, raising questions as to whether or not health benefits may be outweighed by health risks for genetically engineered foods.[22]

In the United States, there are now 20 crops approved for genetic modification under the US Department of Agriculture, with soy and corn being the predominant GMO crops (see Figure 4.2); the number continues to grow. Over 90% of corn and soy grown in the United States is genetically modified under conventional growing standards, and these two high-production crops are turned into thousands of products, including high fructose corn syrup, corn starch, pasta made from corn flour, tofu, soy milk, soy pasta, soy cheese, soy burgers, soy protein powder, soy ice cream, soy yogurt, and soy oil. Many soy derivatives are also added to a wide variety of processed foods, from pudding, to chips and mayonnaise. An estimated 90% of all canola (another GMO crop) grown in the United States and Canada is used to create oil, margarine, and a variety of emulsifiers used in processed foods. A large proportion of GMO corn and alfalfa are also used to feed livestock, which in turn is fed to US consumers in conventional (non-organic) meat products, such as burgers, canned soups, and packaged meat, which are served in restaurants as well as in homes. There are 33 varieties of GMO corn seeds currently commercially available made by a variety of manufacturers (Dow, Monsanto, Syngenta, Bayer, Pioneer, among others), which are designed to resist the ever-expanding list of pesticides used for their growth.[23,24]

Important Takeaway

Foods labeled "USDA Organic" are not allowed to have been genetically engineered or contain GMO ingredients under US regulations. Although the debate on whether or not food labels should openly disclose genetically engineered ingredients is raging, the FDA does not currently require labeling of either GM foods or foods with genetically engineered ingredients.

GMO Health Issues

There are both direct and indirect health risks associated with GMO foods. GMO crops utilize gene modifications that inherently may increase risk for health issues. Gene transfers into the DNA of those who eat GE foods have been linked to increased risk for asthma, allergies, and immune system dysfunction in mice.

Indirectly, GMO foods are associated with a wide variety of toxic pesticide chemical classes, particularly glyphosate (tradename Roundup), the most widely applied herbicide both in the United States and worldwide. Glyphosate is used on a variety of crops, including maize, rice, wheat, soy, and cotton, and its use is growing. Two-thirds of the total volume of glyphosate applied in the United States from 1974 to 2014 was sprayed just since 2010.[25]

Monsanto introduced glyphosate along with their "Roundup Ready" genetically engineered seeds as a combination back in 1996. The seeds were designed to keep the herbicide from killing the seeds themselves—even after multiple applications. Increasing the amount of pesticide sprayed due to a development of resistance to the product in surrounding weed overgrowth has led to a glyphosate overload in many foods in the United States.[26] Glyphosate has now been detected in a large proportion of beer, wine, and honey that was tested.[27-29] Because of weed resistance to glyphosate, the active ingredient in Roundup, Dow now markets "Duo," which combines glyphosate with the herbicide 2,4-D (2,4-dichlorophenoxyacetic acid), a component of Agent Orange, for use on these crops—without any toxicity testing to determine the health consequences. Duo was rapidly approved by the EPA.

GM crops that can resist high levels of pesticides compound the risks that already exist with conventional pesticide use. This is particularly evident with endocrine-disrupting and neurotoxic effects in both animals and humans studied using chlorpyrifos and organophosphate pesticides, especially among children[31] whose brains are developing at an exponential rate.[20,30] In 2015, the International Agency for Research on Cancer (IARC), an arm of WHO, classified glyphosate as class 2B (a "probable human carcinogen"), despite the fact that many researchers and consumer advocates have been pushing to reclassify glyphosate as a class 2A ("known carcinogen").[32] Two major legal settlements were awarded in 2018 and 2019 after juries determined that Monsanto's herbicide glyphosate was responsible for the cancers of two groundskeepers who were regularly exposed to Roundup. These were the first settlements regarding glyphosate; it is predicted that many more lawsuits will follow.

Antibiotic resistance linked to glyphosate exposure has also raised concerns. Although data are still limited, it is believed that increasing glyphosate-resistant bacteria could lead to changes in microbiome diversity, thereby making routine antibiotics ineffective.[33]

Many other commercially available pesticides, such as 2,4-D, organophosphate pesticides, and neonicotinamides, have been studied for neurotoxicity, risks for cancer, and endocrine-disrupting activity, yet despite concerns raised by these studies, their use in US farming remains ongoing, with no end in sight.

Resources for GMO

www.nongmoproject.org
www.responsibletechnology.org/faqs
www.ehn.org/search/?q=GMO

Gut Microbiome and Food Chemicals

The gut bacteria in humans are critical to the normal workings of the entire human body. The human gut, essentially a tube approximately 25 feet long, is lined throughout with almost 5 pounds of microflora, which are made up of bacteria, viruses, and yeast. When made up of robust species and balanced appropriately, microflora are tasked with a variety of critical physiologic activities, including extracting nutrients from food, creating vitamins such as vitamin K, and guarding the gut wall to monitor passage of nutrients through the gut lining into the bloodstream. Much like that bouncer at the hot night club, the gut flora works hard to keep nutrients in and the bad stuff out, such as chemicals, food irritants, and substances that prime the immune system to react.

Produce that has pesticide residues; drinking water that contains chlorinated or fluorinated chemicals; medications, particularly antibiotics, that wipe out both bad and good bacteria; stress that increases acid production; and medications that lower acid production may all reduce, eliminate, or cause an imbalance of flora in the gut, which is known as dysbiosis. Dysbiosis leads to a variety of immune, endocrine, and neuropsychiatric changes. Bacterial resistance from widespread use of antibiotics in agriculture, and the less-than-judicious prescribing of antibiotics in medicine, remains a major public health concern.[34]

Chemicals in Food Packaging ("Food Contact Materials")

If you think the chemicals in processed food are scary, consider the chemicals in the packaging of that food. Most people don't realize that chemicals from food and drink packaging, be it phthalates, styrene (from Styrofoam), lead, or BPA are capable of migrating into the foods and drinks we consume, and ironically, even into what people consider healthy foods. In the United States and around the globe, there are no labels on either food or drink packaging to indicate which chemicals may be in that packaging and thus contributing to toxic exposures. Innovative, sustainable, "green" solutions for packaging should also be labeled; for example, new containers derived from casein (milk protein) can be deadly for those allergic to dairy products.[35]

What do the chemicals in food packaging do—that is, what effects do they have on the body? Many are endocrine disruptors that affect hormone signaling, which can increase the risk for diabetes, infertility, genital defects in newborns, developmental delays in children, attention deficit disorder, and weight gain, and also decrease sperm count and sperm quality.[4–8] If you pack your healthy salad in a plastic container (even if it says "BPA-free"), you are likely being exposed to plastic chemicals that are working against your healthy diet.[36] What about that tea bag placed in a hot cup of boiling water? Many tea bags and sachets contain polyethylene terephthalate (PET), rayon, and other plastic chemicals that have been shown to leach into the healthy green tea you have chosen. Add these to the toxic pesticides and fertilizers used to grow the tea, and you've now created a rather toxic brew.[37]

Recycling Codes

Have you ever wondered what those tiny triangles with a single number in the center on the bottom of plastic food containers are (see Figure 4.3)? In 1988, The Society of the Plastics Industry introduced our current recycling code system, the "plastic resin codes" (Figure 4.4). This coding system was not established by the FDA nor was it intended for the benefit of consumers. It was designed by plastics companies as a marketing gimmick, since

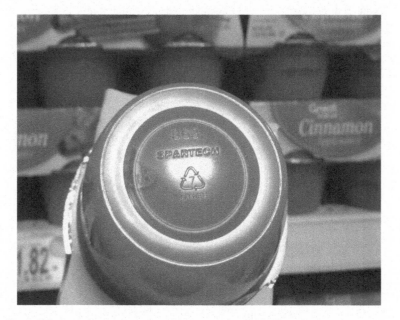

Figure 4.3 Applesauce container with recycling code #7 on the bottom.

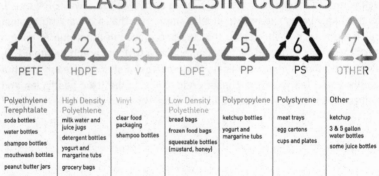

PLASTIC RESIN CODES

PETE	HDPE	V	LDPE	PP	PS	OTHER
Polyethylene Terephtalate	High Density Polyethlene	Vinyl	Low Density Polyethlene	Polypropylene	Polystyrene	Other
soda bottles	milk water and juice jugs	clear food packaging	bread bags	ketchup bottles	meat trays	ketchup
water bottles	detergent bottles	shampoo bottles	frozen food bags	yogurt and margarine tubs	egg cartons	3 & 5 gallon water bottles
shampoo bottles	yogurt and margarine tubs		squeezable bottles (mustard, honey)		cups and plates	some juice bottles
mouthwash bottles	grocery bags					
peanut butter jars						

FIGURE 4.4 Plastic resin codes found on the bottom of plastic food containers and what types of products use these plastic containers.

many plastics (for example, PVC, polycarbonate, polystyrene) are not typically recycled, and overall recycling efforts in the United States have failed. "Recycling is the fig leaf of consumerism," according to Dr. Jane Muncke, managing director of the Food Packaging Forum Foundation.[38] Plastics are labeled #1–#7, but #7 plastics (#7 is "other than #1–6)) often contain BPA and other bisphenol replacements (BPS, BPF, etc.). Plastics labeled #3, polyvinyl chloride plastic (vinyl chloride is a known human carcinogen) contain phthalate plasticer, which make PVC, which is brittle, pliable, and the addition of the plasticizer BPA adds tensile strength; both of these leach out of PVC plastics. We recommend using these codes to decide which plastics to avoid.[39] In general, #1, #2, #5, and #4 are safer than #3, #6, and #7, which are considered more harmful to human health. Remember this jingle: "5, 4, 1 and 2, all the rest are bad for you!" However, since we do not know the actual chemical composition of any plastic, no plastic should be considered to be safe, particularly when heated in a microwave or oven (such as vegetables sold in 'steamer' plastic bags that are marketed to be cooked while in the bag —do not do this).

Tupperware and Other Plastic Containers

Have you ever bought a new set of Tupperware or other plastic containers, washed them in the dishwasher a few times and noticed anything? The plastic changes from see-through to cloudy or opaque after multiple washings.

Why does that happen? Plastic materials are not strong enough to withstand the heat from conventional dishwashers and scratches from routine use, so the materials (known as the matrix) actually breaks down (this is why many dishwasher instructions state that plastic not be placed on the bottom rack where temperatures are higher). The chemicals that make up the plastic can then leach into the food or liquid that they hold, especially if the foods are acidic (e.g., tomatoes, pickles, and fermented foods) or have a high fat content (e.g., olive oil, meat, eggs, and dairy products).

Styrene, a chemical component of Styrofoam, listed as #6 on the recycling codes (although it is not actually recycled), is another packaging material that breaks down at high temperature and can enter the food (think takeout food) and drinks (think coffee cups) it carries. In 2018, the International Agency for Research on Cancer (IARC) classified styrene as "probably carcinogenic to humans"; the National Toxicology Program (NTP) lists styrene as "reasonably anticipated to be a human carcinogen." Styrene can also enter the body through inhalation, as occurs with factory workers working with styrene; it can be detected in blood samples soon after exposure and has been linked to cancer development (such as Hodgkin lymphoma, myeloid leukemia and sinus cancer) in workers regularly exposed.[40]

Paper Food Packaging

Does cardboard packaging pose any threat to human health? Most paper packaging is manufactured from raw organic material using bleaches, glues, and pesticides. Recycled cardboard and paper often accumulates large amounts of BPA (BPA coating of receipt paper contributes much of this), nonstick and antigrease chemicals known as perfluoroalkyls (PFAS), which have been found in high quantities in pizza boxes, newspaper, fast food wrappers, microwave popcorn bags, and recycled toilet paper.[41] Plastic coatings are often added to cups and other containers meant to hold wet materials to reduce the risk of liquids leaking through the absorbent paper (e.g., takeout food containers, coffee cups, frozen dinner containers). Tetra Paks, which are cardboard containers used for boxed soups, juice drinks, milk, and other liquids, contain PET/PETE plastic (#1 on the recycling codes) on the interior to block leakage. PET plastic, which is also used to make one-use plastic water bottles, is currently considered safe, but a metal used in its manufacturing of PET bottles called antimony has raised concerns about health issues, including endocrine system disruption. Ethylene-based plastics degrade when they are thrown away and often end up in lakes and oceans to eventually become microplastic particles, which have been found to cause serious harm to fish and other aquatic organisms.

Canned Foods and Drinks

The United States does not require food packaging to be labeled as to its chemical contents, although we know that many of the chemicals that make up food and drink packaging leach chemicals into the food and liquids that they carry. Take canned foods, for instance. The majority of all canned products in the United States and around the world contain BPA, an epoxy (plastic) resin that lines the interior wall to prevent the contents from contacting the aluminum. However, canned fruit that contains light-colored fruit are an exception, and these cans are typically *not* coated with BPA-containing resin. The tin lining of cans (without BPA) actually prevents fruit discoloration by oxidation. This contradicts assertions by can manufacturers that BPA is essential for the protection of human health, often siting botulism (a rare food pathogen)—as the primary health risk.

Bisphenol A, you may recall, was found to be toxic to human health, so in 2012 it was banned from all baby bottles and sippy cups in the United States. Despite this, the United States has not removed BPA from thousands of other commercial products, such as canned foods and thermal paper (e.g., currency, airline and parking tickets). Because the FDA does not regulate thermal paper, a substantial source of BPA exposure is ignored. Although BPA also gets into humans through dust in the air and skin absorption, the predominant pathway into the body according to the FDA is by consuming BPA in contaminated food, as is often the case when eating and drinking from canned foods and drinks. In one study, 75 participants were served canned soup for lunch over a 2-week period, with all other dietary routines maintained. Then, the same 75 participants were served fresh, unpackaged soup for lunch over the following 2-week period. Testing showed a 1000% increase in urinary BPA levels in participants after eating the canned soup compared with levels found after eating the fresh, unpackaged soup.[42] Thus, BPA as a can liner is a significant, but not the only, source of BPA exposure for humans.

Glazed Pottery

According to the CDC, food should not be stored in glazed pottery originating from outside the United States due to potential lead contamination.[43] Safer choices for food storage and preparation include glass bakeware and food-grade 18/8 (18% chromium and 8% nickel) stainless steel (this should be stamped on the bottom of the container).

Important Takeaway for Food Packaging

- Reduce the use of canned foods and drinks and switch to fresh or frozen foods that can be heated in a glass or metal dish.
- Wherever available as an option, buy food and produce not wrapped in plastic, and buy milk, soda, and other drinks sold in glass containers.
- Carry and store foods in wax paper, glass, or stainless steel, and avoid storing acidic or fatty foods in plastic.
- Avoid microwaving or heating, plastic food containers, and don't wash them in a dishwasher.
- Avoid transporting food in plastic containers in high temperatures or leaving the containers outside when it is hot or in a hot car.
- Avoid water and sports bottles made with ANY plastic, even if labeled "BPA-Free," because harmful BPA substitutes (e.g., BPS, BPF, BPB) are often used, and time, heat, and activity will break down the plastic causing the chemicals in these plastics to leach into the liquids they are carrying.
- Keep a clean set of glass or stainlesss steel glass food containers in your car for takeout food to avoid hot plastics.
- If you do use plastic, choose food containers with the recycling codes #1, #2, #4, and #5. Code #3 is vinyl, #6 is Styrofoam, and #7, or "other," typically contains BPA or equally harmful BPA substitutes.
- Avoid foods that use "grease-proof" chemicals in their packaging, such as microwave popcorn bags, fast food wrappers, and pizza boxes.

Reading Food Labels

Wading through a food label can be confusing and exhausting, so here's a quick way to examine what's in your food.

PLU Codes

According to the Produce Marketing Association (PMA) website, PLU or Price Look Up codes for supermarkets were created in 1990 to make

Table 4.1 How to Read Produce Codes

Ionizing Irradiation Electronically Pasteurized	PLU codes that start with a 3: #3xxxx
Conventionally Grown Sprayed with Pesticides	PLU codes that start with a 4: #4xxxx
Precut Produce Fruits & Vegetables	PLU codes that start with a 6: #6xxx
GMO Genetically Modified Organisms	PLU codes that start with a 8: #8xxxx
Organic Limits the use of synthetic materials during production	PLU codes that start with a 9: #9xxxx

"check-out and inventory control easier, faster, and more accurate" (see Table 4.1). Although PLU codes, similar to recycling codes, were not actually designed with consumers in mind, we can use these codes to identify or confirm how produce was grown. Growers that sell either conventional or organic produce (or both) will have numbers that designate whether that produce is conventional, organic, irradiated, genetically modified or "precut." For instance, the number 9 in front of the other 4-digit code for conventionally grown produce indicates that it is USDA-certified organic. An 8 is placed before the 4-digit conventionally grown code to indicate that the product is genetically modified, but this transparency is not mandatory and, given the controversy surrounding GMO foods, it is interesting that this code does not seem to negatively impact sales. A 3 in front of the 4-digit conventionally grown code indicates that the produce was irradiated to kill bacteria. A 6 in front of a 3-digit code indicates that the produce is precut.

Organic Food Labeling

Organic food labeling standards went into effect in 2002 and apply to fresh, cooked, and processed products. According to USDA standards, these criteria must be met for a food to be labeled as organic:

- Must be free of synthetic additives, artificial preservatives, colors, or flavors, chemical pesticides, chemical fertilizers
- Must not be processed using industrial solvents
- May not be made using bioengineering—no growth hormones or antibiotics (livestock), no GMO ingredients
- Must bear an official USDA label for "organic"
- Must meet above criteria whether the product is grown in the United States or imported
- Producers are inspected annually, and at random, and growers can be fined $10,000+ for each violation

There are specific labeling rules that producers of USDA regulated organic products must follow (see Figure 4.5). There are several organic food stickers, each with a different meaning:

- 100% Organic: products must include solely organic ingredients
- USDA Organic: 95% of the ingredients must be organic

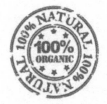 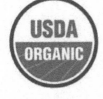 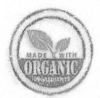

| Products must include all organic ingredients | 95% of the ingredients must be organic | 70% of the ingredients must be organic |

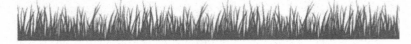

Figure 4.5 Official USDA organic labels. Image credit: USDA.gov.

- "Made with Organic . . .": at least 70% and up to 95% of ingredients (excluding water and salt) must be organic
- <70% organic products can list organic ingredients in the ingredient list, but can't put "organic" on the front label—it is allowed on the back label only

Food Ingredient Labels

- Food ingredients (see Figure 4.6), similar to personal care product ingredients, are listed in order from greatest to least quantity, so the first ingredient is highest in quantity, the second listed ingredient is the next most abundant ingredient in that product, and so on, with the ingredient smallest in quantity (often food coloring and/or a preservative) being last on the list.
- The ingredient list does NOT require that the producer list ingredients that are genetically modified (GMO).
- The ingredient list does not list manufacturing chemicals that end up in food and drink products indirectly, such as pesticides, cleaning agents, food packaging chemicals (styrene, BPA, phthalates, parabens, lead, mercury, cadmium, casein).

Food Preparation and Cooking

Washing Produce

When preparing produce, rinse all produce to help reduce levels of pesticides; use a reputable vegetable cleaner or mix clean warm water with baking soda or white vinegar (in a ratio of 1 part vinegar to 4 parts water). Soak and mildly agitate produce for 5 minutes, then rinse with clean water. Of course, peeling the skin off of produce can also reduce pesticides, but many of the best nutritional benefits of produce will likely be wasted with this approach. Sea salt can also be used as an abrasive agent to clean the skin of produce. If choosing non-organic produce, check the "Dirty Dozen" & "Clean Fifteen" lists from the Environmental Working Group (EWG), which is updated yearly (see Table 4.2 for 2020 lists).

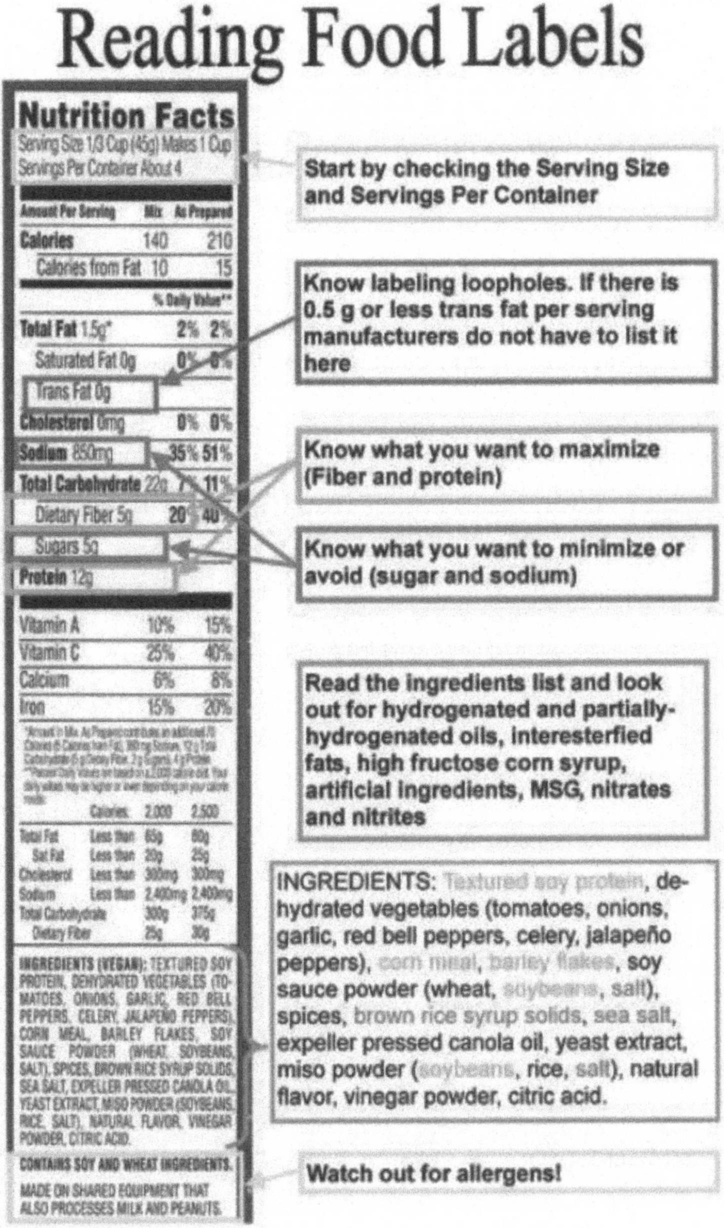

Reading Food Labels

Nutrition Facts

Serving Size 1/3 Cup (45g) Makes 1 Cup
Servings Per Container About 4

Amount Per Serving	Mix	As Prepared
Calories	140	210
Calories from Fat 10		15

	% Daily Value**	
Total Fat 1.5g*	2%	2%
Saturated Fat 0g	0%	0%
Trans Fat 0g		
Cholesterol 0mg	0%	0%
Sodium 850mg	35%	51%
Total Carbohydrate 22g	7%	11%
Dietary Fiber 5g	20%	40%
Sugars 5g		
Protein 12g		

Vitamin A	10%	15%
Vitamin C	25%	40%
Calcium	6%	8%
Iron	15%	20%

*Amount in Mix. As Prepared contributes an additional 70 Calories (5 Calories from Fat), 360mg Sodium, 1g Total Carbohydrate (0g Dietary Fiber, 2g Sugars), 4g Protein.

**Percent Daily Values are based on a 2,000 calorie diet. Your daily values may be higher or lower depending on your calorie needs:

	Calories:	2,000	2,500
Total Fat	Less than	65g	80g
Sat Fat	Less than	20g	25g
Cholesterol	Less than	300mg	300mg
Sodium	Less than	2,400mg	2,400mg
Total Carbohydrate		300g	375g
Dietary Fiber		25g	30g

INGREDIENTS (VEGAN): TEXTURED SOY PROTEIN, DEHYDRATED VEGETABLES (TOMATOES, ONIONS, GARLIC, RED BELL PEPPERS, CELERY, JALAPEÑO PEPPERS), CORN MEAL, BARLEY FLAKES, SOY SAUCE POWDER (WHEAT, SOYBEANS, SALT), SPICES, BROWN RICE SYRUP SOLIDS, SEA SALT, EXPELLER PRESSED CANOLA OIL, YEAST EXTRACT, MISO POWDER (SOYBEANS, RICE, SALT), NATURAL FLAVOR, VINEGAR POWDER, CITRIC ACID.

CONTAINS SOY AND WHEAT INGREDIENTS.

MADE ON SHARED EQUIPMENT THAT ALSO PROCESSES MILK AND PEANUTS.

Start by checking the Serving Size and Servings Per Container

Know labeling loopholes. If there is 0.5 g or less trans fat per serving manufacturers do not have to list it here

Know what you want to maximize (Fiber and protein)

Know what you want to minimize or avoid (sugar and sodium)

Read the ingredients list and look out for hydrogenated and partially-hydrogenated oils, interesterfied fats, high fructose corn syrup, artificial ingredients, MSG, nitrates and nitrites

INGREDIENTS: Textured soy protein, de-hydrated vegetables (tomatoes, onions, garlic, red bell peppers, celery, jalapeño peppers), corn meal, barley flakes, soy sauce powder (wheat, soybeans, salt), spices, brown rice syrup solids, sea salt, expeller pressed canola oil, yeast extract, miso powder (soybeans, rice, salt), natural flavor, vinegar powder, citric acid.

Watch out for allergens!

FIGURE 4.6 How to read food labels.

Grilling

To reduce the risk of exposure to cancer-causing chemicals, steam and broil foods rather than frying or grilling at high heat. Heterocyclic aromatic amines (HCAs) are formed during high-temperature cooking of meat, which occurs with frying and grilling. The levels of HCAs produced in cooked meats vary depending on the cooking method, time of cooking, heat level and type of meat being cooked.

If you do plan on grilling, the application of oregano oil, rosemary oil, black pepper, or several other spices during cooking may reduce the formation of these cancer-causing chemicals.[44] In addition, trimming excess fat off meat can reduce the total concentrations of HCAs and other chemicals in the cooked meat. To reduce exposure to harmful chemicals in fish (such as PCBs and mercury), trim the fat and remove the skin (also fatty) from fish before cooking. Also, choose broiling or baking over frying; these cooking methods allow the PCB-laden fat to cook off the fish.

Cooking foods such as cruciferous vegetables sous vide (under vacuum), or with a pressure cooker, helps retain the most bioactive compounds as compared with steaming and microwaving. Be sure to buy a sous vide or pressure cooker that does not have an interior made with plastic.

Cookware and Utensils

Plastic kitchen utensils have undisclosed chemicals and may be filled with a large number of compounds that can leach into the food you are preparing, especially if the food is fatty and/or cooked at high temperature. As with plastic containers, utensils often contain phthalates and BPA, but may also contain antimicrobial chemicals. Many companies are touting the benefit of antimicrobial chemicals in cooking utensils as a way to thwart food-borne infections, such as salmonella and *E. coli*. Cutting boards, plastic oven mitts, plastic spoons, spatulas, tongs, and bowls are infused with endocrine disruptor antimicrobials, such as triclosan, Bactroban, microban, and many others. Read labels of all kitchenware to avoid these chemicals ending up in your food and your body.

Important Takeaway about Cookware and Utensils

- "Biobased" or "greenware" plastics are typically made from corn and not petroleum-based harmful chemicals, but check with the manufacturers.

- Avoid glazed pottery not made in the USA because of lead exposure risk, according to the CDC.[43] Safer choices for food storage and preparation include glass and food-grade 18/8 stainless steel.
- For a list of PFAS-free products, including nonstick cookware: https://pfascentral.org/pfas-basics/pfas-free-products/.
- Center for Environmental Health (CHE) Report: A Purchaser's Guide to Safer Foodware. https://www.ceh.org/ceh-report-avoiding-hidden-hazards-purchasers-guide-safer-foodware/.

Eating Clean

Healthy dietary recommendations include eating whole, unprocessed foods; produce in an array of natural colors (e.g., carrots, beets, green vegetables, yellow squash, blueberries, strawberries); limiting your intake of sodium, sugar, trans fats, and food additives (e.g., artificial coloring, preservatives, flavoring, emulsifiers/stabilizers); and eating produce that is organic and/or cleaned to removed pesticide residues.

Additional dietary recommendations include the following:

- Choose fresh, unprocessed, organic foods whenever available and affordable. Choosing to eat foods that are truly organic provides the advantage of reducing intake of pesticide (fungicide and herbicide) residues. In addition, one meta-analysis found that organic crops, on average, have higher concentrations of antioxidants and lower concentrations of cadmium than non-organic comparators across regions and production seasons.[45]
- If choosing non-organic produce, check the "Dirty Dozen & Clean Fifteen" lists from the Environmental Working Group (EWG) (Table 4.2), which are updated yearly. EWG sifts through the fruit and vegetable market to find out which types of conventionally grown produce contain the most—and least—chemical pesticides. Research has found that people who eat five fruits and vegetables a day from the Dirty Dozen list consume an average of 10 pesticides a day. Those who eat from the Clean Fifteen ingest fewer pesticides daily.
- If your supermarket or farmers market does not have organic produce, or it's priced too high, reach for something with a thicker peel like avocado, pineapple, or watermelon, which may have fewer pesticides in the actual soft interior.

Table 4.2 EWG's 2020 Shopper's Guide to Pesticides in Produce

Dirty Dozen	Clean Fifteen
(From highest in pesticides to lowest . . . buy these organic)	(Lowest in pesticides . . . Conventional OK)
1. Strawberries	1. Avocados
2. Spinach	2. Sweet corn
3. Kale	3. Pineapples
4. Nectarines	4. Onions
5. Apples	5. Papayas
6. Grapes	6. Frozen sweet peas
7. Peaches	7. Eggplants
8. Cherries	8. Asparagus
9. Pears	9. Cauliflower
10. Tomatoes	10. Cantaloupes
11. Celery	11. Broccoli
12. Potatoes	12. Mushrooms
Dirty Dozen +	13. Cabbages
Hot peppers	14. Honeydew melons
	15. Kiwis

Environmental Working Groups' annual list of produce tested to have the most pesticides (dirty dozen) versus produce tested to have the least pesticide residues (clean fifteen). The "dirty" products are listed with #1 being the worst (even after washing strawberries contained pesticides, in the worst case 23 different pesticides were detected). Copyright © Environmental Working Group www.EWG.org. Adapted with permission from www.FoodNews.org

Seafood

Almost all seafood contains harmful pollutants in varying amounts, including PCBs, mercury, and plastic that has broken down into miniscule pieces (microplastics). Consuming too much seafood can lead to deleterious effects on the brain and nervous system, especially in a growing fetus, because methylmercury and other pollutants can seamlessly cross the human placenta. Other effects from high mercury levels include defects in fine motor coordination, speech, sleep, gait, and neuropathy. PCBs are highly lipophilic—that is, they are concentrated in fat. Mercury is concentrated in muscle.

By cutting away fat (primarily in the skin) before cooking fish and by grilling, broiling, or baking fish, as opposed to sautéing or frying, exposure to these chemicals can be reduced. Choosing fish with lower chemical contaminants is another means of lowering exposure. Larger fish "bioaccumulate" mercury, which means they absorb the mercury from small fish that they consume, so it multiplies as it goes up the food chain. Ingestion of large fish such as shark, swordfish, and tuna should be limited. According to research by the EPA in 2007, canned tuna accounts for 28% of Americans' exposure to mercury (in spite of this information, the FDA blocked for a number of years attempts by the EPA to issue advice to the US public to reduce tuna intake). Many other fish are safer than tuna and can be eaten several times per week without increased health risk. Smaller fish from cold water, for instance, tend to have lower amounts of contaminants; these fish include salmon, mackerel, anchovies, sardines, and herring (i.e., SMASH). Smaller fish retain the same health benefits as larger fish with healthy oils such as docosahexaenoic acid (DHA) and eicosapentaenoic acid (EPA), which have been found to reduce inflammation; reduce risk for some types of arthritis; help with mood and depression, particularly perinatal depression; reduce cholesterol (triglycerides); and reduce risk for heart and neurodegenerative diseases, including Alzheimer's and Parkinson's.[46-48]

Another recommendation is to avoid most farm-raised fish, which contain large amounts of harmful contaminants because of the contaminated feed used in raising them; it is often composed of other contaminated, chopped up seafood, raising the overall contaminant concentration. According to testing by the EWG and other independent groups, farmed salmon contains 5 to 10 times the PCB level of wild salmon.[49] Freshwater fish may contain contaminants from local manufacturing (e.g., PFCs, methylmercury), pesticides, fertilizer, human and animal sewage, and other chemicals from farm runoff. Although the EWG considers farmed-raised US haddock and freshwater trout to have low levels of mercury, it is best, considering our constantly changing environments, to contact your state Fish, Game, and Wildlife Department for important fishing advisories before consuming freshwater fish.

Important Takeaway

Choose fish that are wild-caught, small in size (usually fewer contaminants), responsibly sourced, from less contaminated bodies of water and countries with safer seafood processing (e.g., avoid Atlantic salmon and shrimp from China and Indonesia), and only eat 3–5 servings per week to avoid excessive contaminants. If appropriate and approved by your healthcare provider, take a reputable, vetted omega-3 fish oil supplement daily.

Web Sites and Smart Phone Apps to Help You Choose Healthier Foods and Cookware

Environmental Working Group smartphone apps: Food Scores, Dirty Dozen, Healthy Living

Monterey Aquarium smartphone app: Seafood Watch

SeafoodWatch.org: The Super Green List

The Non-GMO Project: https://www.nongmoproject.org/gmo-facts/

EWG's Seafood Calculator: http://www.ewg/research/ewg-s-consumer-guide-seafood/seafood-calculator

EWG's Consumer Guide to Seafood: http://www.ewg.org/research/ewgs-good-seafood-guide/executive-summary

FDA: Fish—What Pregnant Women and Parents Should Know: http:///www.fda.gov/downloads/Food/Food/FoodborneIllness Contaminants/Metals/UCM400358.pdf

Organic For All: www.OrganicForAll.org

For a list of PFAS-Free Products, including nonstick cookware:

- https://pfascentral.org/pfas-basics/pfas-free-products/
- https://www.ceh.org/ceh-report-avoiding-hidden-hazards-purchasers-guide-safer-foodware/

International Association for Produce Standards, Price Look Up Codes: https://www.ifpsglobal.com/Identification/PLU-Codes

PLU (price look up) produce codes: https://www.ifpsglobal.com/Identification/PLU-Codes

Beer and Wine

One of the world's oldest food-safety laws was created for beer back on April 23, 1516, by Munich's Duke William IX, a Bavarian nobleman. Fearing the amber brew would be adulterated by poisonous plants, soot, and saw-dust, the beer "purity" law, known as "das Rheinheitsgebot," required that beer made in Germany could only contain water, hops, and barley, although yeast was later added to the approved list of ingredients. It was widely speculated that until the 1950s Germany used das Rheinheitsgebot as a pretext, restricting the import of beer from other countries to ward off international competition; however, foreign brands now make up 80% of Germany's annual beer consumption.

The law is still in effect today, to the approval of many health advocates. Unfortunately, although the addition of corn syrup, synthetic flavors, preservatives, or enzymes is not allowed, das Rheinheitsgebot does not regulate the growing and manufacturing of conventional (non-organic) beer ingredients, making German beer just as susceptible to harmful pesticides as the rest of the world's beer.

Beer and wine manufactured and sold in the United States have come under scrutiny for containing impurities. Many studies have shown high levels of a variety of unseemly contaminants, including pesticides like gly-phosate, and other pollutants such as phthalates, BPA (from the lining of metal vats used by wine makers), and microplastics due to manufacturing processing. In one study, 24 German beer brands were analyzed for the presence of microplastic fibers, fragments, and granular material, and contamination was found in every case.[50]

Important Takeaway

There are plenty of organic beer and wine manufacturers, both in the United States and abroad that make excellent products, with the added benefit of reduced chemical and pesticide contaminants. For many, the pleasure of drinking alcohol, especially on a regular basis, is a lifestyle choice that's not going anywhere soon—why not tweak the habit in a healthier direction?

References

1. Simmons AL, Schlezinger JJ, Corkey BE. What are we putting in our food that is making us fat? food additives, contaminants, and other putative contributors to obesity. *Current Obesity Reports.* 2014;3(2):273–285.
2. Rauber F, Campagnolo PD, Hoffman DJ, Vitolo MR. Consumption of ultra-processed food products and its effects on children's lipid profiles: a

longitudinal study. *Nutrition, Metabolism, and Cardiovascular Diseases:* 2015; 25(1):116–122.

3. Manzel A, Muller DN, Hafler DA, Erdman SE, Linker RA, Kleinewietfeld M. Role of "Western diet" in inflammatory autoimmune diseases. *Current Allergy and Asthma Reports.* 2014;14(1):404.

4. World Health Organization and United Nations Environment Programme. State of the Science: Endocrine Disrupting Chemicals—2012. 2012:1–289.

5. The American Academy of Obstetricians and Gynecologists. Committee Opinion; Exposure to Toxic Environmental Agents. 2013(575).

6. Crinnion WJ. Toxic effects of the easily avoidable phthalates and parabens. *Alternative Medicine Review: A Journal of Clinical Therapeutic.* 2010;15(3): 190–196.

7. Collaborative on Health and the Environment. Chemical Contaminants and Human Disease: A Summary of the Evidence. 2006.

8. Diamanti-Kandarakis E, Bourguignon JP, Giudice LC, et al. Endocrine-disrupting chemicals: an Endocrine Society scientific statement. *Endocrine reviews.* 2009;30(4):293–342.

9. Trasande L, Shaffer RM, Sathyanarayana S. Food additives and child health. *Pediatrics.* 2018;142(2).

10. Maffini MV, Neltner TG, Vogel S. We are what we eat: regulatory gaps in the United States that put our health at risk. *PLoS biology.* 2017;15(12):e2003578.

11. Neltner TG, Alger HM, Leonard JE, Maffini MV. Data gaps in toxicity testing of chemicals allowed in food in the United States. *Reproductive Toxicology.* 2013;42:85–94.

12. Neltner, Thomas G., Alger, Heather M., Maffini, Maricel V. Navigating the US food additive regulatory program. *Comprehensive Reviews in Food Science and Food Safety.* 2011;10:342–368.

13. Agriculture USDo. Pesticide Residue Monitoring 2016 Report and Data. https://www.fda.gov/food/pesticides/pesticide-residue-monitoring-2016-report-and-data. Published 2016. Accessed October 28, 2019.

14. Agriculture USDo. USDA Organic Regulations. https://www.ams.usda.gov/rules-regulations/organic. Published 2019. Accessed March 24, 2019.

15. Curl CL, Fenske RA, Elgethun K. Organophosphorus pesticide exposure of urban and suburban preschool children with organic and conventional diets. *Environ Health Perspect.* 2003;111(3):377–382.

16. Oates L, Cohen M, Braun L, Schembri A, Taskova R. Reduction in urinary organophosphate pesticide metabolites in adults after a week-long organic diet. *Environ Res.* 2014;132:105–111.

17. Bradman A, Quiros-Alcala L, Castorina R, et al. Effect of organic diet intervention on pesticide exposures in young children living in low-income urban and agricultural communities. *Environ Health Perspect.* 2015;123(10):1086–1093.

18. Payne-Sturges D, Cohen J, Castorina R, Axelrad DA, Woodruff TJ. Evaluating cumulative organophosphorus pesticide body burden of children: a national case study. *Environmental Science & Technology.* 2009;43(20):7924–7930.

19. Hernandez AF, Gil F, Lacasana M. Toxicological interactions of pesticide mixtures: an update. *Arch Toxicol.* 2017;91(10):3211–3223.

20. Landrigan PJ, Benbrook C. GMOs, herbicides, and public health. *The New England Journal of Medicine.* 2015;373(8):693–695.

21. Landrigan PJ, Belpoggi F. The need for independent research on the health effects of glyphosate-based herbicides. *Environmental Health: A Global Access science source.* 2018;17(1):51.

22. Monastra G, Rossi L. Transgenic foods as a tool for malnutrition elimination and their impact on agricultural systems. *Rivista di biologia.* 2003;96(3):363–384.

23. (USDA) USDoA. Petitions for Determination of Nonregulated Status. https://www.aphis.usda.gov/aphis/ourfocus/biotechnology/permits-notifications-petitions/petitions/petition-status. Published 2019. Updated March 18, 2019. Accessed April 1, 2019.

24. Johnson, David. SOC. These Charts Show Every Genetically Modified Food People Already Eat in the US. http://time.com/3840073/gmo-food-charts/. Published 2015. Accessed April 1, 2019.

25. Benbrook CM. Trends in glyphosate herbicide use in the United States and globally. *Environmental Sciences Europe.* 2016;28(1):3.

26. Vandenberg, L. N.; Blumberg, B.; Antoniou, M. N.; Benbrook, C. M.; Carroll, L.; Colborn, T.; Everett, L. G.; Hansen, M.; Landrigan, P. J.; Lanphear, B. P.; Mesnage, R.; Vom Saal, F. S.; Welshons, W. V.; Myers, J. P., Is it time to reassess current safety standards for glyphosate-based herbicides? *J Epidemiol Community Health* 2017, *71* (6), 613–18.

27. Bai SH, Ogbourne SM. Glyphosate: environmental contamination, toxicity and potential risks to human health via food contamination. *Environmental Science and Pollution Research International.* 2016;23(19):18988–19001.

28. Jansons M, Pugajeva I, Bartkevics V. Occurrence of glyphosate in beer from the Latvian market. *Food Addit Contam Part A Chem Anal Control Expo Risk Assess.* 2018;35(9):1767–1775.

29. Zoller O, Rhyn P, Rupp H, Zarn JA, Geiser C. Glyphosate residues in Swiss market foods: monitoring and risk evaluation. *Food Additives & Contaminants Part B, Surveillance.* 2018;11(2):83–91.

30. Landrigan PJ. What causes autism? Exploring the environmental contribution. *Current Opinion in Pediatrics.* 2010;22(2):219–225.

31. Bouchard MF, Chevrier J, Harley KG, Kogut K, Vedar M, Calderon N, et al. "Prenatal exposure to organophosphate pesticides and IQ in 7-year-old children." *Environ Health Perspect.* 2011;119(8):1189–1195.

32. Davoren MJ, Schiestl RH. Glyphosate-based herbicides and cancer risk: a post-IARC decision review of potential mechanisms, policy and avenues of research. *Carcinogenesis.* 2018;39(10):1207–1215.

33. Van Bruggen AHC, He MM, Shin K, et al. Environmental and health effects of the herbicide glyphosate. *The Science of the Total Environment.* 2018;616–617:255–268.

34. Ritter GD, Acuff GR, Bergeron G, et al. Antimicrobial-resistant bacterial infections from foods of animal origin: understanding and effectively communicating to consumers. *Ann N Y Acad Sci.* 2019;1441(1):40–49.

35. Grob K, Biedermann M, Scherbaum E, Roth M, Rieger K. Food contamination with organic materials in perspective: packaging materials as the largest and least controlled source? A view focusing on the European situation. *Critical Reviews in Food Science and Nutrition.* 2006;46(7):529–535.

36. Heindel JJ, Blumberg B. Environmental obesogens: mechanisms and controversies. *Annu Rev Pharmacol Toxicol.* 2019;59:89–106.

37. *The Atlantic.* Are tea bags turning us into plastic? https://www.theatlantic.com/health/archive/2013/04/are-tea-bags-turning-us-into-plastic/274482/. Published 2013. Accessed April 1, 2019.

38. Myers, J. P. Peering into the Plasticene, our future of plastic and plastic waste. Environmental Health News. https://www.ehn.org/plastic-waste-2595276205.html. Accessed April 18, 2020.

39. Ishak, R. Here's what every plastic recycling symbol actually means. https://hellogiggles.com/lifestyle/how-to-read-plastic-recycling-symbols/. Accessed April 17, 2020.

40. Christensen MS, Hansen J, Ramlau-Hansen CH, Toft G, Kolstad H. Cancer incidence in workers exposed to Styrene in the Danish-reinforced plastics industry, 1968–2012. *Epidemiology (Cambridge, Mass).* 2017;28(2):300–310.

41. Rosenmai AK, Bengtstrom L, Taxvig C, et al. An effect-directed strategy for characterizing emerging chemicals in food contact materials made from paper and board. *Food Chem Toxicol.* 2017;106(Pt A):250259.

42. Carwile JL, Ye X, Zhou X, Calafat AM, Michels KB. Canned soup consumption and urinary bisphenol A: a randomized crossover trial. *JAMA.* 2011;306(20):22182220.

43. Centers for Disease Control and Prevention. *Lead and a Healthy Diet: What You Can Do to Protect Your Child.* 2016.

44. Shabbir MA, Raza A, Anjum FM, Khan MR, Suleria HA. Effect of thermal treatment on meat proteins with special reference to heterocyclic aromatic amines (HAAs). *Critical Reviews in Food Science and Nutrition.* 2015;55(1):8293.

45. Baranski M, Srednicka-Tober D, Volakakis N, et al. Higher antioxidant and lower cadmium concentrations and lower incidence of pesticide residues in organically grown crops: a systematic literature review and meta-analyses. *Br J Nutr.* 2014;112(5):794811.

46. Sanchez-Villegas A, Alvarez-Perez J, Toledo E, et al. Seafood consumption, Omega-3 fatty acids intake, and life-time prevalence of depression in the PREDIMED-Plus Trial. *Nutrients.* 2018;10(12).

47. Ajith TA. A recent update on the effects of Omega-3 fatty acids in Alzheimer's Disease. *Current Clinical Pharmacology.* 2018;13(4):252260.

48. Kamel F, Goldman SM, Umbach DM, et al. Dietary fat intake, pesticide use, and Parkinson's disease. *Parkinsonism & Related Disorders.* 2014;20(1):8287.

49. EWG (2003) PCBs in farmed salmon. https://www.ewg.org/research/pcbs-farmed-salmon, Accessed May 23, 2020.

50. Liebezeit G, Liebezeit E. Synthetic particles as contaminants in German beers. *Food Addit Contam Part A Chem Anal Control Expo Risk Assess.* 2014;31(9):1574–1578.

5

What Is *REALLY* in Our Drinking Water?

There's plenty of water in the universe without life, but nowhere is there life without water.

—Sylvia A. Earle (marine biologist)

What Could Be More Important?

Humans evolved from the earth's vast ocean waters and, as if in tribute, water flows abundantly through human veins (the liquid portion of blood is 92% water). From the time we are born and first bathed to our last cleansing in preparation before burial, we are intricately tied to water (about 60% of the adult human body is water). So important is water to the human body that one would die within days without it. Water sustains us, physically and figuratively. Consumers cling to nostalgic images splashed across plastic drinking bottles and painted on water delivery trucks of crystal clear streams and mountain springs, although the water in these bottles may be taken from the same tap water you drink in your home. This marketing strategy is similar to the idyllic farms with red barns and rolling hills painted across meat packaging and milk cartons, whose contents come from animals housed in overcrowded industrial animal feedlots, referred to as a concentrated animal feeding operation (CAFO), that you would not want to have near where you live.

Bottled water marketed as idyllic, "pure" water in plastic bottles is housed in containers made with toxic, hormone-disrupting chemicals that leach out over time; with only the slightest agitation, temperature change and exposure to sunlight, the matrix of these man-made plastics oozes into our children's drinking water, often while stored for months or waiting in pallets to be loaded aboard a truck in soaring temperatures. Most people will drink any cup of water handed to them, without the slightest knowledge of its origin or contents. In spite of established US regulations and over-sight of municipal water sources, national and worldwide contamination of drinking water has become so pervasive, and its human health effects so profound, it begs the question, why do we take clean drinking water for granted? *What could be more important?*

Safe, Clean Drinking Water

Safe, clean drinking water is greatly misunderstood and undervalued in the United States. As with many environmental topics, we may rely too much on the oversight of government agencies to protect the health of citizens.

A typical American uses 80–100 gallons of water every day, which includes washing dishes and laundry, watering the lawn, taking showers, and flushing toilets. Only 1% of the water coming into people's homes is used for drinking water, but the quality and safety of that water is likely to be unknown to the drinker.

Of course, water quality in the United States far exceeds that of third-world countries—and even some developed countries. Worldwide, more than 650 million people do not have access to safe water, and nearly a thousand children under the age of five die every day from diarrhea caused by poor sanitation, inadequate hygiene, or contaminated water.[1] However, laws intended to protect our water, such as the Safe Drinking Water Act (SDWA) of 1974, have been overwhelmed by the unchecked marketing, distribution, and use of toxic chemicals in the United States. The Toxic Substances Control Act (TSCA) of 1976 has failed to protect our health and environment from manufacturing and releasing toxic chemicals.

Although the law was amended in 2016, it remains unenforceable due to the imbalance of power that gives greater weight to the manufacturer over the consumer. These weak laws and lack of public health oversight allow toxic chemicals to make their way into our water, then into our bodies, impacting our health. The sheer number of chemicals that make their way into US drinking water—and the real health effects that result from acute and cumulative, low-level chemical exposure—should alarm consumers and motivate them to be proactive and aggressive when it comes to obtaining clean drinking water. But as the majority of US citizens neither learn this information in school nor deal with it professionally, it is understandable that they are uninformed about actions they can take to assure clean drinking water for themselves and their children. With knowledge comes power and action. For example, regular folks now have access to water filtration methods that go beyond what the US government has thus far provided through municipal water treatment systems. Using these in-home filtering systems, some of which are not very expensive, can greatly increase the safety of the water we drink, cook with, and bathe in.

Water and the Human Body

When we think of water, we often think of quenching our thirst on a hot summer day. But water is essential for an enormous number of physiologic processes in the human body: it moistens air for breathing, carries nutrients to cells, regulates pH (i.e., acidity/alkalinity), helps maintain our body temperature through sweating, protects and cushions vital organs (e.g., brain, gut), cushions both joints and the discs in our spine, makes tendons flexible, and removes waste and toxins (from, e.g., sweat, urine, feces, mucus, gastrointestinal system, vaginal canal). Water is thus essential for survival (see Figure 5.1).

The National Academies of Sciences, Engineering, and Medicine say that the adequate amount of fluid intake for men is 15.5 cups (3.7 liters) of fluids per day, and 11.5 cups (2.7 liters) for women. Those who live in hot, dry climates, exercise regularly, are experiencing vomiting and/or diarrhea, are prone to kidney stones or blood clots, or are pregnant or breast feeding, will require greater daily fluid intake. About 20% of daily fluids comes from food (extreme examples are watermelon and spinach that are almost 100% water by weight).

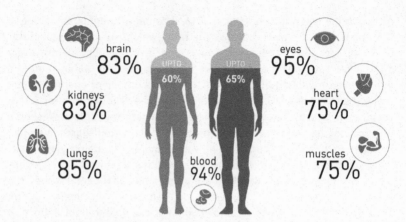

FIGURE 5.1 Water content of organs in the human body.

Water Contamination

Depending on the type of contaminant, water can potentially cause a host of health issues and even irreparable damage, especially for growing fetuses, children, and those with weak immune systems.

How does drinking water become contaminated? First, understand that there are over 90,000 chemical compounds available for commercial use in the United States, and only a handful have been tested for safety or toxicity. These chemicals come from manufacturing, distribution, and chemical disposal processes; trash incinerators; car exhaust and automotive production lines; pesticides; cleaning facilities; and even the bug spray, air freshener, and perfume sprayed into the air in and around homes. Other sources of water contamination are chemicals washed down the drain (think Drano, or toilet cleaners), water filled with microplastics that come from cleaning fleece jackets, rayon and polyester in our washing machines, and pesticides sprayed on or washed off produce. The practice of adding fluoride *intentionally* to drinking water to prevent tooth decay is controversial. The chlorine disinfectant byproducts (called trihalomethanes that are highly toxic) that form when chlorine reacts with organic compounds in water, can all cycle back to the air or end up in soil, in surface water, and eventually in water treatment plants to end up as contaminants in drinking water (see Figure 5.2).

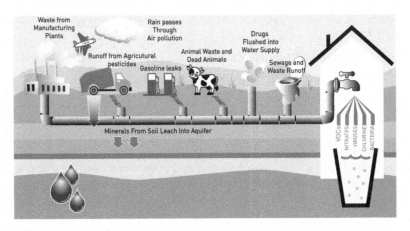

Figure 5.2 How contaminants get into drinking water.

Approximately 80% of U.S drinking water comes from surface sources (lakes, rivers, streams), and approximately 20% comes from groundwater wells, cisterns, and springs.[2]

Pollutants in the air mix with rain water and manufacturing plants may dump chemicals both illegally and legally into water that we drink (using discharge permits). This pollution of water can occur up to allowable levels, which are set without actually determining whether the allowable levels are actually safe, and instead are based on the sensitivity of the analytical systems for measuring the pollutants. Animal feedlot waste (which may contain bacteria such as *E.coli* and salmonella, growth hormones, and antibiotics), fertilizer chemicals from fields and lawns, old plumbing systems (made with lead or copper piping), new plumbing systems (PVC plastic pipes), chemical spills, landfill runoff, natural disasters such as flooding, which disperse greater amounts of industrial chemicals and contaminate wells—all add to the pollutant loads. Even toilet water containing discarded medications (e.g., oral contraceptives, antidepressants, blood pressure medications, illicit drugs) will contribute contaminants to surface and underground waterways, and eventually end up back in drinking water because they are not completely removed by water-treatment systems for municipal water. Waterways, lakes, and streams are too often the vehicle by which chemicals wreak havoc on wildlife and ecosystems as well. These contaminated waterways will eventually reach wells used for drinking water and public water-treatment systems in the United States.

Limitations of the Safe Drinking Water Act (SDWA)

Passed in 1974 (amended in 1996), the SDWA was intended to ensure safe drinking water for citizens by regulating *public* water treatment plants in the United States. The SDWA does not apply to residential wells; it also does not apply to bottled water, which is supposedly overseen by the FDA but in reality is not. The FDA's regulations for bottled-water safety are based on the premise that bottled water is not a potential risk to public health, and this lack of FDA oversight has led some states to pass laws that provide standards for the bottled water industry in the state. The SDWA authorizes the EPA to set "national health-based standards for drinking water to protect against both naturally occurring and man-made contaminants that may be found in drinking water."[3] Under the SDWA, *only 90 contaminants* are screened for and regulated if the contaminant levels exceed EPA-designated cutoffs (see Figure 5.3).[4]

The categories of contaminants the EPA regulates include:

- **Microorganisms**: cryptosporidium, *Giardia lamblia*, coliform, legionella and viruses
- **Disinfectants:** chlorine-based chemicals
- **Disinfection by-products:** Bromate, chlorites, trihalomethanes
- **Organic chemicals:** benzene, chlordane (pesticide), atrazine (pesticide), PCBs, vinyl chloride
- **Inorganic chemicals:** arsenic, asbestos, cadmium, lead, copper, mercury, nitrate and nitrite
- **Radionucleotides:** radium, uranium

Given the limitations of the SDWA, which *currently* screens for and regulates only 90 contaminants, as well as weak regulation and oversight by the EPA, it is critical that individuals be proactive in obtaining clean drinking water for themselves and their families.

National Primary Drinking Water Regulations

Contaminant	MCL or TT[1] (mg/L)[2]	Potential health effects from long-term[3] exposure above the MCL	Common sources of contaminant in drinking water	Public Health Goal (mg/L)[2]
Acrylamide	TT[1]	Nervous system or blood problems; increased risk of caner	Added to water during sewage/ wastewater treatment	zero
Alachlor	0.002	Eye, liver, kidney, or spleen problems, anemia, increased risk of cancer	Runoff from herbicide used on now crops	zero
Alpha/photon emitters	15 picocuries per Liter (pCi/L)	Increased risk of cancer	Erosion of natural deposits of certain minerals that are radioactive and may emit a form of radiation known as alpha radiation	zero
Antimony	0.006	Increase in blood cholesterol; decrease in blood sugar	Discharge from petroleum refineries; fire retardant; ceramics; electronics, solder	0.006
Arsenic	0.010	Skin damage or problems with circulatory systems, and may have increased risk of getting cancer	Erosion of natural depsits, runoff from orchards, runoff from glass & electronics production wastes	0
Asbestos (fibers>10 micrometers)	7 million fibers per Liter (MFL)	Increased risk of developing benign intestinal polyps	Decay of asbestos cement in water mains, erosion of natural deposits	7 MFL
Atrazine	0.003	Cardiovascular systems or reproductive problems	Runoff from herbicide used on row crops	0.003
Barium	2	Increase in blood pressure	Discharge of drilling wastes; discharge from metal refineries, erosion of natural deposits	2
Benzene	0.005	Anemia, decrease in blood platelets, increased risk of cancer	Discharge from factories; leaching from gas storage tanks and landfills	zero
Benzo(alpyrene (PAHs)	0.0002	Reproductive difficulties; increased risk of cancer	Leaching from linings fo water storage tanks and distribution lines	zero
Beryllium	0.004	Intestinal lesions	Discharge from metal refineries and coal-burning factories; discharge from electrical, aerospace, and defense industries	0.004
Beta photon emitters	4 milirems per year	Increased risk of cancer	Decay of natural and man-made deposits of certain minerals that are radioactive and may emit forms of radiation known as photons and beta radiation	zero
Bromate	0.010	Increased risk of cancer	Byproduct of drinking water disinfection	zero
Cadmium	0.005	Kidney damage	Corrosion of galvanized pipes; erosion of natural deposits; discharge from metal refineries; runoff from waster batteries and paints	0.005
Carbofuran	0.04	Problems with blood, nervous systems, or reproductive systems	Leaching of soil fumigant used on rice and alfalfa	0.04

LEGEND

DISINFECTANT · DISINFECTION BYPRODUCT · INORGANIC CHEMICAL · MICROORGANISM · ORGANIC CHEMICAL · RADIONUCLIES

FIGURE 5.3 Fifteen of the 90 contaminants regulated by the EPA under the Safe Drinking Water Act of 1974. For the complete list go to: https://www.epa.gov/sites/production/files/2016-06/documents/npwdr_complete_table.pdf.

How Are Standards for Safe Levels of a Contaminant Designed?

The EPA sets federal "maximum contaminant levels" (MCLs) for the 90 regulated contaminants; an MCL is the highest allowed amount of a specific contaminant that a public water system can legally contain. It takes years and an enormous preponderance of data, testing, and lobbying to have a harmful chemical added to this list and an MCL established. Lead in drinking water, for example, is considered safe by the US EPA at levels of 15 parts per billion, whereas the majority of researchers and physicians agree that there is no safe level for lead in drinking water.[5] The EPA must make available to the public a Contaminant Candidate List (CCL), which specifies unregulated contaminants known to occur in public water systems, for which research may be undertaken by researchers to establish health risk and potential regulation. As of 2020, perchlorate, toluene, several pesticides, and even estrogenic drugs, were still on the CCL list without any federal regulations in place.[6] Do you want these chemicals in YOUR drinking water?

Water Treatment Plants

There are approximately 160,000 public water treatment plants in the United States that provide 86% of Americans with drinking water for their homes, schools, hospitals, and businesses. Water treatment plants may be publicly (by a local government) or privately owned.

By definition, a public water system must serve at least 25 people per day for 60 days out of the year OR have at least 15 service connections.[3] There are 2 different categories of water systems:

- Community water system (there are approximately 54,000 across the US): a public system that serves the same people year-round (such as most residences: homes, apartments, mobile home parks)
- Noncommunity water system: a public water system that does NOT serve the same population year-round. There are two types:
  - Nontransient noncommunity water system (approximately 20,000 across the US). This system **serves** the same people more than 6 months of the year (e.g., a school with its own water supply)

- Transient noncommunity water system (approximately 89,000 across the US). This system **does not serve** the same people for more than 6 months of the year (e.g., campgrounds, highway rest areas)

Different standards apply to these water systems, including the frequency of contaminant testing. Water treatment plants serving smaller populations may conduct weekly testing of particular contaminants, while other plants may conduct monthly testing for those same contaminants. Poor oversight for water treatment plants has come under fire since a 2017 report from the National Resources Defense Council (NRDC) showed that in 2015 alone, there were more than 80,000 reported violations of the Safe Drinking Water Act by community systems; 18,000 of the water systems with violations served nearly 77 million people (25% of the US population). Very small systems found in rural areas account for >50% of all health-based violations. There are often no repercussions for drinking water violations; the report stated that 9 out of 10 violations were subject to no formal action, and only 3.3% faced financial penalties.[7]

- Approximately 86% of the US population relies on water from ~160,000 public water supplies
- EPA: Public water supply has 15 connections or serving at least 25 people
- Public water supply:
  - ~80% surface sources
  - ~20% groundwater wells

More than 97% of the 160,000 US public water systems serve fewer than 10,000 people each.

Several disinfectants and detergents used to clean ground and surface water for drinking use, as well as their byproducts, are also permissible up to enforceable standards. Levels designated as "safe" are based on a grown man who drinks 2 liters of water per day. Many unregulated and regulated chemicals are being identified in thousands of homes, hospitals, and schools throughout the United States. In 2015, extremely high levels of lead found in the drinking water in Flint, Michigan, sounded the alarm for thousands of municipalities across the United States to take a better look and stronger stance on lead identification and remediation. For many it may have been too late; fetuses, infants, and children are most at risk for the irreversible neurologic effects of lead exposure, and contrary to EPA statements, there is no safe level of lead in the human body.[8,9]

It turns out that Flint is only one of dozens of lead-contaminated water systems across the United States; almost every state has been cited for elevated lead levels at one time or another. Lead testing for school water systems is overseen by individual states and is voluntary, and remediation in schools is not mandatory.[7,10,11] States often require children to be screened for lead; New Jersey state law, for instance, currently requires lead screening in children at 12 and 24 months of age, but not at older ages when behavioral changes, cognitive changes, or symptoms of ADHD may begin to appear.[12] Given the increased rate of ADHD diagnosis among school-aged children (and the often reflexive use of ADHD medication), and the pervasiveness of lead contamination from drinking water and other sources, testing blood lead levels in children is warranted.[13]

In addition to lead, hundreds of other harmful chemicals are pervasive in municipal water systems and are not filtered out at water treatment plants. Among them are PFAS chemicals, which are commonly called "forever chemicals" because they do not degrade. This class of chemicals include PFOS and PFOA (used for waterproofing and nonstick products) (see Box 5.1),[14–16] but nearly 5,000 chemically related PFAS have been produced and used by industry. Hundreds of these chemicals have been detected in the environment, and dozens have been detected in human blood. So far, the EPA has issued nonbinding health advisories for just two chemicals in this class—but it took over 50 years from the first evidence in 1965 that PFOA was harmful to human health to phase out PFOA in 2015. This class of chemicals is known to have endocrine-disrupting effects that can result in early menopause, kidney and testicular cancers, liver dysfunction, delayed puberty, obesity, and reduced vaccine response in children, resulting in less protection to some infections.

Glyphosate (i.e., Roundup) is the most widely used herbicide in the United States followed by atrazine; these have made their way into underground and surface waters across the United States. Atrazine was not re-registered for use in the European Union (essentially it is banned), but in the United States atrazine has been detected and flagged at "unacceptable" levels in areas throughout the country. In animal studies using exposure levels comparable to human exposure, atrazine has been found to

> **Box 5.1 List of chemicals not removed from conventional water treatment plant processing**
>
> Contaminants commonly found in public drinking water after "treatment" (these chemicals are NOT removed):
> - Disinfectants and disinfection byproducts
> - Discarded medicines (e.g., antidepressants, antibiotics, blood pressure, oral contraceptive meds)
> - Plasticizers such as BPA and phthalates
> - Nonstick/grease-proofing/waterproofing chemicals such as PFOS, PFOA (PFAS)
> - Antimicrobials, such as triclosan
> - Industrial chemicals such as benzene, toluene, vinyl chloride, carbon tetrachloride, and styrene (the main ingredient of Styrofoam)
> - Coal ash and fracking chemicals
> - Fragrance chemicals
> - Agricultural chemicals, pesticides, fertilizers, and herbicides (e.g., Roundup)
> - Chemicals from discarded cosmetics, beauty products, and hair dyes
> - PCBs
> - Plastic microfibers/microplastics
> - Nanoparticles used in sunscreens, anti-odor fabrics, and as a method to treat drinking water for viruses

turn young male bull frogs into female frogs. Studies show that exposure to atrazine in drinking water during early and mid-pregnancy may be most critical for its toxic effects on the fetus.[17,18] In humans, atrazine exposure during pregnancy is associated with low birth weight, preterm delivery, developmental delays, and increased risk for autism. In March 2015, the International Agency for Research on Cancer (IARC), an arm of the World Health Organization, classified glyphosate as "probably carcinogenic to humans." In a growing trend, municipalities across the United States are voluntarily restricting its use in parks and public areas.

Microplastics found in drinking water are also of great concern. Microplastics are plastic fibers that come from polyester, rayon, and other synthetic fabrics as well as from larger plastic pieces that breakdown through sun, heat, and mechanical exposure. Research shows billions of people globally are drinking water contaminated by microplastics, with 83% of samples found to be polluted.[19,20]

Important Takeaway

As previously mentioned, thousands of untested, unregulated industrial, pharmaceutical, and farming chemicals, bacteria, viruses, radionucleotides, microplastics, metals from old plumbing, fracking runoff, fecal waste, and medications are capable of ending up at public water treatment plants across the United States. Only 90 chemicals are actually monitored and regulated under US law, and the frequency of contaminant testing varies from water system to water system based on the population it serves. If levels of chemicals in drinking water are tested and found to be too high, there are steps that can be taken to reduce those levels to concentrations that meet the EPA's standards as safe for the public. However, the EPA's standards for "safe" for many of the chemicals listed in the SDWA are disputed by researchers. Not only does that mean thousands of potentially harmful chemicals can—and do—get into our drinking water, but some of the 90 chemicals that *are* regulated are "allowable" at levels far higher than may be safe for a healthy adult, let alone for small children whose safety is not considered when the EPA sets its safety levels. Also at risk are those with impaired immune systems, and the elderly. (See Box 5.1) for a list of chemicals not typically removed from the treatment plant filtering process.)

Municipal Water Testing

Like many people reading this book, one of us (AC) receives a monthly water bill from a privately owned water treatment company that delivers their tap water from 50 miles away. How can customer know how safe their munic-ipal water supply is? Commercial water testing kits are often ineffective, and having household water tested by a certified laboratory can be very expensive if the lab charges for each chemical tested. Often, commercial laboratories are not equipped to test for chemicals that are biologically ac-tive at low levels. The EPA requires most community water systems to pro-vide customers with an annual water quality report or consumer confidence report (CCR) that provides detailed information about the quality of your drinking water during the past year. Reports can be obtained by contacting your water company directly, and resources such as the National Sanitation Foundation (NSF) can help interpret the report (see link below). However, the yearly report that you receive only presents the average level of the chemicals that were measured. Periodically, the water treatment plant may hyperchlorinate the water, and there will be a strong chlorine or other chemical smell from tap water, but when averaged over the year, these high exposure events are not obvious to the public.

One can also look up contaminants through the Environmental Working Group's tap water database, where you can look up your municipal tap water testing results by zip code.

https://www.ewg.org/tapwater/#.W5QcBS2ZO34

National Sanitation Foundation (NSF):

http://www.nsf.org/consumer-resources/water-quality/water-filters-testing-treatment/consumer-confidence-reports

Wells

In the United States, approximately 15 million households rely on private wells for drinking water. Domestic wells do not fall under any governmental supervision; thus, the SDWA does NOT apply to residential well water and requires NO water testing for corrosive or toxic chemicals (lead, mercury, arsenic, or other pesticides) until or unless the property is sold, at which time only limited chemical testing is mandated.

Although the CDC *recommends* testing individual home wells for bacteria and other contaminants (e.g., arsenic, benzene, lead) at least once per year, testing can be costly and finding certified water specialists may be difficult. By the time an annual or biannual water analysis is completed, often by paying for each individual contaminant of interest, a reputable "point-of-use" water filtration system could be installed, saving both time and expense.

Common contaminants of domestic wells include pesticides: arsenic, organophosphates, glyphosate and atrazine (in the Midwest farm belt), fluoride, metals, nitrates and phosphorous from farming fertilizers, radionucleotides (radon, uranium), and legacy chemicals that were banned decades ago but are highly persistent in the environment (PCBs, lindane, DDT). In the United States, more than 500 million pounds (230 million kg) of herbicides, fungicides, and insecticides are used annually. Chemical pesticides are capable of traveling for miles in the air, through underground aquifers, and along surface waters to contaminate drinking wells; they often go undetected through wastewater treatment plants. In areas where hydrofracking for oil and natural gas extraction is occurring, groundwater aquifers are showing contamination by hydrofracking fluids. An important issue to consider when testing for herbicides is to be aware of farming practices and what herbicides are being used, and test for them during the time of year that they are being applied to nearby fields (for instance, if you live in the Midwest where use of atrazine spikes in the spring).

Homeowners with residential well water, who choose not to filter their drinking water, should undergo water testing at least once per year for carcinogenic ground contaminants such as nitrates and arsenic, as well as for heavy metals from plumbing contamination (lead, copper, mercury). Well water should also be tested after natural disasters such as flooding or tornados, as recommended by most water regulators as well as the American Academy of Pediatrics (AAP).

Know where your home water comes from as well as the water in your children's schools and day care centers. If you live in an area where agricultural or concentrated animal feeding operations are present, be aware of the increased risk of nitrates in groundwater, which may directly affect well water safety.

Well Water: Resources

For more information on well maintenance and testing, visit
http://water.epa.gov/drink/info/well/index.cfm
www.cdc.gov/healthywater/drinking/private/wells
www.cdc.gov/healthywater/drinking/private/wells/testing.html

Types of Water Filtration

Water filters can selectively remove unwanted materials from drinking water. Filters vary by cost, type of technology, type of contaminant removed, size, and certification for effectiveness, such as "National Sanitation Foundation (NSF) certified." It is important to remember that, in addition to ingesting contaminants from drinking water, breathing moist air during showering or washing dishes and clothing can provide exposure to contaminants. In addition, chemicals are often able to cross the skin and be absorbed into the body through direct contact while bathing.

Water filters for home use include water pitcher filters, carbon filters on refrigerator doors or attached to the faucet, countertop filters, undercounter reverse osmotic water filter systems and whole home water filtration systems (see Table 5.1).

Table 5.1 Examples of Filtration Systems to Create Clean Drinking Water from EWG.org[21]

This option...	Is used at home...	To remove...
Carbon/Activated carbon	In water pitchers, on the head of a faucet, on a shower head, or under the sink connecting to a separate faucet.	Chlorine, several chlorinated byproducts from water treatment plants, some pesticides
Ultraviolet	As part of a whole house system	Bacteria and other microbes
Reverse Osmosis (RO)	Under sinks or in whole house systems	Bacteria, medications, chlorine, fluoride, and radioactive particles
Water softener	In faucets or whole house system	Dissolved minerals from rock: calcium, iron, magnesium carbonate and manganese. Sodium is often used for mineral exchange, so check with your doctor. Use a separate pipe for gardening/watering plants
Mechanical (ex. ceramic)	Countertop	Has small holes to block sediment but will not remove chemical contaminants
Distillers	Countertop; heats water to high temperature to vaporize, and then condenses the steam back into water	Removes minerals, many bacteria and viruses, and chemicals with high boiling point. Does not remove chlorine, trihalomethanes or VOCs from water
Ion-Exchange	Whole house system; water passes over a resin that exchanges ions	Removes mineral salts and other charged particles. Does not remove microorganisms, trihalomethanes, and other common VOCs
Ozone	Whole house system	Bacteria and other microbes

TIP: Be aware that all filters require replacement after a specific period of use, so pay attention to filter-change dates (record the installation date on the filter with a magic marker) as well as the annual cost of filter replacements. For the pros and cons of various consumer water filters, go to the Environmental Working Group's Updated Water Filter Buying Guide.[21]

TIP: Only reverse osmotic, ion exchange filters, and some carbon filters can remove appreciable amounts of lead from tap water. Search the NSF database by type of filter, brand, and the substance you want to filter out at http://info.nsf.org/Certified/DWTU.

Consumer Reports has a free online buying guide: http://www.consumerreports.org/cro/water-filters/buying-guide.htm

Environmental Working Group: https://www.ewg.org/tapwater/water-filter-guide.php#.W5P0_y2Z034

EPA Filtration Facts PDF: https://www.epa.gov/sites/production/files/2015-11/documents/2005_11_17_faq_fs_healthseries_filtration.pdf

Water Quality Association: https://www.wqa.org

Reverse Osmosis Filters

Reverse Osmosis (RO), also called hyperfiltration by the filtration industry, is the most thorough water cleaning method available to the public. RO filters can be installed by most plumbers, and their use likely provides cleaner water than what you purchase in a disposable bottle; RO systems dramatically reduce the use of plastic water bottles that add waste to our environment. This filtration system was developed in the late 1950s as a method of taking salt out of seawater (desalination). RO filters force water through a semipermeable membrane. Pores in the membrane block and trap contaminants such as chemicals, bacteria, and heavy metals (see Figure 5.4). The smaller the pore size, the more contaminants are trapped and filtered out. Carbon filters are part of or can be added to an RO system to remove specific volatile industrial and agricultural chemicals, such as pesticides. The greater the filtration, the slower the flow of water; this is why RO filters require a small tank that stores the filtered water for on-demand use once it has been slowly forced through the series of filters.

The "heart" and most important part of a RO system is its membrane filter. Membrane filters are rated and priced by their quality and flow rates of water (gallons per day [GPD]). RO systems have to be serviced regularly or when the water pressure begins to drop indicating

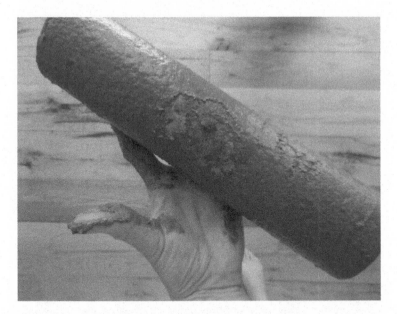

Figure 5.4 Image of author's own old RO filter during replacement (taken by author AC, fall of 2018).

that the filters need changing. Like all filtration systems, the filter must be replaced regularly, and the tubing cleaned annually to remove bacteria that may collect inside. RO filters can be cleaned by flushing the system with hydrogen peroxide annually. Testing of RO performance, based on chemical analysis, can be performed by a certified water testing company that should have experience purifying the system if contaminants are found. Look for a "Certified Water Specialist" in your area to service the RO system. From a sustainability perspective, RO filters on average waste 1–3 gallons of water in order to create 1 gallon of filtered drinking water, so this may increase water usage costs in areas of severe drought or where water restrictions are in effect. However, if the RO system is only used for drinking and cooking, this may be a tradeoff that is worth the extra cost.

Important Takeaway: Your RO water system is only as effective as the membrane filters that come with it. Many big box stores outsource the manufacture of the membrane filter to other countries while still carrying a "Made in America" label. Look for a Consumer Reports–rated RO filter with NSF certification.

Bottled Water

In the 1980s, one might have thought it absurd to bottle drinking water and sell it at a high price. Then fear of tap water contamination began to set in, and marketing companies spent billions on harnessing the idea that drinking bottled water was cleaner, safer, and healthier. Within a single generation, buying water in a bottle became normal and routine rather than something done in response to a natural disaster. (See Figure 5.5.)

What costs more in North America, gasoline or bottled water? Surprise, it's water! Bottled water costs up to $9 per gallon, and gasoline ranges

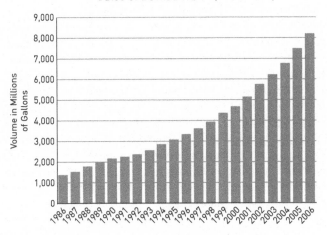

Figure 5.5 Worldwide sales of bottled water over time.

between $2 and $4 per gallon. Hydration is the third largest global industry behind oil and electricity. Americans spend almost $8 billion per year on bottled water, and over 47 million barrels of oil per year are used to produce plastic bottles.[22]

Bottled Water and Environmental Pollution

We now know that the use of bottled water is complicated, with a vast array of downstream pollution consequences for both the environment and the human body. The mantra that for routine use bottled water is safer for human health than tap water must be reevaluated. To begin with, most bottled water that you buy in the store is just packaged tap water. According to the Beverage Marketing Corporation's annual report for 2009, municipal tap water is the source for 47.8% of bottled water, and you *now* know how many contaminants can be in municipal tap water! In addition, chemicals from the plastic bottle itself routinely leach into the water it is holding, especially when it is hot.

Needless to say, the contribution of plastics (particularly single-use plastic water bottles) to environmental contamination is enormous and daunting. The consequences of waste from one-use plastics is extraordinary, not only for land debris, but for the astounding contribution that it makes to contaminating ocean waters. According to researchers, 275 million metric tons (MT) of plastic waste was generated in 192 coastal countries in 2010, with 4.8 to 12.7 million MT entering the ocean. Single-use plastic bottles are a major source of this ocean garbage, contributing up to 1.5 million tons of plastic waste into ocean waters every year. These bottles break down into smaller pieces over time, and sun exposure directly acts as a catalyst for further breakdown, harming wildlife and their ecological systems worldwide.[23] In 2006, Americans consumed an astounding 30 billion bottles of water in one-use plastic bottles, more than 80% of which ended up in landfills or were incinerated. From an economic perspective, bottled water costs up to1000-times more than tap water, not including the energy and pollution costs for transport nationally and internationally.[24] Recycling efforts have failed, rendering our environment grossly disfigured, as pointed out in chapter 4.

Regulation of Bottled Water

Bottled water is regulated by the FDA, and therefore, the water content undergoes less overall testing for contaminants than most municipal water systems. In addition, bottled water companies (except those selling water in California, as of 2007 [SB 220]) are not required to disclose the ingredients of their water nor are they required to answer three key questions:

- Where does the water come from?
- Is it purified? How?
- Have tests found any contaminants?

Both state and federal bottled-water regulation programs are severely underfunded; it is rare that FDA inspectors visit bottled-water plants. In 2002, the agency's own website acknowledged that "bottled water plants generally are assigned low priority for inspection," and nothing has changed since then.[25]

Bottled Drinking Water and Human Health

What is the impact on human health of contaminants that may be coming from the plastic packaging used for bottled water? The main plastic in most clear plastic containers used for beverages (e.g., bottles for water, soda, sports drinks), condiments (e.g., vinegar and salad dressing), and cosmetics (shampoo bottles) worldwide is PET, or polyethylene terephthalate (recycling code #1). The major chemical constituents in the synthesis of PET are terephthalic acid (TPA) and ethylene glycol. TPA has been implicated in increasing the ratio of estrogen receptors (ERα:ERβ) in high-risk donor breast epithelial cells (HRBECs), suggesting an estrogen receptor-disrupting effect.[26] Other additives in PET plastics include the EDCs known as phthalates (e.g., DEHP, DEP) as well as the unintended additive antimony, a naturally occurring element often widely used as a catalyst in the production of PET and has also been found to have estrogenic properties.[27] Studies show that depending on the manufacturer and country of origin, the quantities of ingredients used to make PET resin, such as various phthalates and antimony, vary greatly.[28,29]

Many studies have been undertaken to understand whether estrogen-like chemicals (xenoestrogens) leach from these bottles into the substances that they hold. In 2009, researchers observed that New Zealand mudsnails, *Potamopyrgus antipodarum*, incubated for 56 days in PET bottles produced significantly more embryos, an estrogenic effect, compared to those incubated in glass bottles.[30]

This same group of researchers later supported their findings by exposing cells from a human cancer cell line (MCF7) to PET chemicals via bottled mineral water manufactured in France, Germany, and Italy. They compared water from the same spring packed in glass versus water packed in plastic bottles made of PET, and found estrogenic activity to be three times higher in water from the plastic bottles. These data, along with other studies, continues to build the concept that PET packaging materials are a source of estrogen-like compounds. The findings showed that the contamination of bottled water with chemicals known to affect the human endocrine system is a global phenomenon.[31]

Where has *your* water been before landing in your local supermarket's refrigerator? Bottled water may sit in a hot warehouse for months or even years, or wait for shipment on loading docks in 100-degree weather, before ending up on store shelves. Studies show estrogen-like chemicals and antimony may leach out at faster rates, depending on environmental conditions and time from manufacture. These levels may also differ between brands.[32] (See Figure 5.6.)

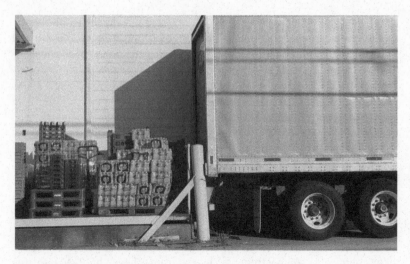

Figure 5.6 Plastic water bottles waiting for shipment in 100 degree heat (taken by author AC in Cape May, NJ—summer 2018).

Important Takeaway: Create Your Own Water Purification System

The most important message from this chapter is to create a "system" for intake of clean drinking water that you understand, can operate effectively, and that reduces your household chemical exposure from drinking, skin absorption, and inhalation of contaminants in water over the long term. No matter whether you have a domestic well or use municipal tap water, having point-of-use filtration for drinking water and cooking will be invaluable for your health. Overall, tap water costs far less than bottled water and doesn't come in plastic bottles to clog landfills, clutter streams and rivers, and build up in the ocean.

Carry Your Water Safely

Once you have created filtered drinking water at home and plan to take it with you, what is the safest way to carry it? Choose glass, US-made ceramic (to avoid lead from foreign ceramics), or stainless steel containers to hold and store your drinking water. BUT, make sure the containers don't have a plastic lid, plastic flip straws, or a plastic interior, which is added to some stainless steel and glass containers. Avoid commercial sports bottles, even if labeled "BPA-free"; often BPA is replaced by other harmful plasticizers/epoxy resins such as BPS, BPF, and BPSIP. Plastic chemicals in a bottle can leach into the water it is carrying (particularly on a hot day), so avoid drinking out of plastic sports bottles left in the heat. Try using single-use paper straws if they are necessary. Plastic straws are now banned in many countries worldwide.

Additional recommendations include:

- Try to understand where your water comes from and do not assume it is entirely safe. Most plastic bottled water sits for days, weeks, or months in hot warehouses and on loading docks for delivery, leaching plastic chemicals into the water they are holding.
- Understand the water source for your children's daycare and schools. If the water source is a well, ask about scheduled water testing and inquire about results.
- Try to use a water filter, ANY filter available (e.g., activated carbon pitcher filters), to help improve the safety and quality of this substance that is vital for life. With so much water ingested during one's lifetime, it makes sense to set up a system that is safe, easy to manage, and cost effective for you and your family.

Remember: You will have the most control over water that comes out of your home faucet by designing an in-home filtering system, also known as a point-of-use system. Water can travel many miles from a treatment plant before it arrives at your faucet, which allows for possible contamination along the way (water typically flows to your house through PVC pipes that leach phthalates and BPA). Bottled water costs 1000 times more than tap water, so filtering at home is most cost efficient, even counting the cost of a filtration system.

- If you buy single-use plastic water bottles, do not store them in the heat or leave them in the hot sun or in hot cars, and do not reuse them, because of bacterial contamination risk.
- It's smart to avoid drinking from the outside water hose in the summer, especially when the hose is hot from the sun because the plasticizers, phthalates and BPA, have been found to migrate into water from garden hoses made from PVC.

- Avoid water from the 5-gallon blue carboy water containers often found in office water coolers; they likely are polycarbonate, which is made from chains of BPA molecules that break apart and release BPA into the water (check for the recycle code #7 in a triangle).
- Bottled water should *only* be used if elevated levels of harmful chemicals are found in municipal or well drinking water, and only until effective filtration has been put into place.

Drinking Water Resources

Environmental Protection Agency: https://www.epa.gov/sites/production/files/2016-06/documents/npwdr_complete_table.pdf

National drinking water contaminant occurrence database:

http://water.epa.gov/scitech/datait/databases/drink/ncod/databases-index.cfm

http://water.epa.gov/drink/contact.cfm

Safe Drinking Water hotline at (800) 426-4791

US Geological Survey: www.usgs.gov

Environmental Working Group (EWG) National Drinking Water Database: www.ewg.org/search/site/water

Centers for Disease Control (CDC): http://www.cdc.gov/healthywater/drinking

Agency for Toxic Substances and Disease Registry: http://www.atdsr.cdc.gov

National Resource Defense Council: http://www.nrdc.org/water/ and http://www.nrdc.org/living/waterair/select-right-filter.asp

NSF international: www.nsf.org

Private well information/management: http://www.epa.gov/privatewells.

Direct patients to Environmental Working Groups website for additional information on filter options: www.EWG.org

EPA Safe Drinking Water Hotline: https://www.epa.gov/ground-water-and-drinking-water/safe-drinking-water-hotline.

Environmental Health News: https://www.ehn.org/search/?q=water%20quality

References

1. World Health Organization. Preventing disease through healthy environments: a global assessment of the burden of disease from environmental risks. http://

apps.who.int/iris/bitstream/10665/204585/1/9789241565196_eng.pdf?ua=1. Published 2016. Accessed September 2018.

2. Environmental Protection Agency (EPA). Private drinking water wells. https://www.epa.gov/privatewells. Published 2016. Accessed September, 2018.

3. EPA. Understanding the Safe Drinking Water Act. https://www.epa.gov/sites/production/files/2015-04/documents/epa816f04030.pdf. Published 2004. Accessed September 8, 2018.

4. EPA. Table of Regulated Drinking Contaminants. http://www.epa.gov/your-drinking-water/table-regulated-drinking-water-contaminants. Published 2016. Accessed February 2016.

5. Levallois P, Barn P, Valcke M, Gauvin D, Kosatsky T. Public health consequences of lead in drinking water. *Current Environmental Health Reports.* 2018;5(2):255–262.

6. EPA. Drinking water contaminant candidate list (CCL) and regulatory determination. https://www.epa.gov/ccl. Published 2017. Updated February 27, 2020. Accessed April 18, 2020.

7. Natural Resources Defense Council (NRDC). Threats on tap: widespread violations highlight need for investment in water infrastructure and protections. https://www.nrdc.org/resources/threats-tap-widespread-violations- water-infrastructure. Published 2017. Accessed April 18, 2020.

8. EPA. Drinking Water Requirements for Lead. 2016.

9. American Academy of Pediatrics Committee on Environmental Health. Lead exposure in children: prevention, detection, and management. *Pediatrics.* 2005;116(4):1036–1046.

10. Copp T. New database: water sources in 43 states contain potentially unsafe chemical levels. https://www.mcclatchydc.com/latest-news/article230009434.html. Published 2019. Accessed July 2, 2019.

11. Dore E, Deshommes E, Andrews RC, Nour S, Prevost M. Sampling in schools and large institutional buildings: Implications for regulations, exposure and management of lead and copper. *Water Research.* 2018;140:110–122.

12. State of New Jersey Department of Health. Childhood Lead: Testing for Lead Exposure. https://www.state.nj.us/health/childhoodlead/testing.shtml. Published 2019. Accessed January 1, 2020.

13. Huang S, Hu H, Sanchez BN, et al. Childhood blood lead levels and symptoms of attention deficit hyperactivity disorder (ADHD): a cross-sectional study of Mexican children. *Environ Health Perspect.* 2016;124(6):868–874.

14. Bartell SM, Calafat AM, Lyu C, Kato K, Ryan PB, Steenland K. Rate of decline in serum PFOA concentrations after granular activated carbon filtration at two public water systems in Ohio and West Virginia. *Environ Health Perspect.* 2010;118(2):222–228.

15. Centers for Disease Control and Prevention. Fourth National Report on Human Exposure to Environmental Chemicals. 2013 (March).

16. Perfluoroalkyl and Polyfluoroalkyl Substances (PFAS). National Institute of Environmental Health Sciences (NIEHS). Last reviewed April 15, 2020. https://www.niehs.nih.gov/health/topics/agents/pfc/index.cfm. Accessed April 24, 2020.

17. Almberg KS, Turyk ME, Jones RM, Rankin K, Freels S, Stayner LT. Atrazine contamination of drinking water and adverse birth outcomes in community water systems with elevated atrazine in Ohio, 2006–2008. *Int J Environ Res Public Health.* 2018;15(9).

18. Carter CJ, Blizard, BR. Autism genes are selectively targeted by environmental pollutants including pesticides, heavy metals, bisphenol A, phthalates and many others in food, cosmetics or household products. *Neurochem Int.* 2017;16:30197–30198.

19. Pivokonsky, M., Cermakova, K., et. al. Occurrence of microplastics in raw and treated drinking water. *Sci Total Environ.* 2018(643):1644–1651.

20. Mintenig SM, Löder MGJ, Primpke S, Gerdts G. Low numbers of microplastics detected in drinking water from ground water sources. *Sci Total Environ.* 2018(648):631–635.

21. Environmental Working Group (EWG). EWG's updated water filter buying guide. https://www.ewg.org/tapwater/water-filter-guide.php#.W51qBi2ZO34. Published 2018. Accessed September 15, 2018.

22. Royte, E. *Bottlemania: How Water Went on Sale and Why We Bought It.* Bloomsbury, London, 2008.

23. Jambeck J, Geyer R, Wilcox C, et al. Plastic waste inputs from land into the ocean. *Science* 2015(347):768–771.

24. Galgani F, Fleet D, Van Franeker J, et al. Marine strategy framework directive task team 10 report. Marine Litter. *JRC (EC Joint Research Centre) Scientific and Technical Reports.* 2010.

25. EWG. Is your bottled water worth it?: bottle vs tap—double standard. http://www.ewg.org/research/your-bottled-water-worth-it/bottle-vs-tap-double-standard. Published 2009. Accessed October 3, 2016.

26. Luciani-Torres MG, Moore DH, Goodson WH, 3rd, Dairkee SH. Exposure to the polyester PET precursor—terephthalic acid induces and perpetuates DNA damage-harboring non-malignant human breast cells. *Carcinogenesis.* 2015;36(1):168–176.

27. Choe SY, Kim SJ, Kim HG, et al. Evaluation of estrogenicity of major heavy metals. *The Science of the Total Environment.* 2003;312(1–3):15–21.

28. Sax L. Polyethylene terephthalate may yield endocrine disruptors. *Environ Health Perspect.* 2010;118(4):445–448.

29. Shotyk W, Krachler M. Contamination of bottled waters with antimony leaching from polyethylene terephthalate (PET) increases upon storage. *Environmental Science & Technology.* 2007;41(5):1560–1563.

30. Wagner M, Oehlmann J. Endocrine disruptors in bottled mineral water: total estrogenic burden and migration from plastic bottles. *Environmental Science and Pollution Research International.* 2009;16(3):278–286.

31. Wagner M, Oehlmann J. Endocrine disruptors in bottled mineral water: estrogenic activity in the E-Screen. *The Journal of Steroid Biochemistry and Molecular Biology.* 2011;127(1–2):128–135.

32. Westerhoff P, Prapaipong P, Shock E, Hillaireau A. Antimony leaching from polyethylene terephthalate (PET) plastic used for bottled drinking water. *Water Research.* 2008;42(3):551–556.

6

Medications Are Chemicals Too

Though the doctors treated him, let his blood, and gave him medications to drink, he nevertheless recovered.
—Leo Tolstoy, *War and Peace* (1828–1910)

By all accounts, billions of human lives have been saved by the advent of modern medicine and pharmaceuticals. Antibiotics for infection, insulin for diabetes, pain medications for cancer patients, medications for blood pressure control, immune system modulators for autoimmune diseases, blood thinning medications to prevent stroke, and medications that seem to magically flip cancer into remission. These medications, along with thousands of others, when used judiciously, conservatively, and under careful supervision, have indisputably benefited humankind and contributed to countless added years of human life.

That Being Said . . .

The US pharmaceutical industry is a behemoth enterprise, representing more than 45% of the global pharmaceutical market, with an estimated $209 billion dollars in sales annually from 2010 to 2014. Generic medications, which now comprise over 70% of all pharmaceutical sales, add to the exponential growth of this industry. There is an estimated $50 billion spent annually on research and development (R&D) of new drugs.[1]

Despite such factors as the ever-changing health needs of the US population, new clinical guidelines, treatment advances, the addition or removal of medications from the US market, ingredient-contamination issues, and policy changes regarding drug promotion and marketing, consumers continue to spend a large proportion of their income on medications. Using data collected from the biannual, nationally representative, cross-sectional survey of civilians in the United States (the NHANES data) by the CDC, an article published in the *Journal of the American Medical Association* concluded that overall prescription drug use continues to increase significantly, and this increase is occurring across almost all classes of medication, particularly those for treating blood pressure, diabetes, acid reflux, psychiatric disorders, and high cholesterol.[2] As the US population becomes sicker from chronic health conditions, the race to create innovative medications to treat these conditions continues to grow. Add slick pharmaceutical marketing and positive framing of medications by prescribers, and you have fertile ground for medication overload.[3]

The True Cost of Medication Overload: Side Effects

Most of us would agree that for life-threatening conditions, the benefits of medical therapy often far outweigh the side effects and/or downstream problems that may result. But for hundreds of *other* medications, the short- and long-term health risks may far outweigh the benefits. Medication side effects often lead to *additional prescriptions* to mitigate those side effects, a process known as a "prescribing cascade."

Let's say Mrs. Jones comes in to see her doctor for knee pain. Instead of a simple approach, such as physical therapy, topical pain relievers applied to the injured joint, massage, acupuncture, reasonable weight loss, and even localized steroid injection, any of which may have solved her knee pain, Mrs. Jones is prescribed an anti-inflammatory pain medication, such as ibuprofen or naproxen sodium. Many anti-inflammatory medications can raise blood pressure, which may lead the same or another physician to add a blood pressure–lowering medication, such as a calcium-channel blocker. Some calcium-channel blockers cause water retention, triggering a prescription for a diuretic, or "water pill." Some anti-inflammatory medications can also cause stomach irritation or burning, which may lead to a prescription for an acid reflux medication called a proton pump inhibitor (or PPI), and so on. Pretty soon, Mrs. Jones, who came in to the doctor for routine knee pain and who was taking no medications at the time, is now on 3 or 4 medications, prescribed over the course of a few months. Of course, if you are selling these drugs you are happy to reap the profits.

How much medication are Americans taking? According to reports from Express Scripts, a US pharmacy management organization, Americans consume approximately 80% of the world's opiate supply despite representing only 5% of the world's population.[4] Ten percent of the general population and 30% of older adults in the United States are taking five or more different pharmaceutical drugs simultaneously (termed polypharmacy), and this trend continues to increase.[2] According to a 2016 study, 36% of unassisted community–dwelling older adults (ages 62–85 years) were taking 5 or more prescription medications in 2010 to 2011—up from 31% in 2005 to 2006. In another study, among frail older US citizens, 40% were prescribed *9 or more* medications at hospital discharge, with 44% of these patients receiving at least one unnecessary drug.[5] As you might predict, when multiple drugs are prescribed by the same or multiple physicians simultaneously, problems such as adverse interactions between the drugs can *and do* occur. Between 2000 and 2014, drug overdoses involving opioids rose 200%; that many of these overdoses and deaths were attributed to legal opioids prescribed by physicians was a wakeup call.[6,7] Adverse drug reactions, in general, cause 4 hospitalizations per 1000 people each year and are among the top 4 reasons for emergency room visits. In addition, adverse drug reactions are among the 10 most common causes of death, and they result in an estimated $30–180 billion annually in lost wages and hospital costs.[8] Combining medications, whether prescription or over-the-counter (OTC), pose another threat—a number of them may contain the same ingredients (e.g., acetaminophen), and without supervision, the user may exceed the maximum safe dose.

Unintended New Diseases Caused by Pharmaceuticals

Statins

Medications used to *treat* one illness may *cause* another as discussed above. The class of medications called statins (generic names: atorvastatin, lovastatin, rosuvastatin, etc.), is widely used both in the United States and worldwide to help lower a specific type of cholesterol, low density lipoprotein (or LDL), which has been linked to an increased risk for atherosclerosis, stroke, and heart attack. Statin prescriptions have been on the rise ever since they hit the consumer market in the late 1980s, but there is now growing concern about their widespread use. Statins have been shown to increase the risk of developing new-onset type 2 diabetes (NOD), particularly in high doses and with more aggressive statins, and while some mechanisms, such as increased blood glucose levels and insulin resistance have been proposed, the exact mechanism is currently unknown.

Many cardiologists argue that the benefits for heart protection far outweigh the risks of statins, and for patients with a history of heart attack, stroke, or blocked arteries on vascular testing, or who are at high risk for these conditions, that may be true. Some cardiologists also feel that "patients at risk for the development of *diabetes* should be prescribed statins with caution."[9] Wouldn't it appear that in the United States where approximately 30 million people are living with diabetes and 84 million currently have *pre*diabetes (and are therefore at high risk for developing full blown type 2 diabetes), prescribing statins with abandon is a foolish undertaking?

Statins may also increase the risk of developing autoimmune diseases such as rheumatoid arthritis. Using an electronic database with 511,620 patient records, one recent study compared patients 40 years or older taking at least one prescribed statin to non–statin users. The study found that statin users had an increased risk of developing rheumatoid arthritis, especially during the first year after starting the medication.[10]

Gastroesophageal Reflux Disease (GERD) Medications

Many of us have experienced some degree of "heartburn" (generally caused by overproduction of stomach acid) in our lives, particularly after eating a meal that was too large, spicy, fried, or perhaps unhealthy. But as gastroesophageal reflux (GERD) or heartburn incidence has increased, often due to other factors than food choices (e.g., stress), the pharmaceutical industry has capitalized on heartburn and created a powerful new class of drugs called proton-pump inhibitors (PPIs) to block acid production in the stomach. PPIs are so powerful that they can decrease acid in the stomach by up to 99%. The problem is that humans *need* the stomach to produce acid; stomach acid lowers pH levels, thereby enabling the gut to perform a whole host of activities that have evolved in humans over millions of years. Protein digestion, absorption of key vitamins (e.g., vitamin B12) and minerals (e.g., iron, magnesium, calcium), and protecting the gut from infections, are just a few of these important activities. The term "gut microbiome" refers to the trillions of bacteria, fungi, and viruses that have evolved in a cooperative (commensal) relationship with humans to protect the intestines and maintain gut lining integrity. The gut microbiome influences all aspects of human health; this too becomes disrupted and unbalanced with the long-term use of PPIs.

Thus, it was not surprising when people taking PPIs for long periods of time were found to have nutrient deficiencies—including high rates of osteoporosis and hip fractures from reduced calcium absorption.[11-13] Low magnesium levels were putting patients at risk for seizures and arrhythmias to the point that in 2011, the FDA issued a safety warning advising doctors to check blood magnesium levels prior to initiating treatment with a PPI and to monitor levels throughout therapy. Diarrheal infections from overgrowth of the bacteria *Clostridium difficile*, which is often unresponsive to conventional antibiotic treatment, began to rise in patients on long-term PPIs, as did new cases of chronic kidney disease (CKD), progression of CKD, and increase in end-stage kidney disease (ESRD).[14-16] New data show an elevated risk for heart attack in long-term PPI users and increases in dementia risk in the elderly.[17,18] Despite the multitude of downstream effects from chronic PPI use and the availability of safe and effective alternatives for symptomatic GERD (e.g., dietary and lifestyle modifications, coating agents, antacids, herbal medicine), as of 2017, the American Gastroenterological Society continues to recommend long-term use of PPIs for symptomatic GERD.[19]

Drug-Induced Lupus

Over 90 commonly prescribed medications are implicated in causing a syndrome that looks and feels like a very serious autoimmune disease called systemic lupus erythematosus or SLE. Some of these medications are used to treat common problems such as high blood pressure (e.g., hydralazine, procainamide), skin acne in teenagers (minocycline), and rheumatoid arthritis (TNF-alpha inhibitors).[20] "Lupus-like" symptoms include joint pain, joint swelling, hair loss, and facial rash. Of concern, is that blood testing for antinuclear antibody (ANA) indicative of autoimmune disease, can lead to results that are falsely positive. Fortunately, drug-induced lupus rarely causes life-threatening complications or organ damage, and responds well to stopping the medication.[21]

Cancer Therapies

There are hundreds of cancer therapies, and although the benefits of treatment may far outweigh the health risks that may result from their use for those with cancers, we include this example to further illustrate the consequences that can arise from medication use. Cancer treatments that utilize the human immune system to fight cancer cells, called check-point inhibitors (CPIs), are now considered to be the cornerstone of cancer treatment. However, new findings show that some of these medications are associated with a host of side effects called immune-related adverse events (irAEs), including the development of autoimmune diseases and endocrine disorders.[22-25] A commonly used therapy for prostate cancer, known as androgen deprivation therapy (ADT), is associated with increased risk for developing rheumatoid arthritis (RA). Researchers found a 25% higher risk for developing RA in ADT users overall, but the longer the ADT continued, the greater the risk.[26] Androgens also play an important role in mood, energy level, and libido, and ADT use can depress all of these.

Opioid Pain Medications

If you live in the United States, you'd be hard pressed not to know about the ongoing opioid crisis. Years of heavy pharmaceutical lobbying and marketing, aggressive drug distribution throughout the United States, and overprescribing by physicians and dentists, has created one of the greatest preventable man-made epidemics the United States has ever seen. In 2016, opioid-related deaths approached 42,000, of which approximately 17,000 were due to prescription opioids and 15,000 due to heroin. In 2016, a staggering 116 people died every day in the United States due to opioid abuse, and the economic costs nationally were estimated to be $506 billion.[27] Without the use of effective alternatives to *medicinal* pain-control methods (see integrative medicine approaches below), prescribers will continue to use a limited number of tools that they have been taught in training, and potentially create escalating dosing to stronger, more addicting opioids to alleviate pain.

Medications in Drinking Water

How do medications get into drinking water? Quite simply, medications being excreted in urine and feces into toilet water will make their way into sewage systems or into large bodies of natural water that feed into the 160,000 water treatment plants across the country. From there they will likely pass through the treatment process without being removed. There are no laws that require detection of medications in drinking water, and there is thus no system to detect medications, nor are there ways to effectively filter out medications as they travel through the water treatment system.[28,29]

Agricultural animal production in the United States, particularly concentrated animal feeding operations (CAFOs), adds to this exposure of pharmaceuticals among humans and wildlife through the pervasive use of antibiotics in animal feed. Farming activities represent the largest use of antibiotics, with millions of tons added to feed to make animals grow larger at faster rates, as well as to prevent infection among animals that live in undersized lots and in close quarters, where infections can spread rapidly. This, of course, results in the development of antibiotic resistance in the pathogens being targeted. In addition, as much as 80% of the antibiotics fed to livestock are found in their waste unchanged—waste which is then used as fertilizer for growing crops. As a result of the widespread use of pharmaceuticals among humans and livestock, more and more prescription medications are being found in our soil, sediment, and water.[30]

Medications and the Gut Microbiome

The human gastrointestinal system is home to over 100 trillion microorganisms, such as bacteria, fungi, and viruses that are vital to the normal, healthy workings of their human host. These microscopic organisms, also known as microbes, or flora, are scattered throughout the approximately 25 feet of bowel (21 feet of small bowel and 4 feet of large bowel or colon) and cumulatively weighs almost 5 pounds. As we have already noted, these tiny wonders have a multitude of important functions: extracting nutrients from the food we eat, manufacturing vitamins, such as vitamin K, keeping the lining of the gut impenetrable to harmful irritants, and many more vital activities that have evolved over millions of years to maintain human health.

Despite their enormity in number and species, and their versatility in adjusting to changes in diet (e.g., fiber, fats, proteins, carbohydrates), microbes of the gut are vulnerable to a whole host of exposures, including food chemicals (preservatives, coloring, artificial sweeteners), overproduction of stomach acid from stress, drinking water contaminants (e.g., chlorine, lead, arsenic, pesticides), and most notably, exposure to medications such as antibiotics from prescriptions as well as those used in US food animal manufacturing. It is estimated that over 80% of all antibiotics produced in the United States are for the meat and poultry industry.[31]

Antibiotics are not the only medications that disturb the human gut microbes. Many other common medications are harmful to the thriving "zoo" in our gut. Medications for blood pressure and acid reflux management are among the classes of medications shown to wreak havoc, reducing the number and diversity of the gut flora, creating an imbalance of bacteria that can lead to overgrowth of harmful bacteria such as *C. difficile*, and even increase risk for antibiotic resistance.

One team of researchers used special screening tests to map the effects of 1,197 pharmaceuticals on 38 common bacteria species. The drugs studied included all of the main therapeutic classes, including diabetes, blood pressure, and psychiatric medications. They found that 24% of the medications blocked the growth of at least one important gut bacterial species. Metformin, a widely used diabetes drug, inhibited 3 of the 22 tested bacterial strains. The results showed an increasing risk of acquiring antibiotic resistance by being exposed to *non*-antibiotic drugs.[32] Why is this an issue? Most pharmaceutical spending in the United States goes toward non-antibiotic drugs. A 2016 *Pharmacy Times* report on medication use indicated that, ranked by number of prescriptions, antihypertensives, diabetes medications, antipsychotics, and pain-relieving drugs are more widely used than antibiotics,[33] and these widely used drugs can alter the gut microbiome. Antibiotics, while a problem, are not the only concern for the health of your digestive system.

Medications That Affect Hormones: Endocrine Disruptors

Common over-the-counter pain medications also have the ability to disrupt hormone activity in the human body. Yes, that Tylenol (acetaminophen) you just popped for a headache may help your throbbing head, but it may also act as an endocrine disruptor, altering production of the male hormone testosterone, interfering with release of insulin (a hormone necessary to regulate blood sugar levels), and promoting the growth of "hormone-sensitive" cancers such as endometrial, breast, or prostate cancer.

The idea that a medication, prescribed with good intention, may have harmful effects on hormones is not new. Between the early 1940s and 1971, an FDA-approved medication was regularly prescribed by doctors to pregnant women to prevent miscarriage and premature births, particularly during the first and second trimesters when miscarriage rate is highest. Approximately 5-10 million women were thought to have taken the medication DES, or diethylstilbestrol. DES was later discovered to cause a whole host of health issues in the daughters and sons of women who took this medication while pregnant. Female offspring (DES daughters) were discovered to be at increased risk for developing cancer of the vagina (adenocarcinoma), and many decades later, other types of cancers (squamous cell and breast cancer), as well as increased occurrence of structural abnormalities of the reproductive tract and infertility. Sons of pregnant women who took DES were found to be at increased risk for noncancerous cysts of the epididymis later in life. Both sons and daughters were later found to have increased rates of heart disease.[34-36]

DES was eventually taken off of the market, but sadly, the effects from exposure during fetal life are both lasting and irreparable and serve as a warning of the potential for harm from future use during pregnancy of medications and other chemicals that affect the normal workings of the endocrine system. The long latency period before effects of DES on the developing reproductive system become apparent—not until the DES-exposed fetus reached reproductive age—contrasts with the highly visible devastating effects of another drug, thalidomide, which was prescribed to women by physicians as an antidepressant. In nonpregnant women, thalidomide did not cause overt harm, but it turned out to be a teratogen for the unborn fetus—that is, a drug that produced dramatic physical and functional defects in limb and neural development in embryos (including lack of arms and legs) if administered in early pregnancy.

Vulnerable Periods of Exposure

As we have learned from DES and thalidomide, some periods of growth and development are more vulnerable than others, a concept so important that it earns the right to be repeated. Pregnancy, the infant and toddler years, puberty, and menopause are all periods of tremendous changes in hormone production, and these periods are particularly vulnerable to the hormone-disrupting effects from many common chemicals that act as endocrine system disruptors (see chapter 3). We now have evidence that many OTC pain medications, such as acetaminophen and ibuprofen, are no exception. Mixtures of OTC pain meds that have hormone-disrupting capability, along with exposure to endocrine-disrupting chemicals in everyday products, can compound and even synergize the hormone disruption effects.[37]

First Trimester: A Critical Window for Medication Exposure

Although the environment for fetal growth is critical throughout pregnancy, the first and into the second trimesters of pregnancy pose specific issues when it comes to exposures of any kind, be they chemical, stress, nutritional, or pharmaceutical. Medications used during pregnancy cause particular concern, not only because there is typically limited or no information for drug effects and interactions in pregnant women, but because so many vital changes to the embryo/fetus are taking place at this early stage of development. Brain, heart, and reproductive organs all begin to take form during this critical time period (see Figure 6.1).[38] We now know that many chemicals and prescription medications are capable of seamlessly crossing the placenta into the growing fetus; unfortunately, studies have described that more than 50% of pregnant women reported taking at least one medication in the first trimester.[39]

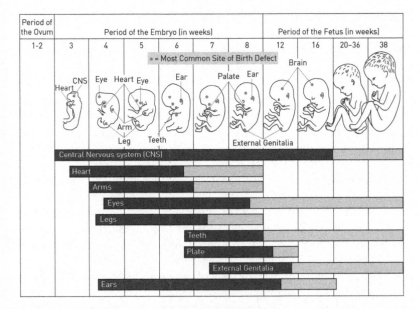

Period of the Ovum	Period of the Embryo (in weeks)						Period of the Fetus (in weeks)			
1-2	3	4	5	6	7	8	12	16	20–36	38

● = Most Common Site of Birth Defect

Figure 6.1 Fetal Development Chart in Weeks: Vulnerability of the fetus to defects during different periods of development, in this case fetal alcohol exposure. The black portion of the bars represents the most sensitive periods of development, during which alcohol-induced (i.e., teratogenic) effects on the sites listed would result in major structural abnormalities in the child. The gray portion of the bars represents periods of development during which physiological defects and minor structural abnormalities would occur. Adapted from Moore and Persaud 1993.[38]

Pregnancy and Pain Medications

One area of concern during pregnancy is OTC pain killers. Pain medications are the most widely used medications worldwide, and they often do not require a prescription. The OTC pain relievers include nonsteroidal anti-inflammatory drugs (NSAIDS); salicylates (including aspirin); and acetaminophen (N-acetyl-p-aminophenol or APAP), which is marketed under the brand name, Tylenol, Paracetamol, and dipyrone or generically as acetaminophen. These medications are often used for pain or reducing inflammation from a back strain, for instance, or for reducing fever.

Healthcare practitioners have recommended the use of OTC pain killers for decades because of the low risk to adults, based on both animal and human studies. These studies only looked at higher doses of exposure because classical toxicology dictated that increasing risk comes from increasing exposures. However, similar to what we now know about commercial and industrial chemicals, OTC pain relievers can have harmful effects on the hormones of the human endocrine system at miniscule doses; this is a shocking revelation, given the pervasiveness of the use worldwide of pain medications.

Acetaminophen (N-acetyl-p-aminophenol or APAP or Tylenol) and ibuprofen are able to relieve pain by decreasing inflammatory substances, prostaglandins, COX-1 and COX-2 enzymes, and arachidonic acid in the body. These substances, however, are critical for normal fetal development, including development of male reproductive organs and the brain. Use of acetaminophen during pregnancy is linked to changes in testosterone levels and insulin-like growth factor-3 that can lead to changes to the male fetuses' reproductive tract and sex differences in the developing brain, as well as increased risk for asthma, ADHD, reduced IQ, and disruption of male testes maturation in toddlers.[40-43] These OTC pain relievers, similar to the plastic chemicals (i.e., phthalates) used in PVC plastic, cosmetics, and other products, are able to disrupt the balance between androgens and estrogens that is essential for normal male and female development.[44] The most common birth defect of the male genital tract, cryptorchidism, is the failure of one or both testes to descend into the scrotum; the condition affects more than 200,000 babies per year in the United States. Acetaminophen and ibuprofen are both associated with increased risk for cryptorchidism in babies born to mothers who used these drugs, especially during the first trimester of pregnancy.[45,46] Thus, the effects from hormone-disrupting medications such as acetaminophen and ibuprofen, when added to the known hormone effects from ubiquitous, everyday chemicals (e.g., phthalates), substantially increases risk for harmful health effects in developing fetuses. Some of these effects, unlike cryptorchidism, do not become apparent until reproductive defects and infertility are identified in adulthood, decades after the actual fetal exposure and with no treatment available to undo the damage.[47,48]

It was discovered that women use a surprisingly large amount of medication throughout their pregnancy; greater than 90% of women take at least one medication during pregnancy. One study looked at 9,546 participants and found that, after excluding vitamins, supplements, and vaccines, 73.4% of women took a medication during their pregnancy, with 13.0% reporting polypharmacy (the use of 5 or more medications). Pain relievers made up 23.7% of medications used, with 19.9% of those being acetaminophen (Tylenol) and 6.6% other NSAIDs. Overall, 15.6% of the pregnant women reported using pain medications during the first trimester.[39] Another study showed that 56% of US women used acetaminophen at some point during their first trimester.[49] Clearly, the healthcare industry and medical professionals have given pregnant women the message that OTC pain medications are effective and safe. What we now know, however, is that there is inherent risk to the fetus with any medication taken during pregnancy; educating women and healthcare professionals on all other available options for pain control is the best approach.

Integrative Medicine Approaches to Pain Control

What can be used for pain when the common OTC pain medications we've grown up taking prove to be harmful to fetuses? What can pregnant women do to relieve back pain, muscle stiffness, breast tenderness, and other common causes of pain?

Here are some effective suggestions:

RICE: Rest, Ice, Compression, and Elevation

RICE is often used for acute injuries, such as sprained ankle or pulled muscle, to help reduce swelling and pain and speed up recovery.

Dietary and Lifestyle Changes

Anti-inflammatory diet

This diet consists of a variety of fruits and vegetables; whole grains like barley, brown rice, whole wheat; healthy fats (extra virgin olive oil, avocado); oily fish and shellfish (preferably wild-caught; see chapter 4 seafood section), seeds; nuts; limited sugar, caffeine, and alcohol (preferably red wine); and occasional sweets like 70% (or greater) dark chocolate. In addition, filter your drinking water, and remove pesticide residues by soaking produce in white vinegar mixed with warm water (1:4 ratio) or wash produce with a safe vegetable detergent, and/or buy organic produce.

Smoking cessation

Smoking is associated with chronic pain, particularly with chronic low back pain. Aside from many other health benefits, quitting smoking may result in significant pain relief.[50]

Stress reduction

Both long- and short-term stress is associated with pain and exacerbation of ongoing pain. Make an effort to reduce stress, be it social, financial, school, or work-related; this can have a large impact on pain reduction.

Sleep

Restful sleep can have a dramatic effect on pain and pain perception, so it is always a good idea for those in pain to improve both the quantity and quality of sleep.[51] Create a routine that includes a regular bedtime, maintaining a comfortable room temperature, remove stressful paperwork or homework from the bedroom, add blackout shades for window covering and avoid exposure to bright light before trying to sleep, reduce EMF [Electromagnetic Field] radiation by removing electric (plug in) alarm clocks, cell phones and tablets, reduce use of technology at night, and avoid pharmaceutical "sleeping pills" whenever possible.

Exercise

Aerobic exercise, yoga, Tai Chi, or Pilates can help improve chronic pain. After an acute injury with resulting pain, exercise should only be attempted when swelling is resolved.

Topical Pain Relievers

Arnica (from the plant *Arnica montana*)
Capsaicin (from hot peppers)

When used on unbroken skin, both arnica tincture or gel and capsaicin can help reduce pain, swelling, and in the case of arnica, prevent bruising.

Safe, Evidence-Based Supplements for Pain and Inflammation

Omega-3 fish oil
Curcumin (active ingredient in turmeric)

Both curcumin and omega-3 supplementation (from plant or fish sources), can help to reduce inflammation, which is linked with pain. Always consult your healthcare provider for safe dosing, vetted brands, and contraindications for use with certain medications and medical conditions.

Hot/Cold Therapy

Using regular, intermittent topical heat (especially *moist* heat) for muscle strains or chronic joint pain, and cold packs for acute injuries that have swelling, can be very helpful in reducing pain from musculoskeletal injury.

Mind-Body Approaches

Breathing exercises

Breathing is fundamental to all normal functions of the human body and focused breathing is therefore helpful for pain reduction. Popular examples include Lamaze techniques used for pain during pregnancy and childbirth and 4:7:8 breathing. With 4:7:8 breathing, you breathe in through the nose for a count of 4 seconds, hold for 7 seconds, and then exhale through the mouth for a count of 8 seconds.

Meditation

A technique by which a person focuses on a particular object, place, thought, or activity, to train their attention and awareness, in order to clear stressful thoughts, clear the mind, and reduce pain perception.

Guided meditation

A process by which one meditates using guidance from a trained practitioner, whether in-person or via video or audio recordings, utilizing music, verbal instruction, or both.

Guided imagery

Uses words and music to evoke positive imaginary scenarios in a subject to bring about relaxation, manage stress, and reduce tension.

Hypnosis

The induction of a state of consciousness in which a person loses power of voluntary action and is highly responsive to suggestion or commands.

Hypnosis is often used to help people recover suppressed memories, but it is also used to reduce pain perception and aid with pain management.

Journaling

Keeping a diary or journal that explores thoughts and feelings surrounding events, social connections, and health issues. Journaling can help those with chronic pain manage their emotions, document pain levels, evaluate pain control therapies, and make plans for further pain intervention.[52]

The Arts

Includes drawing, sculpture, poetry, dance, and music and/or song, which are all capable of improving spiritual well-being and health, as well as pain reduction.[52]

Manual Therapies

Acupuncture

Many effective methods for controlling pain have been around for thousands of years. Acupuncture is a part of traditional Chinese medicine that dates back to the Han dynasty (206 BC–220 AD). It is most commonly used to relieve musculoskeletal pain, such as back, shoulder, and knee pain, but is also used for a wide range of other conditions, including headache, nausea, and even improving fertility. Acupuncture entails the use of small needles that are inserted into the top layers of the skin to manipulate the electrical currents that flow through the body.

Massage

Effective in loosening up tight muscles after a strain or injury, particularly around the site of injury. Massage is also valuable in reducing anxiety, and for the benefits of human touch.

Chiropractic Manipulation

Often used for musculoskeletal pain, particularly back and neck pain, shoulder injury, and osteoarthritis. Under the care of a well-trained chiropractor, many patients experience reduced pain, increased function, and flexibility.

Osteopathic Manipulation (OMT)

Involves a set of hands-on techniques used by osteopathic physicians (DOs) for stretching, resistance, and gentle pressure.

The Bottom Line

Pharmaceutical medications should be prescribed and taken with much consideration due to the many known—and most importantly, unknown—downstream effects on the immune system, gut microbiome, brain and endocrine system. Pregnancy creates another set of problems, because generally little is known about the effects medications might have on fetuses during critical windows of development. Medications can and often do have risks for side effects, and these risks increase with the use of multiple medications and with the potential synergistic effects with pervasive environmental chemicals. Talk with your healthcare provider and ask these simple questions:

- Are there nondrug methods to solving my medical problem?
- Why am I taking this medication? What are the endpoints for judging success of this medication?
- Is this medication absolutely necessary? At some point can I stop and/or taper off of it safely?
- How long is this medication recommended to be taken?
- What is known about effects on fetuses when taking the medication during pregnancy?
- Has the medication done its job?

WARNING: Never stop or change any prescription medication without first discussing with your physician or the prescribing healthcare provider.

References

1. Paul SM, Mytelka DS, Dunwiddie CT, et al. How to improve R&D productivity: the pharmaceutical industry's grand challenge. *Nature Reviews Drug Discovery.* 2010;9:203–214.

2. Kantor ED, Rehm CD, Haas JS, Chan AT, Giovannucci EL. Trends in prescription drug use among adults in the United States from 1999–2012. *JAMA*. 2015;314(17):1818–1831.
3. Brown WA. Expectation, the placebo effect and the response to treatment. *Rhode Island Medical Journal (2013)*. 2015;98(5):19–21.
4. Express Scripts. *A Nation in Pain U.S. Opioid Trends*. December 9, 2014. https://www.express-scripts.com/corporate/drug-trend-report/nation-pain-us-opioid-trends. Accessed April 24, 2020.
5. McGrath K, Hajjar ER, Kumar C, Hwang C, Salzman B. Deprescribing: a simple method for reducing polypharmacy. *The Journal of Family Practice*. 2017;66(7):436–445.
6. Sutherland JJ, Daly TM, Liu X, Goldstein K, Johnston JA, Ryan TP. Co-prescription trends in a large cohort of subjects predict substantial drug-drug interactions. *PLoS One*. 2015;10(3):e0118991.
7. Schnell M, Currie J. Addressing the opioid epidemic: is there a role for physician education? *American Journal of Health Economics*. 2018;4(3):383–410.
8. Quinn K. Shah N. Data descriptor: A dataset quantifying polypharmacy in the United States. *Nature: Scientific Data*. 2017.
9. Agouridis AP, Kostapanos MS, Elisaf MS. Statins and their increased risk of inducing diabetes. *Expert Opinion on Drug Safety*. 2015;14(12):1835–1844.
10. de Jong HJI, Cohen Tervaert JW, Lalmohamed A, et al. Pattern of risks of rheumatoid arthritis among patients using statins: A cohort study with the clinical practice research datalink. *PLoS One*. 2018;13(2):e0193297.
11. Hussain S, Siddiqui AN, Habib A, Hussain MS, Najmi AK. Proton pump inhibitors' use and risk of hip fracture: a systematic review and meta-analysis. *Rheumatology International*. 2018;38(11):1999–2014.
12. Poly TN, Islam MM, Yang HC, Wu CC, Li YJ. Proton pump inhibitors and risk of hip fracture: a meta-analysis of observational studies. *Osteoporosis International: A Journal Established as Result of Cooperation between the European Foundation for Osteoporosis and the National Osteoporosis Foundation of the USA*. 2018.
13. Skjodt MK, Ostadahmadli Y, Abrahamsen B. Long term time trends in use of medications associated with risk of developing osteoporosis: nationwide data for Denmark from 1999 to 2016. *Bone*. 2018;120:94–100.
14. Xie Y, Bowe B, Li T, Xian H, Balasubramanian S, Al-Aly Z. Proton pump inhibitors and risk of incident CKD and progression to ESRD. *Journal of the American Society of Nephrology:* 2016;27(10):3153–3163.
15. Freedberg DE, Salmasian H, Friedman C, Abrams JA. Proton pump inhibitors and risk for recurrent *Clostridium difficile* infection among inpatients. *The American Journal of Gastroenterology*. 2013;108:1794.

16. Trifan A, Stanciu C, Girleanu I, et al. Proton pump inhibitors therapy and risk of Clostridium difficile infection: Systematic review and meta-analysis. *World J Gastroenterol.* 2017;23(35):6500–6515.
17. Kawada T. Proton pump inhibitors and dementia incidence. *JAMA Neurology.* 2016;73(8):1025–1026.
18. Shah NH, LePendu P, Bauer-Mehren A, et al. Proton pump inhibitor usage and the risk of myocardial infarction in the general population. *PLoS One.* 2015;10(6):e0124653.
19. Freedberg DE, Kim LS, Yang YX. The risks and benefits of long-term use of proton pump inhibitors: expert review and best practice advice from the American Gastroenterological Association. *Gastroenterology.* 2017;152(4):706–715.
20. Vaglio A, Grayson PC, Fenaroli P, et al. Drug-induced lupus: traditional and new concepts. *Autoimmunity Reviews.* 2018;17(9):912–918.
21. Araujo-Fernandez S, Ahijon-Lana M, Isenberg DA. Drug-induced lupus: Including anti-tumour necrosis factor and interferon induced. *Lupus.* 2014;23(6):545–553.
22. Calabrese LH, Calabrese C, Cappelli LC. Rheumatic immune-related adverse events from cancer immunotherapy. *Nat Rev Rheumatol.* 2018;14(10):569–579.
23. Sapalidis K, Kosmidis C, Michalopoulos N, et al. Psoriatic arthritis due to nivolumab administration a case report and review of the literature. *Respiratory Medicine Case Reports.* 2018;23:182–187.
24. Bukhari M. Drug-induced rheumatic diseases: a review of published case reports from the last two years. *Current Opinion in Rheumatology.* 2012;24(2):182–186.
25. Tan MH, Iyengar R, Mizokami-Stout K, et al. Spectrum of immune checkpoint inhibitors-induced endocrinopathies in cancer patients: a scoping review of case reports. *Clin Diabetes Endocrinol.* 2019;5:1.
26. Yang DD, Krasnova A, Nead KT, et al. Androgen deprivation therapy and risk of rheumatoid arthritis in patients with localized prostate cancer. *Annals of Oncology: Official Journal of the European Society for Medical Oncology.* 2018;29(2):386–391.
27. Kochanek KD, Murphy SL, Xu J, Arias E. Mortality in the United States, 2016. In: Statistics. NCHS Data Brief, #293, 2017.
28. Yang Y, Ok YS, Kim KH, Kwon EE, Tsang YF. Occurrences and removal of pharmaceuticals and personal care products (PPCPs) in drinking water and water/sewage treatment plants: a review. *The Science of the Total Environment.* 2017;596–597:303–320.
29. Elliott SM, Erickson ML, Krall AL, Adams BA. Concentrations of pharmaceuticals and other micropollutants in groundwater downgradient from large on-site wastewater discharges. *PLoS One.* 2018;13(11):e0206004.

30. Administration FaD. *FDA Annual Summary Report on Antimicrobials Sold or Distributed in 2013 for Use in Food-Producing Animals.* 2015.

31. Watkins RR, Bonomo RA. Overview: Global and local impact of antibiotic resistance. *Infect Dis Clin North Am.* 2016;30(2):313–322.

32. Maier L, Pruteanu M, Kuhn M, et al. Extensive impact of non-antibiotic drugs on human gut bacteria. *Nature.* 2018;555(7698):623–628.

33. Gilchrist, A. Top 10 drug spending categories by traditional therapeutic class: *Pharmacy Times;* 2016. Available from: https://www.pharmacytimes.com/news/top-10-drug-spending-categories-by-traditional-therapeutic-class.

34. Troisi R, Hatch EE, Palmer JR, et al. Prenatal diethylstilbestrol exposure and high-grade squamous cell neoplasia of the lower genital tract. *American Journal of Obstetrics and Gynecology.* 2016;215(3):322.e321–328.

35. Hilakivi-Clarke L. Maternal exposure to diethylstilbestrol during pregnancy and increased breast cancer risk in daughters. *Breast Cancer Research:* 2014;16(2):208.

36. Troisi R, Titus L, Hatch EE, et al. A prospective cohort study of prenatal diethylstilbestrol exposure and cardiovascular disease risk. *J Clin Endocrinol Metab.* 2018;103(1):206–212.

37. Drakvik E, Altenburger R, Aoki Y, et al. Statement on advancing the assessment of chemical mixtures and their risks for human health and the environment. *Environ Int.* 2019;134:105267.

38. Moore K, Persaud TVN. *The Developing Human: Clinically Oriented Embryology.* Philadelphia: W.B. Saunders; 1993.

39. Haas DM, Marsh DJ, Dang DT, et al. Prescription and other medication use in pregnancy. *Obstetrics and Gynecology.* 2018;131(5):789–798.

40. Liew Z, Ritz B, Virk J, Arah OA, Olsen J. Prenatal use of acetaminophen and child IQ: a Danish cohort study. *Epidemiology (Cambridge, Mass).* 2016;27(6):912–918.

41. Liew Z, Ritz B, Rebordosa C, Lee PC, Olsen J. Acetaminophen use during pregnancy, behavioral problems, and hyperkinetic disorders. *JAMA Pediatrics.* 2014;168(4):313–320.

42. Sordillo JE, Scirica CV, Rifas-Shiman SL, et al. Prenatal and infant exposure to acetaminophen and ibuprofen and the risk for wheeze and asthma in children. *The Journal of Allergy and Clinical Immunology.* 2015;135(2):441–448.

43. Sato T, Matsumoto T, Kawano H, et al. Brain masculinization requires androgen receptor function. *Proceedings of the National Academy of Sciences of the United States of America.* 2004;101(6):1673–1678.

44. Swan SH, Sathyanarayana S, Barrett ES, et al. First trimester phthalate exposure and anogenital distance in newborns. *Human Reproduction (Oxford, England).* 2015;30(4):963–972.

45. Snijder CA, Kortenkamp A, Steegers EA, et al. Intrauterine exposure to mild analgesics during pregnancy and the occurrence of cryptorchidism and hypospadia in the offspring: the Generation R Study. *Human Reproduction (Oxford, England).* 2012;27(4):1191–1201.

46. Jensen MS, Rebordosa C, Thulstrup AM, et al. Maternal use of acetaminophen, ibuprofen, and acetylsalicylic acid during pregnancy and risk of cryptorchidism. *Epidemiology (Cambridge, Mass).* 2010;21(6):779–785.

47. Kristensen DM, Skalkam ML, Audouze K, et al. Many putative endocrine disruptors inhibit prostaglandin synthesis. *Environ Health Perspect.* 2011;119(4):534–541.

48. Toppari, J, Virtanen, HE, Main, KM, and Skakkebaek, NE, (2010). Cryptorchidism and hypospadias as a sign of testicular dysgenesis syndrome (TDS): environmental connection. *Birth Defects Res A Clin Mol Teratol* 88: 910–919.

49. Thorpe PG, Gilboa SM, Hernandez-Diaz S, et al. Medications in the first trimester of pregnancy: most common exposures and critical gaps in understanding fetal risk. *Pharmacoepidemiology and Drug Safety.* 2013;22(9):1013–1018.

50. Petre B, Torbey S, Griffith JW, et al. Smoking increases risk of pain chronification through shared corticostriatal circuitry. *Human Brain Mapping.* 2015;36(2):683–694.

51. Sivertsen B, Lallukka T, Petrie KJ, Steingrimsdottir OA, Stubhaug A, Nielsen CS. Sleep and pain sensitivity in adults. *Pain.* 2015;156(8):1433–1439.

52. Ettun R, Schultz M, Bar-Sela G. Transforming pain into beauty: on art, healing, and care for the spirit. *Evidence-based Complementary and Alternative Medicine:* 2014;2014:789852.

7

The Air We Breathe
Indoor and Outdoor Air Quality

Take a course in good water and air; and in the eternal youth of Nature you may renew your own. Go quietly, alone; no harm will befall you.
—John Muir, American engineer, environmentalist writer
(1838–1914)

Air is essential for human life and needs to be clean and free of contaminants. Even if no odor is apparent, contaminants may be present in the air.[1] The fastest route of entry into the human bloodstream, aside from injection into a vein, is via inhalation. Inhalation substantially bypasses the detoxifying enzymes in the liver and directly exposes all cells in the body to air-borne toxins. Fortunately, we have more control over the quality and safety of the air we breathe in our homes compared to air outside the home, and the main focus of this chapter will be on controlling and thus improving the quality of indoor air in homes. Practical changes to air filtration, furnishings, cleaning products, and air freshening activities can greatly mitigate the risk of exacerbating asthma, allergy symptoms, and long-term exposures in your home.

At work, school, or other buildings outside of the home in which you spend time, it is important to promote, speak up, and demand changes if there are sources of contamination not being addressed (such as the use of cleaning chemicals or pesticides). This is also true for the outside air you breathe. The Clean Air Act of 1970 was instrumental in putting stricter standards on pollutants in outdoor air, and outdoor air quality has improved in the United States over the last 50 years. However, there is concern that environmental laws such as the Clean Air Act (as well as the Clean Water Act) have become partisan political issues rather than public health issues. Actions to reduce pollutant exposure that are mandated by these acts are being systematically rolled back to the "good-old days" of high pollutant levels, which threaten the health of everyone in the name of increased profits for shareholders in polluting businesses.

Throughout the world, a large number of people live in places where outdoor air is highly polluted, with the consequence, according to the WHO, being premature deaths. According to the WHO, ambient air pollution contributed to 7.6% of all deaths worldwide in 2016.[2] Airborne pollutants can travel via wind currents from China to the United States in a few days, so pollutants emitted by Chinese industries can impact the air quality and health of those living in the United States and other countries. Air pollution is thus a global problem.

Both indoor and outdoor air pollutants have contributed to the rise in chronic obstructive pulmonary disease (COPD) and cancers among adults, as well as asthma, particularly in children.[3,4] Studies show that long-term exposure to air pollution is associated with lower scores on learning and memory tests. In one study researchers followed 998 women ages 78–87, not suffering from dementia, over an 11-year period, using cognitive testing and MRI, and found that, "women who were exposed to higher levels of fine particle air pollution had more Alzheimer's-like changes in brain structure and greater memory declines than those with less exposure to such pollution."[5]

In addition, the high death rate caused by COVID-19 in areas with the worst air pollution [6] has drawn attention to air pollution as a serious public health issue in that it creates the chronic inflammation in otherwise healthy people that results in them being likely to die when their damaged lungs and impaired immune system are challenged by a respiratory virus such as the novel coronavirus.[62] Researchers from Harvard School of Public Health reported that prolonged exposure to *any degree of air pollution* increased susceptibility to contracting COVID-19, resulting in a higher percentage of hospitalizations and death. The study found that an increase of particulate count as low as 1 microgram per cubic meter correlates to a 15% rise in number of deaths.[7]

Indoor Air Pollution

Indoor air quality (IAQ) is influenced by many factors; some examples include chemicals released from building materials (carpeting, vinyl flooring,[8] paint, interior walls)[9,10,12]; home furnishings (particle board resins, furniture glues[11]); overall dust levels including pet dander, dust mites, mold spores, insect parts and fecal matter; and rodent droppings. Cleaning chemicals and air fresheners, gas ranges, and insecticide use are also problems. The incidence of asthma, allergy, and sinusitis has been increasing for decades.[4] Household air and dust has been found to contain phthalates, alkylphenols, pesticides, polybrominated diphenyl ethers, and other endocrine-disrupting compounds.[11,13] The accumulation of dust anywhere in the place that you live thus poses a direct threat to your health. Occupation also plays a key role in asthma prevalence: workers in the healthcare and social assistance industries have some of the highest asthma rates nationally,[14] as do hairdressers, manicurists, and allied professionals due to chemicals they are exposed to at work.[15-20]

Of course, there are also social determinants of health, which include poverty and housing segregation, which often force people to live in highly polluted environments, such as old houses with lead-containing paint (built prior to the lead paint ban in the United States in 1978), mold, rodent infestation, and so on. There are dramatic differences in life expectancy across the United States depending on where you were born and where you now live. The places with highest longevity tend to be in the Northeast and West and the lowest in the South. Some have argued that "ZIP code, race, and class trump genetics and healthcare as predictors of health."[21-23]

> We don't inherit the earth from our ancestors, we borrow it from our children
>
> —Native American Proverb

One key problem with regulatory limits, including those related to air quality, is that the exposure standards are based on studies conducted only on adults. Children, however, consume more food and water and have higher inhalation rates per pound of body weight than adults. If medications, for instance, are designed for efficacy as well as side effect risks based on age and weight, it would seem appropriate that children be protected by air pollution regulations not soley based on adult exposure standards.

Recommendations to Improve Indoor Air Quality

We can all make simple changes to improve indoor air quality for adults, children, and growing fetuses. Here are some recommendations:

Smoking/E-cigarettes/Vaping. In addition to nicotine, which is a carcinogen and highly addictive, tobacco smoke contains 300 or more individual chemicals (e.g., benzene, toluene, BPA, lead, mercury) that are present in each cigarette and filter. The term *firsthand smoke* describes inhalation by the person who is smoking; *secondhand smoke* refers to those inhaling smoke from a smoker nearby; and *thirdhand smoke* refers to the residual chemicals that land on clothing, furnishings, and objects in the environment of a smoker, which results in exposure of those not directly inhaling tobacco smoke. Smoking cessation, along with other lifestyle changes (e.g., weight loss, exercise, reduced alcohol consumption), could prevent roughly half of all cancer deaths in the United States.[24] In fact, a significant decrease in smoking-related cancers since the release and online posting of internal documents from tobacco companies, which has led to a substantial decrease in smoking in the United States, proves that smoking and cancer are linked. Sadly, smoking has been replaced by vaping, which uses a handheld, battery-powered vaporizer or e-cigarette to simulate the act of smoking, and has attracted and on-boarded a new generation of children addicted to nicotine.[25] Despite the fact that e-cigarettes are marketed as a safer option to conventional cigarettes, the liquid filling cartridges contain many undisclosed, unregulated chemicals that are proving to be highly toxic and can cause severe lung injury, even death, in both short- and long-term users.[26] It is therefore advisable to make every effort possible to reduce cigarette/vaping/e-cigarette smoke and its residue in homes, especially around pregnant women, children, and teens. The lifelong health consequences of developmental exposure to chemicals in both cigarette smoke and vaping include obesity and other metabolic diseases, respiratory diseases, and cancer.[27] Secondhand smoke is linked to increased risk for ear infections and asthma in children as well as for Sudden Infant Death Syndrome (SIDS).[28,29]

Radon. Radon is an invisible, odorless gas produced by the decay of naturally occurring uranium in soil and water. Inhalation of radon gas is likely to be the single largest contributor to an individual's background radiation exposure. Because this risk depends on where you live, you should determine whether exposure to radon gas is an issue in your area and in your home. Radon gas can enter any building through cracks in the foundations or construction seams. It is responsible for about 22,000 lung cancer deaths every year and is the number one cause of cancer among *non*-smokers and the second leading cause of lung cancer overall.[30] Radon gas can be detected using widely available commercial kits. The EPA recommends taking steps to remove radon at levels above 4 picocuries/liter, but this does not account for sources of radiation exposures other than in-home—such as from cell phones, tablets, and other radiation-emitting devices discussed in chapter 12.

Mold. Mold can grow in any damp or wet area and reproduce by means of tiny spores that float through the air. Use a dehumidifier for humid areas of a home or other building, particularly basements. If there is an identifiable source of the high moisture, such as a crack in the foundation, it needs to be fixed, as dehumidifiers cannot compensate for excessive moisture. The ideal humidity for best air quality is 45%. If a humidifier is used to add moisture in dry areas, inspect and clean it regularly. Inspect and clean home heating-system filters regularly as well. Inspecting the heating/air conditioning ductwork is more complicated, but accumulation of mold in the ducts can be a source of health problems, so this should be investigated if respiratory symptoms persist after other actions are taken.

Carbon Monoxide (CO). CO is a colorless, odorless gas that interferes with the delivery of oxygen throughout the body. CO exposure can cause dizziness, weakness, headache, nausea, and even lead to death. The most common source of CO is a poorly vented heat source: woodstoves, leaking furnaces, gas or kerosene space heaters, and automobile exhaust. Appliances such as dryers, water heaters, and gas stoves can also release CO, and it is an ingredient in cigarette smoke. Proper ventilation is *essential* to decreasing risk for CO poisoning or death. However, the most critical, and easiest, protection we can recommend is investing in carbon monoxide monitors and placing them near potential sources of CO. Monitors for use in the home or workplace are inexpensive and widely available in hardware or big-box stores and could save your life.

Furnishings. Many furnishings (dressers, cabinets, shelving), bought assembled or to be assembled, contain wood made with medium-density fiberboard. This fiberboard, also known as pressboard, often contains urea-formaldehyde resins that off-gas (migrate out of the product) as formaldehyde into the surrounding spaces. The National Cancer Institute has listed formaldehyde as a known carcinogen. Without appropriate ventilation, formaldehyde concentrations in indoor air can reach high levels and produce symptoms such as headache, nausea, rash, and confusion. Other sources of formaldehyde include permanent-press or dry-cleaned clothing, draperies, wrinkle-free linens, glues and adhesives, and some cleaning and personal care products. Dry-cleaned garments should be allowed to "off-gas" the toxic cleaning chemicals *outside*, in a garage or back porch, before being put in a closet. You should avoid furniture made of pressboard. If formaldehyde-treated furniture is purchased, it should be aired out for several days in a well-ventilated garage or basement before use. Alternatively, one can use exterior-grade pressed wood products, which contain lower concentrations of phenol-formaldehyde resins.

Children, dust, and vinyl floors. Avoid letting children play or eat on vinyl (PVC) floors, which break down over time and off-gas formaldehyde.[12] In addition, PVC flooring and wall coverings contain BPA and phthalates, with the phthalates softening the PVC (which is otherwise brittle) and then BPA making it harder but not brittle. BPA and phthalates, which are both endocrine disruptors, migrate from vinyl and then stick to dust particles in the air—the more dust, the more BPA, phthalates, and other airborne pollutants you will be breathing in your home. Phthalates and BPA can penetrate skin; they also act as allergens and are implicated in respiratory symptoms, asthma, and allergies, as well as obesity.

Personal care products. Avoid hair-straightening treatments (e.g., Brazilian, keratin) with constituents containing formaldehyde or breakdown products such as quaternium 15, bronopol (or 2-bromo-2-nitropane-1,3-diol) diazolidinyl urea, DMDM hydantoin, imidazoliidinyl urea, and sodium hydroxymethlglycinate. These products are banned in Canada and the European Union but not in the United States, as discussed in chapter 1.

Cleaning products. Avoid using cleaning products with bleach or other lung irritants and products containing fragrance or perfume. Limonene and other citrus fragrances are often added to cleaning products but should be avoided because of their ability to form formaldehyde when interacting with ozone in air. Avoid using carpet powders, stain-guard sprays, and toxic floor cleaners. Keep children's play areas free of dust and products that contain toxic chemicals, such as Lysol, Febreze, and other commercial cleaners and air fresheners. Due to their constant hand-to-mouth behaviors and smaller size relative to adults, children will absorb greater amounts of these toxic chemicals that bind to dust. Use natural cleaning products in areas where children play, such as vinegar, filtered water, lemon juice, and baking soda.

Candles and air fresheners. Avoid synthetic candles made with substances such as limonene, which is used to make citrus fragrance. Choose organic candles made with 100% beeswax. Soy candles, although found to release fewer harmful chemicals when burned than typical of petroleum wax candles, may be adulterated with synthetic fragrance and should also be avoided unless all information about the composition is available.

Vacuum. Vacuum often to remove dust, which is a major source of toxic chemicals, including flame-retardant chemicals (see chapter 11). Many vacuum cleaners stir up more dust than they pick up, so use a vacuum with a HEPA (High Efficiency Particulate Air) filter which reduces the amount of dust recycling back into the air.[31] Filters that meet HEPA filter standards remove 99.7% of particles greater than 0.3 μm in size, which includes removal of dust particles that commonly carry toxic chemicals. Remember to vacuum drapes, under beds, behind bookshelves, around stoves and fireplaces, and inside closets. Remove shoes at the door to reduce dirt and chemicals they bring into the home; this is particularly important if you have been someplace that has been sprayed with a disinfectant or lawn chemicals.

Ventilation. If you live in an area with clean outside air and with no nearby polluting industries or highways that are sources of vehicle emissions, open windows to increase airflow and air circulation in indoor spaces whenever the weather permits. This can reduce exposure to home and workplace chemicals that off-gas from furniture, flooring, carpeting, and cleaning products.[32] Many workers complain of "sick building syndrome" (SBS), which is characterized by nonspecific complaints such as mucous membrane irritation, skin symptoms, headache, and dizziness due to a chemical exposures and time spent within a contaminated work space.[33,34] If you work in this type of environment, go outside for work breaks, open office windows if possible, and limit time spent in closed, poorly ventilated areas.

Air quality in cars. Those who commute on heavily trafficked roads often experience greater exposure to engine fumes containing pollutants such as ozone, benzene, mercury, dioxins, and furans. Americans typically spend more than 1.5 hours per day in their cars, putting them at increased risk for headache, COPD, and asthma exacerbation. You can reduce exposure to exhaust by closing your car's air vents, thereby blocking outside air from entering the car's interior.[35] Look for the recirculation button on your air conditioning controls (see Figure 13.1), and open or close car air vents based on outdoor air quality (e.g., ozone level), exposure to traffic, and pollen counts. Use the smartphone apps listed in the section on Outdoor Air Quality to check air quality levels.

Aeration of new products and dry cleaning. That new car smell is actually phthalates off-gassing from synthetic materials (e.g., vinyl, plastics, tanning chemicals, flame-retardant chemicals). Try to aerate a new car before spending time in it. Leave dry-cleaning, new mattresses, carpeting, and home furnishings outside on the porch, or in a garage or other uninhabited space before use.

Air Filter & Purifier. Use a quality air purifier to help reduce indoor fine particulate matter (particles <2.5 μm diameter ($PM_{2.5}$)). The purifier should meet HEPA filter standards (99.7% of particles greater than 0.3 μm in size are removed).[36] HVAC systems are typically installed in the modern home or workplace and require a high-quality filter that is checked regularly and changed as needed. Air filters have a minimum efficiency reporting value (MERV) rating to assess their effectiveness for HVAC systems. The MERV rating (from 1 to 16) identifies the size of the particles trapped. The higher the MERV rating, the greater the percentage of particles captured with each pass of air. Check Consumer Reports for recommendations of reputable, certified air purifiers.

Humidity Control. To minimize the growth of mold as well as the infiltration of dust mites and other insects, maintaining an airtight home at a humidity level not over 45% is key. Do not keep boxes and paper products in areas where there is moisture to avoid the growth of mold. Also remember that if humidity is too low, irritation of the respiratory system can occur.

Plants. Plants can be enormously helpful in creating better air quality. They convert carbon dioxide into oxygen through photosynthesis. The more plants in a space, the greater the effect on air quality. Plus, the leaves of plants have a large surface area and act to catch dust and particulate matter (take the plant outside to remove the dust if possible). Several researchers and NASA scientists have studied plants to see which were most capable of reducing harmful chemicals from the air and found a variety of common, available plants were effective.[37-40] Here are a few:

- Areca palm
- Money plant
- Peace lily
- English ivy
- Spider plant
- Dracaena (many varieties including mother-in-law's tongue)

Home Remodeling. Take steps to minimize air pollution when remodeling, particularly with sanding and paint removal. Ensure adequate protective equipment and ventilation, use materials with reduced volatile organic compounds (VOCs), aerate newly installed materials, and keep pregnant women, children, and pets away from remodeling areas to prevent inhalation of particulate matter.

Outdoor Air Pollution

Taking action to create cleaner outdoor air today is challenging. Decades of industrialization have fostered fossil fuel combustion, the manufacture of chemicals that are persistent organic pollutants (POPs), such as chlorinated pesticides (e.g., DDT) and brominated flame retardants (e.g., PBDEs), VOCs (e.g., formaldehyde, gasoline), ozone, carbon monoxide, sulfur dioxide, nitric oxide, lead and particulate matter (eg, $PM_{2.5}$), and other toxic man-made chemicals.

Diseases Related to Outdoor Air Pollution

Ambient fine particulate matter is linked to increased risk for developing atherosclerotic disease, acute coronary events, stroke, diabetes, and obesity.[41-43] Depression, mood changes, and increased rate of emergency room visits for suicide attempts are all associated with poor air quality.[44-51] Fine particulate matter exposure during pregnancy is implicated in the development of autism spectrum disorder, gestational diabetes, adverse birth outcomes, and obesity and asthma later in life,[48-52] while infant through childhood exposure is linked to reduced lung function in adolescence, autism spectrum disorder, and reduced cognitive development. Some of the above illnesses are part of "executive function disorder," in which a child's ability to analyze, organize, and complete tasks is impaired.[57-60] One group of researchers in the United Kingdom found that the rise of cancer is most apparent in exposed teenagers and young adults aged between 15 and 24.[61] Clearly, the degree to which people have access to unpolluted air broadly impacts their health, beyond the known effects on asthma and allergy.

Monitoring your outdoor air quality is as easy a pulling up a website on your computer or app on your phone that checks air quality by zip code. Check out these easy free apps and websites to help decide if outdoor air is clean enough to open windows for air circulation!

- The EPA website: https://airnow.gov/ allows you to check air quality index forecast and alerts by zip code
- EPA smartphone app: Air Now
- EPA Indoor Air Quality: https://www.epa.gov/indoor-air-quality-iaq
- EPA AirCompare: https://www3.epa.gov
- World Air Quality Index website: https://waqi.info.
- App: Air Quality Live
- App: AirVisual (from IQAir): https:www.//iqair.com
- App: Air Matters
- App: Air Quality—PM2.5 Index

Additional Indoor and Outdoor Air Resources:

EPA Transportation, Air Pollution, and Climate Change: https://www.epa.gov/air-pollution-transportation

Watch this TED talk, "How to Grow Fresh Air," by Kamal Meattle:

https://www.ted.com/talks/kamal_meattle_on_how_to_grow_your_own_fresh_air

Healthy Materials & Sustainable Building Certificate: HealthyMaterialsLab.org:

https://healthymaterialslab.org/education/e-learning-online-certificate-program?utm_source=Keep+in+Touch%21&utm_campaign=ac310ca73d-EMAIL_CAMPAIGN_2018_08_01_04_58&utm_medium=email&utm_term=0_0b37213cb4-ac310ca73d-206911529&utm_source=September+2018+FRI&utm_campaign=Constant+Contact+Analytics&utm_medium=email

Outdoor air pollution video: https://www.youtube.com/watch?v=_dTtvtlct9k

References

1. Guxens M, Aguilera I, Ballester F, et al. Prenatal exposure to residential air pollution and infant mental development: modulation by antioxidants and detoxification factors. *Environ Health Perspect.* 2012;120(1):144–149.
2. World Health Organization (WHO). Mortality and burden of disease from ambient air pollution. https://www.who.int/gho/phe/outdoor_air_pollution/burden/en/. Published 2019. Accessed April 18, 2020.
3. Khreis H, Kelly C, Tate J, Parslow R, Lucas K, Nieuwenhuijsen M. Exposure to traffic-related air pollution and risk of development of childhood asthma: a systematic review and meta-analysis. *Environ Int.* 2016.
4. Centers for Disease Control and Prevention (CDC). Asthma: data, statistics and surveillance. http://www.cdc.gov/asthma/asthmadata.htm. Published 2016. Accessed April 18, 2020.

5. Younan D, Petkus AJ, Widaman KF, et al. Particulate matter and epi-sodic memory decline mediated by early neuroanatomic biomarkers of Alzheimer's disease. *Brain.* 2019;143(1):289–302.

6. Conticini, E, Frediani, B and Caro, D (2020). Can atmospheric pollution be considered a co-factor in extremely high level of SARS-CoV-2 lethality in Northern Italy? Environ Pollut114465.

7. Wu XM, Sabath B, Nethery RC, Braun D, Dominici F. Exposure to air pollution and COVID-19 mortality in the United States. medRxiv 2020. doi: https://doi.org/10.1101/2020.04.05.20054502

8. Shu H, Jonsson BA, Larsson M, Nanberg E, Bornehag CG. PVC flooring at home and development of asthma among young children in Sweden, a 10-year follow-up. *Indoor Air.* 2014;24(3):227–235.

9. Walls KL, Boulic M, Boddy JW. The built environment-a missing "Cause of the Causes" of non-communicable diseases. *Int J Environ Res Public Health.* 2016;13(10).

10. Schon P, Ctistis G, Bakker W, Luthe G. Nanoparticular surface-bound PCBs, PCDDs, and PCDFs—a novel class of potentially higher toxic POPs. *Environmental Science and Pollution Research International.* 2016.

11. Bornehag CG, Sundell J, Weschler CJ, et al. The association be-tween asthma and allergic symptoms in children and phthalates in house dust: a nested case-control study. *Environ Health Perspect.* 2004;112(14):1393–1397.

12. Amiri A, Turner-Henson A. The roles of formaldehyde exposure and oxi-dative stress in fetal growth in the second trimester. *Journal of Obstetric, Gynecologic, and Neonatal Nursing:* 2016.

13. Rudel RA, Camann DE, Spengler JD, Korn LR, Brody JG. Phthalates, alkylphenols, pesticides, polybrominated diphenyl ethers, and other endocrine-disrupting compounds in indoor air and dust. *Environ Sci Technol.* 2003;37(20):4543–4553.

14. CDC. Morbidity and Mortality Weekly Report: Asthma Among Employed Adults, by Industry and Occupation—21 States, 2013. http://www.cdc.gov/mmwr/volumes/65/wr/mm6547a1.htm?s_cid=mm6547a1_w. Published 2016. Accessed December 4, 2016.

15. Takkouche B, Regueira-Mendez C, Montes-Martinez A. Risk of cancer among hairdressers and related workers: a meta-analysis. *International Journal of Epidemiology.* 2009;38(6):1512–1531.

16. Garbaccio JL, de Oliveira AC. Adherence to and knowledge of best practices and occupational biohazards among manicurists/pedicurists. *American Journal of Infection Control.* 2014;42(7):791–795.

17. Garbaccio JL, de Oliveira AC. Adherence and knowledge about the use of personal protective equipment among manicurists. *Revista brasileira de enfermagem.* 2015;68(1):46–53, 52–49.

18. Kiec-Swierczynska M, Chomiczewska-Skora D, Swierczynska-Machura D, Krecisz B. [Manicurists and pedicurists—occupation group at high risk of work-related dermatoses]. *Medycyna Pracy.* 2013;64(4):579–591.

19. Kreiss K, Esfahani RS, Antao VC, Odencrantz J, Lezotte DC, Hoffman RE. Risk factors for asthma among cosmetology professionals in Colorado. *Journal of Occupational and Environmental Medicine / American College of Occupational and Environmental Medicine.* 2006;48(10):1062–1069.

20. Kwapniewski R, Kozaczka S, Hauser R, Silva MJ, Calafat AM, Duty SM. Occupational exposure to dibutyl phthalate among manicurists. *Journal of Occupational and Environmental Medicine / American College of Occupational and Environmental Medicine.* 2008;50(6):705–711.

21. Hindery R. Zip code, race class trump genetics and healthcare as predictors of public health. UCSF News. http://www.ucsf.edu/news/2009/01/8246/zip-code-may-predict-health-expert-says. Published 2009. Accessed April 18, 2020.

22. GBD Risk Factors Collaborators. Global, regional, and national comparative risk assessment of 79 behavioural, environmental and occupational, and metabolic risks or clusters of risks, 1990-2015: a systematic analysis for the Global Burden of Disease Study 2015. *Lancet* 2016;388(10053):1659–1724.

23. Shirinde J, Wichmann J, Voyi K. Allergic rhinitis, rhinoconjunctivitis and hayfever symptoms among children are associated with frequency of truck traffic near residences: a cross sectional study. *Environmental Health: A Global Access Science Source.* 2015;14:84.

24. Song M, Giovannucci E. Preventable incidence and mortality of carcinoma associated with lifestyle factors among white adults in the United States. *JAMA Oncology.* 2016.

25. Kaplan S. Teenage vaping rises sharply again this year. New York Times Web site. https://www.nytimes.com/2019/09/18/health/vaping-teens-e-cigarettes.html. Published 2019. Accessed October 4, 2019.

26. Salzman GA, Alqawasma M, Asad H. Vaping associated lung injury (EVALI): an explosive United States epidemic. *Mo Med.* 2019;116(6):492–496.

27. Heindel JJ, Blumberg B, Cave M, et al. Metabolism disrupting chemicals and metabolic disorders. *Reproductive Toxicology (Elmsford, NY).* 2016.

28. Zhou S, Rosenthal DG, Sherman S, Zelikoff J, Gordon T, Weitzman M. Physical, behavioral, and cognitive effects of prenatal tobacco and postnatal second-hand smoke exposure. *Current Problems in Pediatric and Adolescent health care.* 2014;44(8):219-241.

29. Boldo E, Medina S, Oberg M, et al. Health impact assessment of environmental tobacco smoke in European children: sudden infant death syndrome and asthma episodes. *Public Health Reports (Washington, DC: 1974).* 2010;125(3):478-487.

30. Environmental Protection Agency (EPA). Radon. https://www.epa.gov/radon. Published 2016. Accessed January 8, 2017.

31. Sulser C, Schulz G, Wagner P, et al. Can the use of HEPA cleaners in homes of asthmatic children and adolescents sensitized to cat and dog allergens decrease bronchial hyperresponsiveness and allergen contents in solid dust? *International Archives of Allergy and Immunology.* 2009;148(1):23-30.

32. Asikainen A, Carrer P, Kephalopoulos S, Fernandes Ede O, Wargocki P, Hanninen O. Reducing burden of disease from residential indoor air exposures in Europe (HEALTHVENT project). *Environmental Health: A Global Access Science Source.* 2016;15 Suppl 1:35.

33. Burge PS. Sick building syndrome. *Occupational and Environmental Medicine.* 2004;61(2):185-190.

34. Miyajima E, Tsunoda M, Sugiura Y, et al. The diagnosis of sick house syndrome: the contribution of diagnostic criteria and determination of chemicals in an indoor environment. *The Tokai Journal of Experimental and Clinical Medicine.* 2015;40(2):69-75.

35. Hudda N, Fruin SA. Models for predicting the ratio of particulate pollutant concentrations inside vehicles to roadways. *Environmental Science & Technology.* 2013;47(19):11048-11055.

36. Park HK, Cheng KC, Tetteh AO, Hildemann LM, Nadeau KC. Effectiveness of air purifier on health outcomes and indoor particles in homes of children with allergic diseases in Fresno, California: A pilot study. *J Asthma.* 2017;54(4):341-346.

37. Dela Cruz M, Christensen JH, Thomsen JD, Muller R. Can ornamental potted plants remove volatile organic compounds from indoor air? A review. *Environmental Science and Pollution Research International.* 2014;21(24):13909-13928.

38. Wolverton BC, Johnson A, Bounds K. Interior landscape plants for indoor air pollution abatement. NASA Technical Reports Server. https://ntrs.nasa.gov/search.jsp?R=19930073077. Published 1989. Accessed April 24, 2020.

39. Deng L, Deng Q. The basic roles of indoor plants in human health and comfort. *Environmental Science and Pollution Research International.* 2018;25(36):36087-36101.

40. Wikipedia. NASA clean air study. https://en.wikipedia.org/wiki/NASA_Clean_Air_Study. Published 2019. Updated May 1, 2019. Accessed May 5, 2019.

41. Sun Q, Yue P, Deiuliis JA, et al. Ambient air pollution exaggerates adipose inflammation and insulin resistance in a mouse model of diet-induced obesity. *Circulation.* 2009;119(4):538-546.

42. Matsuo R, Michikawa T, Ueda K, et al. Short-term exposure to fine particulate matter and risk of ischemic stroke. *Stroke.* 2016;47(12):3032-3034.

43. Pope CA, Bhatnagar A, McCracken J, Abplanalp WT, Conklin DJ, O'Toole TE. Exposure to fine particulate air pollution is associated with endothelial injury and systemic inflammation. *Circ Res.* 2016.

44. Kim KN, Lim YH, Bae HJ, Kim M, Jung K, Hong YC. Long-term fine particulate matter exposure and major depressive disorder in a community-based urban cohort. *Environ Health Perspect.* 2016;124(10):1547-1553.

45. Air Pollution and Depression [press release]. 2016.

46. Lim YH, Kim H, Kim JH, Bae S, Park HY, Hong YC. Air pollution and symptoms of depression in elderly adults. *Environ Health Perspect.* 2012;120(7):1023-1028.

47. Fonken LK, Xu X, Weil ZM, et al. Air pollution impairs cognition, provokes depressive-like behaviors and alters hippocampal cytokine expression and morphology. *Molecular Psychiatry.* 2011;16(10):987-995, 973.

48. Felger JC, Lotrich FE. Inflammatory cytokines in depression: neurobiological mechanisms and therapeutic implications. *Neuroscience.* 2013;246:199-229.

49. Gladka A, Rymaszewska J, Zatonski T. Impact of air pollution on depression and suicide. *International Journal of Occupational Medicine and Environmental Health.* 2018;31(6):711-721.

50. Yang CY, Weng YH, Chiu YW. Relationship between ozone air pollution and daily suicide mortality: a time-stratified case-crossover study in Taipei. *Journal of toxicology and environmental health Part A.* 2019;82(4):261-267.

51. Gu X, Liu Q, Deng F, et al. Association between particulate matter air pollution and risk of depression and suicide: systematic review and meta-analysis. *The British Journal of Psychiatry: The Journal of Mental Science.* 2019:1-12.

52. Flores-Pajot MC, Ofner M, Do MT, Lavigne E, Villeneuve PJ. Childhood autism spectrum disorders and exposure to nitrogen dioxide, and particulate matter air pollution: A review and meta-analysis. *Environ Res.* 2016;151:763-776.

53. Mao G, Nachman RM, Sun Q, et al. Individual and joint effects of early-life ambient PM2.5 exposure and maternal pre-pregnancy obesity on childhood overweight or obesity. *Environ Health Perspect.* 2016.

54. Lavigne E, Yasseen AS, 3rd, Stieb DM, et al. Ambient air pollution and adverse birth outcomes: differences by maternal comorbidities. *Environ Res.* 2016;148:457–466.

55. Stieb DM, Chen L, Beckerman BS, et al. Associations of pregnancy outcomes and PM2.5 in a national Canadian study. *Environ Health Perspect.* 2016;124(2):243–249.

56. Jedrychowski WA, Perera FP, Maugeri U, et al. Effect of prenatal exposure to fine particulate matter on ventilatory lung function of preschool children of non-smoking mothers. *Paediatric and Perinatal Epidemiology.* 2010;24(5):492–501.

57. Talbott EO, Arena VC, Rager JR, et al. Fine particulate matter and the risk of autism spectrum disorder. *Environ Res.* 2015;140:414–420.

58. Harris MH, Gold DR, Rifas-Shiman SL, et al. Prenatal and childhood traffic-related pollution exposure and childhood cognition in the Project Viva cohort (Massachusetts, USA). *Environ Health Perspect.* 2015;123(10):1072–1078.

59. Harris MH, Gold DR, Rifas-Shiman SL, et al. Prenatal and childhood traffic-related air pollution exposure and childhood executive function and behavior. *Neurotoxicology and Teratology.* 2016;57:60–70.

60. Schultz ES, Hallberg J, Bellander T, et al. Early-life exposure to traffic-related air pollution and lung function in adolescence. *American Journal of Respiratory and Critical Care Medicine.* 2016;193(2):171–177.

61. Knapton S. Modern life is killing our children: cancer rate in young people up 40 per cent in 16 years http://www.telegraph.co.uk/science/2016/09/03/modern-life-is-killing-our-children-cancer-rate-in-young-people/. The Telegraph, Published 2016. Accessed April 24, 2020.

62. vom Saal, FS and Cohen, A (2020). How toxic chemicals contribute to COVID-19 deaths. Environmental Health News. https:// www.ehn.org/ toxic-chemicals-coronavirus-2645713170.html?ct=t(RSS_EMAIL_CAMPAIGN. Accessed April 17, 2020.

8

Is My Antiperspirant Harming Me?

Personal Care Products and Chemicals

The most beautiful makeup of a woman is passion. But cosmetics are easier to buy.

—Yves Saint Laurent (1936–2008)

Throughout history, the desire to achieve beauty and cover physical flaws has been embraced by all cultures and societies. Greeks, Romans, and Egyptians used foundations made from lead and tin and brushed minerals on their faces to add color and definition. War paint, tribal markings, and other visual expressions of celebration and ritual all used topical concoctions made from available resources. Many people born into caste systems and societal hierarchies that weighted fair complexions as superior would employ skin-lightening techniques to change their natural skin color. From generation to generation, aesthetic traditions, beauty secrets, and recipes were passed down, often with the blind assumption that the practices were safe and free of any health risks.

Today, people still want to look and feel attractive and will often pay greatly for it, both financially and emotionally, by using trendy applications, unvetted products, and risky medical procedures. According to *Forbes* magazine, the beauty industry is currently worth over $445 billion in annual sales and continues to grow at a steady rate.[1] Consumers want to make their skin silky smooth, create luscious lips, and make wrinkles, gray hair, and acne disappear. The personal care product industry spends billions every year to convince you that the money you invest in their products will ensure a beautiful return on your investment.

What products do *you* use every day? There are plenty of products to choose from: shampoo, body spray, cologne, hair gel, deodorant, antiperspirant, sunscreen, foot cream, hair dye, lipstick, mascara, tampons, bug spray, toilet paper, face powder, and nail polish, just to name a few. Did you know that, on average, adult women in the United States use 12 different personal care products per day and adult males use 6 products per day? Teenagers use the most personal care products daily of any demographic in the United States, with an average use of 15 such products daily.

Lash Lure and the Food, Drug, and Cosmetic Act of 1938

Despite all of the promises of eternal youth and glamor, the history of harm from personal care products is long and problematic. In 1933, a young mother in Dayton, Ohio, Mrs. J. W. Musser, casually decided to apply a new eyelash and eyebrow dye called Lash Lure. She was heading to a PTA banquet to be honored for her volunteer work for the school. It was a new kind of product, and Mrs. Musser found the application messy and awkward, but continued with the process nonetheless. At first she experienced burning in her eyes, but the pain quickly grew worse, and she woke the next morning to find that her eyes had swollen shut and ulcers had formed on her corneas (see Figure 8.1). Her eyes oozed pus for days, and eventually she lost her vision.

Lash Lure eyelash-darkening treatment contained a toxic ingredient called paraphenylenediamine (PPD). Still used today in many dark hair dyes, temporary tattoos, and construction materials, PPD is made from

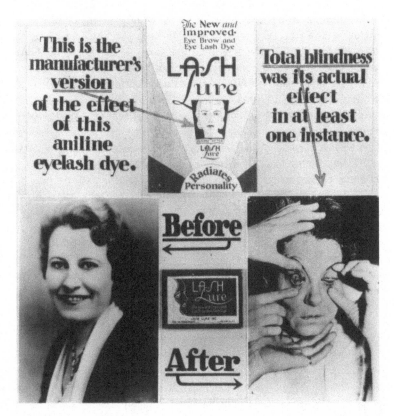

The New and
Improved·
Eye Brow and
Eye Lash Dye

LAƧH
ure

Radiates
Personality

This is the manufacturer's version of the effect of this aniline eyelash dye.

Total blindness was its actual effect in at least one instance.

Before

After

FIGURE 8.1 Eye ulcerations after reacting to her mascara which contained, paraphenylenediamine (PPD). Congress has not updated cosmetics legislation since 1938. Courtesy of the FDA.

aniline coal tar, a hydrocarbon-based organic chemical. PPD causes many health problems and particularly, allergic reactions. In 2006, it was listed as "Allergen of the Year" by the American Contact Dermatitis Society.[2]

In the early 1930s, sixteen women were seriously injured, and some blinded, after applying Lash Lure. The cases were documented in medical journals, including the November 11, 1933, issue of the *Journal of American Medicine*. Mrs. Musser's 10-year-old daughter, Hazel Fay, wrote a heart-breaking letter to President Franklin Delano Roosevelt about her mother's tragedy. In response to this and other tragedies resulting from the toxic chemicals found in Lash Lure and other "elixirs" and "beautifying" agents, Congress set out to improve consumer protections. What developed was

Is My Antiperspirant Harming Me?

173

a weak attempt, at best, to regulate the safety of cosmetics. Congress ultimately added just 1½ pages to the 345-page Federal Food, Drug, and Cosmetic Act of 1938, demonstrating the power of the Cosmetic Industry Association to control members of Congress. The critical issue regarding this legislation is that there was no mandate for any testing for health effects for any chemical used in products.[3,4]

Although the Food, Drug, and Cosmetic Act has been in place for nearly a century, as of 2020 meaningful regulatory action regarding safety and disclosure of ingredients in personal care products has never been adequately addressed in the United States. Most Americans assume, as did Mrs. Musser in 1933, that when they pull a personal care product off the shelf, its ingredients have been rigorously tested for safety or health risks and that there is some oversight by US regulators. In fact, as of this writing, there are almost *no* regulations covering the safety of ingredients used in personal care products in the United States.

After much wrangling on both sides of the political aisle, the Toxic Substances Control Act (TSCA) was signed into law in 1976. The TSCA exempted all existing chemicals from regulation, and all existing chemicals were considered to be safe for use (the "grandfather" clause). This 1976 law remained in effect until 2016 when it was amended by Congress. In reality, chemical industry lobbyists dictated the language of the 2016 legislation, and consequently, federal agencies remain unable to require chemical corporations to determine if chemicals are actually safe prior to using them in products. One of this Act's most egregious errors is that it *does not require chemicals used commercially in the United States to be tested for safety related to reproductive health, developmental issues in children, cancers, or endocrine disorders prior to being used in products.* In fact, on its website the EPA states that the amended 2016 TSCA grandfathered in 83,000 chemicals that were already available for commercial use without requiring any additional safety testing (of course, no safety testing had been previously required).

Under the revised 2016 TSCA, the FDA has *no* authority to pull cosmetics or personal care products from store shelves should independent research show that they pose a health risk. Manufacturers may decide to remove a potentially harmful product *voluntarily*, but this typically means that removal of a chemical occurs only as a consequence of litigation (i.e., as a result of financial penalties awarded by juries) rather than action by federal regulatory agencies (as occurred with Johnson and Johnson ceasing sale of baby powder in the United States but not abroad). Since some states have tried to pass laws regulating these hazardous products, industry lobbyists have focused on getting Congress to pass laws requiring "federal preemption" of state laws, meaning that federal regulators—who never take action—would be the sole source of protection of the public health from these dangerous products.

In 1976, manufacturers and chemical industry scientists created the Cosmetic Ingredients Review Panel to investigate product ingredients and *tell the FDA* if there were any safety issues. To no one's surprise, given the panel's biases due to many members being paid by cosmetics corporations, only 11 chemicals have been removed from cosmetics in the United States since 1976. The European Union (EU), which has greater oversight and much stricter regulations for cosmetic and food safety, has restricted 1,200 chemicals in products since the 1970s, most of which *we still use* in the United States every day. European governments, as well as the government of Canada, far surpass the United States on chemical regulations and con- sumer protections. Thousands of potentially harmful chemicals remain in products we soak in, and lather and spray onto our skin every day, yet the general public has no idea of the short- and long-term health risks these products may cause.

Health Issues

An estimated 11,000 different chemicals are used in cosmetics, make-up, and other personal care products, including lead, parabens, phthalates, hy- droquinone, nitrosamines, and 1,4 dioxane.[5] Many carcinogenic chemicals reside in personal care products. In fact, 1,4 dioxane, a probable carcinogen, is found in almost a quarter of all personal care products as a contaminant.[6]

Human skin is the largest organ in the human body; it acts like a sponge, absorbing substances directly through its many intricate layers right into the bloodstream (see Figure 8.2). As consumers, whether consciously or not, this is what we're hoping for, that these products will be absorbed into the body in order to make a desired change. Similarly, we rely on this skin-transport property to take medications that are purposely designed to enter the body through the skin via patches, sprays, ointments, lotions, and gels. OTC medications, such as seasickness, nicotine, and pain patches ap- plied to the skin, topical arthritis sprays, wart creams, and rash ointments, regularly fly off of drugstore shelves.

Ironically, when harnessing the absorbent property of the skin for aes- thetic and medicinal improvement, many harmful chemicals go along for the ride. The chemicals in personal care products, for example, can seri- ously compromise your body's defense against other toxic environmental chemicals due to the fact that personal care product allow other chemicals

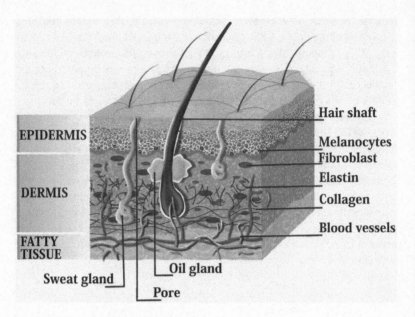

Figure 8.2 The structure of human skin.

to pass through the barrier layer of the skin. Many chemicals have been developed with so-called permeation enhancers or penetration enhancers designed primarily by the pharmaceutical industry to deliver medication into the body. This class of chemicals is capable of maneuvering through the epidermis layer of skin, which has evolved over millions of years to be a relatively impermeable protector for the human body. For example, chemical names with the prefix "peg-" (denoting pegylated chemicals), which are found on the labels of many personal care products—particularly skin-softening lotions and hand sanitizers—are designed to degrade the epidermal barrier layer and cross through skin seamlessly. And if one chemical isn't bad enough, studies show that combining these permeating chemicals may synergize to better allow chemical pollutants to cross through the fatty layers of human skin and stealthily enter the body.[7] Researchers have found that the more personal care products used, the greater the amount of harmful chemicals such as phthalates are found. People using no personal care products had the lowest level of phthalates and their breakdown products in their urine (see Figure 8.3); the level was much higher when more products were added, such as, for example, after-shave, hair gel, deodorant, and lotion.[8]

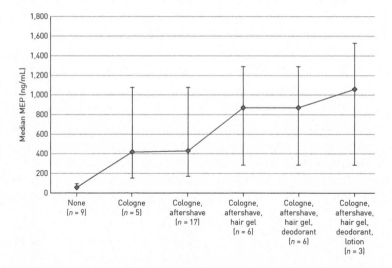

FIGURE 8.3 Number of personal care products used vs. a phthalate breakdown product in the human body (mono-ethyl phthalate or MEP) in Urine (ng/mL). From Duty et al with permission.[8]

Pregnant Moms and Personal Care Products

Many of the chemicals in personal care products that get absorbed by the mother can cross the placenta and into a growing fetus. In fact, a 2005 study by the Environmental Working Group analyzed the umbilical cord blood of 10 newborns and found over 200 total industrial chemicals among all of the children tested.[9] Humans are, in effect, born polluted!

Chemicals such as phthalates (used in fragrance), parabens, mercury (used as a preservative), and formaldehyde have been shown to affect normal brain growth and development, including disrupting the development of the genitals, which are regulated by testosterone and other sex hormones in the growing male fetus.[10-17] Even breast milk can carry many harmful toxins, such as phthalates, but the health benefits of breastfeeding generally outweigh the risks from transferring chemicals compared to the use of commercial infant formulas.[12] However, there are occupational situations, for example lactating women working on farms where pesticides are being sprayed, in which women are so contaminated by endocrine-disrupting pesticides, that breastfeeding could lead to substantial contamination of their nursing infant.

***

A critical time to reduce (and preferably eliminate) the use of cosmetics and other personal care products is the period prior to, during, and after pregnancy while breast feeding.

Children and Personal Care Products

Parents are the key deciders for which personal care products are used for their newborn, infant, and child, so it seems reasonable that they be well informed about the multitude of harmful chemicals that exist in infant and children's personal care products. Children's products are cleverly *marketed* as safe, but, as with adult personal care products, there are no regulations, required safety testing, or oversight for ingredients used in children's personal care products under current US laws.[13]

As we mentioned in chapter 3, pound-for-pound, infants and small children have greater surface area exposure (relative to body weight) to all chemicals than do adults, which effects total absorption of those chemicals. Infants have a limited ability to break chemical pollutants down (due to still developing detoxification systems in the liver) and thus a limited ability to detoxify pollutants and rid them from their bodies. Nutrition also plays a key role in chemical exposure: children are often picky eaters and thus may not consume foods known to "detox" the body (leafy green vegetables, whole fruits and vegetables, probiotic-rich foods). In addition, the younger the exposure to harmful chemicals starts, the greater the cumulative exposure over a lifetime. Although skin reactions, such as rash, are the most common *visible reaction* to any ingredient in personal care products, it's best to introduce safe, vetted personal care products (e.g., skin lotion, shampoo, detangler, soap) into children's lives at an early age, to lower total life-long exposure to unnecessary and often "unseen" harmful chemicals.[14]

Teens and Personal Care Products

Teenagers have many harmful chemicals in their bodies. In 2008, the Environmental Working Group evaluated a group of 20 teen girls aged 14–19 from across the United States, from different socioeconomic and cultural backgrounds. The EWG detected 16 chemical breakdown products from 4 chemical families—phthalates, triclosan, parabens, and musks—in blood and urine samples. The young women were widely exposed to parabens, a common class of preservatives often found in personal care products;

methylparaben and propylparaben, in particular, were detected in every single girl tested. All of the girls together were exposed to an estimated 174 combined unique cosmetic ingredients. Each young woman had between 10 and 15 chemicals in her body, 9 of which were found in every single teen tested.[21]

Feminine care products, whose use is often initiated when young girls jump into womanhood with the start of menstruation, can contain a variety of harmful chemicals; for example, tampons may contain chlorine and pesticides used in cotton production, synthetic plastics like rayon and polyester, fragrance containing phthalates, and added antibacterial chemicals. With 10–20 tampons used monthly by the average teen, how many tampons does a typical woman use over her lifetime? And, the mucosal lining of the vaginal canal, similar to tissue lining the mouth and gastrointestinal tract, can rapidly absorb chemicals and medications into the blood stream.

It's important to understand that teens are not just small adults; their bodies are continuing to develop. Teens are unique in that they experience a tremendous growth spurt, and surge of hormone release, that will define their stature, fertility, and even cognitive maturity.

So many vital and yet vulnerable hormone-sensitive glands "turn on" during the teenage years, signaling bone and muscle growth, cartilage hardening, and brain development.[22–24] In girls, puberty is commonly defined as the period of growth of pubic hair and breasts, overall growth, and ultimately the beginning of menstrual cycles (that are often initially not regular as the endocrine control systems are still maturing). Greater exposure to pollution overall and, in particular endocrine-disrupting chemicals, is implicated in a variety of physiologic changes in teens, including an enormous rise in obesity. There is concern that the age at which girls begin puberty has been decreasing, which research suggests can be caused by ongoing, pervasive exposure to endocrine-disrupting chemicals, particularly those that mimic the activity of estrogen.[25]

Environmental Health Education for Teens

It seems ironic that the teen demographic, whose endocrine system is on overdrive, uses more personal care products with endocrine-disrupting chemicals daily than any other age group. But, we can actively reduce the amount of harmful chemicals in the body, and this begins with what we *choose* to put onto our skin. In 2015, 100 Latina teens from across the United States swapped out their personal care products for safer versions of the same products over a 3-day period.[26] The results from this study showed a dramatic drop in urinary metabolites of specific harmful chemicals, including chemicals that affect and manipulate estrogen in women (phthalates, BPA, parabens, triclosan, and benzophenone-3).

Teenagers in the United States represent a unique and critical demographic for environmental health education. Based on several pilot projects with high school students, author AC discovered that teens are "body aware" and hungry for vetted health and beauty information. Many teens are tech savvy and can use online educational apps and resources effectively. Given the sheer buying power of their demographic, teens have the ability to move the consumer market toward safer, less toxic products. Additionally teens are approaching the age to vote, and will be able to use the power of their demographic to positively shape the political landscape to deal with environmental health issues. Perhaps most importantly, today's teenagers may one day have children and will be more knowledgable and thus empowered than previous generations to keep their children's bodies "clean" and protect them from chemicals that could potentially cause harm to *their* offspring and the generations to follow.

With all that we now know about chemical exposures increasing risks for a variety of chronic health conditions, it seems foolish not to integrate this critical information into the curricula of elementary, middle, and high school students. There are over 160,000 private and public schools in the United States, presenting an enormous opportunity to educate and empower our next generation to make safer, smarter choices for their bodies and to help keep them healthy now and into the future.

To view author AC's TEDx talk on this topic, go to YouTube and search Aly Cohen.

Breast Cancer Risk from Personal Care Products

The number of new cases of breast cancer has been increasing among American women over the past several decades, and researchers have found strong links to environmental exposures, such as pesticides, industrial chemicals, and chemicals commonly found in personal care products.[27-33] Additional evidence shows that breast cancer rates among younger women may be of particular concern. In 2016, the *Journal of the American Medical Association* (*JAMA*) published data showing a statistically significant rise in the incidence of breast cancer with metastasis among women aged 25–39 in the United States over the past 40 years, without a corresponding increase in the incidence in older women.[67] Researchers believe endocrine-disrupting chemicals play a major role in this increase.[34] Another important study showed that, when breast cancer tissue from mice was "treated" with the chemical BPA, a broad range of chemotherapy treatments were ineffective at stopping the cancer growth.[35]

African American Personal Care Products and Health Issues

African American women and teens may experience more adverse health effects than whites and other ethnic groups from harmful personal care product ingredients because of the formulations created and marketed to African American consumers. Each year, this market segment spends about $9 billion on beauty products, twice as much as any other ethnic group. African American women and girls use a proportionally greater number of hair products in particular, such as detangle products, oils, hair moisturizers, "perm" chemicals, and relaxers. Many of these products contain eye and lung irritants, carcinogens such as lye, and estrogen-like chemicals present in ingredients such as animal placenta extract, used to soften and strengthen hair.[34,37] A recent study looking at chemical levels in the blood and urine of African American women and children, found multiple chemicals associated with both endocrine system changes and asthma. Parabens and DEP (a phthalate) are two classes of endocrine disruptors found at higher levels in African American women than in white women.[36] Exposure to these chemicals is thought to contribute to increased rates of uterine fibroids, menstrual cycle irregularities, and early age onset of menstruation (which is associated with increased risk for breast cancer because of increased lifetime exposure to estrogen) in women of this ethnic group.[38-42] In a recent comprehensive study looking at the association between hair dye and chemical relaxer/straightener use and breast cancer risk by ethnicity, it was discovered that a higher breast cancer risk was associated with *any* use of straightener or permanent dye, *especially* among African American women.[43] It is also known that African American women are experiencing increased rates of *aggressive* forms of breast cancer.[44] What's most concerning about this is that these aggressive cancers are occurring well before the recommended age for routine mammogram screening, which is generally not covered by most health insurance companies before age 45.

Education will play a key role in reducing exposure to harmful chemicals among African American women and their daughters. Organizations such as Black Women for Wellness are instrumental in bringing health issues to light and working to reduce exposures through product disclosure for the benefit of the next generation of African American women.[42]

Occupational Risks and Personal Care Products

In 1970, the United States Congress and President Richard Nixon created the Occupational Safety and Health Administration (OSHA), a national public health agency dedicated to the basic proposition that no worker should have to "choose between their life and their job." The OSHA mission statement makes it clear that "the right to a safe workplace is a basic human right." It further states, "OSHA is committed to protecting workers from toxic chemicals and deadly safety hazards at work, ensuring that vulnerable workers in high-risk jobs have access to critical information and education about job hazards."[45] While this is the lofty intent of OSHA, the reality is far different.

"Aestheticians" (such as manicurists, cosmetologists, makeup artists, and hair salon workers) are some of the occupations in the United States in which workers are most exposed to hazardous chemicals. Thousands of chemicals are used by these workers on a daily, weekly, monthly, and yearly basis, often starting at young ages. As female-dominated occupations, aestheticians are often exposed even while pregnant. Many of these workers are immigrants, many may be undocumented, and they often do not have healthcare insurance to cover routine medical care or physical complaints. Beauty industry workers, in general, are unaware of the chemicals that they are handling (often without gloves) and breathing in during the workday. For manicurists, air quality poses a particular risk due to the volatile organic compounds (VOCs) that they inhale while at work, including toluene, formaldehyde, dibutyl phthalate (DBP, used to make nail polish

Table 8.1 Harmful Chemicals Found in Nail Products

Compounds	Nail Care Use[1]	Potential Health Effects[2]	Route(s) of Exposure
Ethyl acetate	Nail polish, nail polish remover	Eye, nose, throat irritant; dermatitis	Inhalation
Formaldehyde	Nail hardener, tool disinfectant[1]	Known carcinogen	Inhalation, dermal
Silica (quartz or crystobalite)	Acrylic nail powder	Known carcinogen	Inhalation
Methylene Chloride	Artificial nail solvent	Possible carcinogen	Inhalation, dermal
Titanium Dioxide	Acrylic nail powder[1]	Possible carcinogen	Inhalation
Isopropyl acetate	Nail polish	Eye, nose, skin, lung irritant	Inhalation
DiButyl Phthalate	Nail polish	Endocrine disruptor	Inhalation, dermal
Toluene	Nail polish, nail adhesives[1]	Suspected teratogen	Inhalation, dermal

[1] US EPA Pollution Prevention Practices for Nail Salons: A Guide to Protect the Health of Nail Salon Workers and their Environment, 2007.
[2] Agency for Toxic Substances Disease Registry (ATSDR), Toxicological Profile Information Sheet [web page], 2006.

less brittle), and ethyl acetate (acetone) (see Table 8.1). Sadly, some of the most vulnerable workers in the United States are at great risk for occupational exposure to harmful chemicals at levels far greater than deemed safe by federal regulations (which are not really protective of health). There are approximately 54,000 nail salons across the United States, and regular inspection and oversight for healthy air quality, flow, and filtration is limited. Given the magnitude of aerosolized and volatile chemicals present in these spaces, proper air duct design, appropriate rate of air exchanges, installation, cleaning, and ongoing maintenance is a must to ensure good air quality for the workers inside.

Hairdressers also handle many toxic chemicals, including permanent hair dyes containing paraphenylenediamine (PPD; see above section "Lash Lure and the Food, Drug, and Cosmetic Act of 1938"), which is linked to liver cancer and immune system dysfunction.[46] According to studies, human urothelial and bladder cancers, induced by these toxic chemicals (known as aromatic amines), may remain dormant for more than 20 years before causing noticeable health issues. Researchers subsequently found higher rates of bladder cancer developing in hairdressers who had worked with permanent hair dyes prior to the 1980s. This finding reiterates the concept that chemical exposures earlier in life could have an impact decades later. [47,48]

Cosmetologists handle and apply makeup containing harmful metals such as lead, mercury, and cadmium; cosmetics with fragrance (phthalates); and chemical makeup removers with solvents. Actually, mercury is often added intentionally to these products to reduce bacterial contamination. In 2013, researchers showed that lead is pervasive in lipstick, even among the expensive brands. Of the 32 lipsticks analyzed, 75% contained lead at levels exceeding the acceptable daily intakes (ADIs) from all sources, which, as discussed previously, are arbitrarily set high levels not based on current science. High levels of manganese, titanium, aluminum, chromium, and cadmium were also found.[49] Since it has been estimated that women swallow an average of about 5 pounds of lipstick over a lifetime, that is a big problem, and *still*, the FDA has not set limits for lead levels in cosmetics.

How to Choose Safe Personal Care Products

Choosing safer personal care products requires some knowledge about what ingredients to avoid, which can be acquired through the use of computer technology and available phone apps, such as the EWG's Healthy Living app and website, www.EWG.org/SkinDeep. These sites offer easy-to-navigate safety ratings for almost 90,000 products, along with available ingredient data and related health risks. You will then be equipped to read labels such as that shown in Figure 8.4 and learn which products to avoid. If you choose to search the web for information rather than rely on the EWG database, which is independent of industry influence, be aware that the cosmetics industry spends millions of dollars

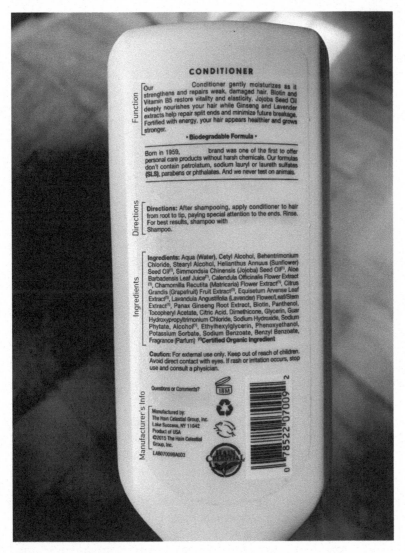

FIGURE 8.4 Interpreting personal care product label.

on advertising to promote as completely safe what are actually dangerous products. These industry-funded sites often have names that might make you think that they are consumer-oriented rather than product-protection sites.

Steer clear of these ingredients in your products:

- Parabens (ethyl, propyl, butyl, and methyl)
- Lead acetate
- Sodium lauryl sulfate (SLS)
- Mercury (thimerosal)
- Diethanolamine (DEA)
- Propylene glycol (PG)
- Coal tar
- Toluene
- Phenylenediamine (PPD)
- Petrolatum
- Synthetic color pigments
- Fragrance or perfume (unless well-vetted for synthetic and undisclosed ingredients and/or listed as a product with 100% organic ingredients)

Products that release formaldehyde (bad stuff!):

- Quaternium 15
- DMDM hydantoin
- Imidazolidinyl urea
- Diazolidinyl urea
- 2-bromo-2-nitropropane-1,3-diol
- Pegylated ingredients (denoted by peg-)

General recommendations:

- Use fewer products overall, *especially* during the 6 months before becoming pregnant, and then during pregnancy and while nursing.
- Check ingredients in personal care products you and your family use, and change out hazardous products.
- Avoid products with "perfume" or "fragrance" listed as ingredients, as these may have 300 or more undisclosed, proprietary chemicals that may pose an allergy and/or cancer risk, but which are considered to be trade secrets and are thus not disclosed.
- Avoid personal care products that contain dermal penetration enhancers that increase dermal absorption of toxic chemicals. They break down the protective barrier in the epidermis; this is why they are used in drugs designed for transdermal absorption. Among the most commonly used enhancers are isopropyl myristate, propylene glycol, and various alcohols.[7]

Body/Facial Soap

- Avoid products with antimicrobial ingredients, such as triclosan, bactroban, microban, and triclocarban (bar soap), which can result in endocrine disruption and antibiotic resistance.

Shampoo/Conditioner

- Avoid shampoo and conditioner with fragrance, polyethylene glycol (PEG) and polyethylene, ceteareth, DMDM hydantoin, and parabens (e.g., propylparaben, isopropylparaben, butylparaben, isobutylparaben), which increase cancer and developmental risks.

Sunscreens

- Look for sunscreens labeled as "skin blocks," which contain chemicals that remain on top of the skin and are not absorbed, such as zinc or titanium dioxide (see Table 8.2).
- Avoid suncreens with nanoparticles, tiny particles that can penetrate skin more efficiently and enter the blood stream.
- Avoid products with "perfume" or "fragrance."
- Avoid retinyl palmitate or retinol in moisturizing and lip products and sunscreens, which increase risk for skin cancers.
- Do NOT use sunscreens with added insect repellant!
- Avoid SPF >50, which is misleading because it gives users a false sense of security that the higher SPF level may not require application of sunscreen at the recommended 60- to 80-minute intervals recommended for all SPF levels. An SPF level higher than 50 does not add additional protection; it is the reapplication interval of 60- to 80-minutes that is most effective in preventing sun damage to skin.
- Water resistant does not mean waterproof. There is no such thing. Reapply every 60- to 80-minutes, especially when swimming or sweating.
- UVA rays are longer waves and penetrates the skin deeply, while UVB rays are shorter and damage the outer layer of skin and cause sunburn. Both UVA and UVB rays can cause skin cancers and melanoma, so look for products that adequately block both.

Makeup

- Avoid retinyl palmitate or retinol in moisturizing and lip products.
- Lipstick has been found to contain heavy metals, such as lead and mercury, regardless of cost or brand.[49-51] Given the quantity of lip products

Table 8.2 Tips for Choosing Safe Sunscreens

1. Quick tips for a good sunscreen

	🚫 Avoid these	✔ Look for these
Ingredients	Oxybenzone Vitamin A (retinyl palmitate) Added insect repellent	Zinc oxide Titanium dioxide Avobenzone or Mexoryl SX
Products	Sprays Powders SPF above 50+	Cream Broad-spectrum protection Water-resistant for beach, pool & exercise SPF 30+ for beach & pool

that are ingested annually through eating, and the potential health effects of cumulative doses of heavy metal exposure, reduce the use of colored lipstick when possible.

Nail Polish/Base Coat

• Avoid nail polish and base coat containing formaldehyde, formalin, toluene, dibutyl phthalate (DBP), which pose risks for allergy, developmental issues, and cancer. These chemicals are volatile and end up in the air and are thus inhaled, especially when appropriate ventilation is not in place.

Tampons and Other Feminine Care Products

• Given that the use of these products begins in adolescence, women and young girls should try to use tampons and feminine care products that are 100% cotton; are chlorine, phthalate, and pesticide-free; and are preferably organic, whenever possible, due to the rapid absorption of chemicals through the vaginal lining into the bloodstream.[52–60] Avoid products with plastic applicators, which are designated as "medical waste," are not recyclable, and contribute to plastic pollution globally.

Hair Dyes/Hair Spray

- Look up darkening hair dye products for safety risks on EWG.org/skindeep database and contact the manufacturer to inquire about harmful ingredients. Hair dyes, containing dozens of undisclosed chemicals, may cause irritation to skin and scalp as well as increased risk for development of autoimmune disease and cancer by aromatic amines, even decades after regular use.[46,61–65]
- Consider an alternative to hair dying; in a recent comprehensive study looking at the association between hair dye and chemical relaxer/straightener use and breast cancer risk by ethnicity, it was discovered that a higher breast cancer risk was associated with use of *any* straightener or permanent dye, especially among African American women.
- Avoid cosmetics and hair products that are aerosolized due to inhalation risk. Hairsprays often contain propellant chemicals, alcohol, formaldehyde, artificial fragrance, and polyvinylpyrrolidone (PVP), all of which can cause cough, sore throat, eye and nasal irritation, and long-term health issues.

Deodorant versus Antiperspirant

- Antiperspirants stop sweat by coating the armpit with particles (often aluminum chlorohydrate or aluminum zirconium) that are so small that they can enter into the sweat glands beneath the outer skin. These particles hold onto sweat *inside* of the skin because of the osmotic effect (flow of water from weak solution (no aluminum) to strong solution (with aluminum)). Aerosolized antiperspirant is often inhaled, causing respiratory issues such as cough and throat irritation as well as absorption into the body through the lungs.
- Aluminum is effective, but not necessarily safe, and should be avoided as an antiperspirant, especially because of its use so close to vulnerable breast tissue. Aluminum is a metalloestrogen and has the potential to adversely effect human breast cells by contributing to cyst formation and cancer risk.[66]
- Antibacterial chemicals, such as triclosan, triclocarban, cloflucarban, phenol, and chloroxylenol, are often added to antiperspirants as well as

deodorants. These chemicals are readily absorbed through the skin and have been detected in blood samples.

- Deodorants are not specifically designed to get absorbed into sweat glands like antiperspirants, so in general they have fewer health risks.

***

Both deodorant and antiperspirant may still contain fragrance and other potentially harmful chemicals, so research deodorant brands from reliable databases such as the Environmental Working Group (EWG.org/skindeep).

Toothpaste

- Many toothpastes contain unnecessary ingredients such as artificial coloring, titanium dioxide for whitening, abrasive ingredients, fluoride which can be toxic if swallowed, and sodium laurel sulfate (SLS) which can cause canker sores.

Make Your Own Personal Care Products

Many personal care products can be made using simple, safe ingredients, such as baking soda, essential oils, bentonite clay, and organic coconut oil. Do It Yourself (DIY) products can be safe, simple, economical, long-lasting, and customizable.

DIY Deodorant

2½ teaspoons of unrefined coconut oil (helps kill fungi, yeast, and bacteria)

2½ teaspoons of unrefined shea butter

2 teaspoons baking soda

¼ cup arrowroot starch/flour (absorbs moisture)

6 drops of essential oil (lavender or orange)

6 drops of grapefruit essential oil

2 drops of tea tree oil (helps kill bacteria)

1. Place coconut oil and shea butter in a glass bowl or jar and place the bowl or jar inside a medium sauce pan (creating a double cooker for even heating)

2. Add water to the saucepan halfway up (enough to surround the bowl/jar) and bring to a boil
3. As the water is heating up, stir coconut oil and shea butter until melted
4. Add in arrowroot starch, baking soda, and essential oils
5. Transfer to a 3-ounce jar and allow to cool at room temp or in fridge
6. Cover with lid until use

Total time: 10 minutes
Yield: 3 ounce jar, will last 3 to 4 months
Coconut oil melts at temperatures greater than 75 degrees F, so store in a cool location.

Alternate DIY Deodorant

¼ cup of coconut oil
1/8 cup of baking soda
1/8 cup of arrowroot starch
15–20 drops of essential oils (e.g., lavender, tea tree, red grapefruit)

Mix all ingredients together and store in a cool dry place
You can find additional DIY recipes here:
Tree Hugger: https://www.treehugger.com
The Free Spirited: http://www.thefreespirited.co/beauty/

Bottom Line

Exposure to harmful chemicals in personal care products poses real health risks, both short- and long-term, even in very low doses, and particularly among fetuses (exposed via the mother), infants, toddlers, and teens whose bodies and brains are developing rapidly. Chemicals are absorbed through skin, are inhaled through the air, and even absorbed through the thin tissue of the vaginal canal and anus. Use fewer products and check the safety of those that you do use through reliable resources.

Activity

Go to EWG's Skin Deep Guide to Cosmetics and look up your brand of shampoo or other personal care products (e.g., shaving cream, aftershave, toothpaste, deodorant, nail polish, foundation, skin lotion, lipstick, self-tanner)

1. Describe the rating system for products vetted by EWG (0-10): what number implies the least number of toxic ingredients and what number implies the greatest number of toxic ingredients?
2. What was the rating given by EWG for your product?
3. What health concerns are associated with this product?
4. List 3 ingredients that have been found in this product.
5. Go back to the main page for the SkinDeep database and look up a "cleaner"/ less-toxic shampoo brand or other personal care product (i.e., has a lower EWG rating for toxic chemicals).

Resources

- The Story of Cosmetics, released on July 21, 2010, examines the pervasive use of toxic chemicals in our everyday personal care products, from lipstick to baby shampoo. https://www.youtube.com/watch?v=pfq000AF1i8
- Safe Cosmetics Tips Sheet https://donate.ewg.org/images/Quick%20Tips%20for%20Choosing%20Safer%20Pesonal%20Care%20Products.pdf
- More information can be obtained from the EWG's cosmetics database: http://www.ewg.org/skindeep/ and Healthy Living smartphone app.
- Campaign for safe Cosmetics: www.safecosmetics.org/
- Black Women for Wellness: www.bwwla.org
- The Smart Human: TheSmartHuman.com
- Women's Voices for the Earth: https://www.womensvoices.org/

References

1. Sorvino C. Why the $445 billion beauty industry is a gold mine for self-made women. *Forbes Magazine*. https://www.forbes.com/sites/chloesorvino/2017/05/18/self-made-women-wealth-beauty-gold-mine/#233e78022a3a. Published 2017. Accessed October 21, 2018.
2. American Contact Dermatitis Society. Allergen of the Year. 2006. Wikipedia. https://en.wikipedia.org/wiki/Allergen_of_the_Year. Accessed April 24, 2020.

3. Baker N. *The Body Toxic: How the Hazardous Chemistry of Everyday Things Threatens Our Health and Well-being.* New York: North Point Press; 2008.

4. Food and Drug Administration (FDA). Part II: 1938, Food, Drug, and Cosmetic Act. FDA.gov. https://www.fda.gov/about-fda/fdas-evolving-regulatory-powers/part-ii-1938-food-drug-cosmetic-act. Published 2018. Accessed November 22, 2019.

5. FDA. Cosmetics: proucts and ingredient safety. https://www.fda.gov/cosmetics/productsingredients/default.htm. Published 2018. Accessed October 26, 2018.

6. Nudelman J, Taylor B, Evans N, et al. Policy and research recommendations emerging from the scientific evidence connecting environmental factors and breast cancer. *International Journal of Occupational and Environmental Health.* 2009;15(1):79–101.

7. Karande P, Mitragotri S. Enhancement of transdermal drug delivery via synergistic action of chemicals. *Biochim Biophys Acta.* 2009;1788(11):2362–2373.

8. Duty SM, Ackerman RM, Calafat AM, Hauser R. Personal care product use predicts urinary concentrations of some phthalate monoesters. *Environmental Health Perspectives.* 2005;113(11):1530–1535.

9. Environmental Working Group (EWG). Body burden: the pollution in newborns: a benchmark investigation of industrial chemicals, pollutants and pesticides in umbilical cord blood. 2005.

10. Genuis SJ. Nowhere to hide: chemical toxicants and the unborn child. *Reproductive Toxicology (Elmsford, NY).* 2009;28(1):115–116.

11. Herdt-Losavio ML, Lin S, Chapman BR, et al. Maternal occupation and the risk of birth defects: an overview from the National Birth Defects Prevention Study. *Occupational and Environmental Medicine.* 2010;67(1):58–66.

12. Hines EP, Calafat AM, Silva MJ, Mendola P, Fenton SE. Concentrations of phthalate metabolites in milk, urine, saliva, and serum of lactating North Carolina women. *Environ Health Perspect.* 2009;117(1):86–92.

13. Bonchak JG, Prouty ME, de la Feld SF. Prevalence of contact allergens in personal care products for babies and children. *Dermatitis.* 2018;29(2):81–84.

14. Cornell E, Kwa M, Paller AS, Xu S. Adverse events reported to the Food and Drug Administration from 2004 to 2016 for cosmetics and personal care products marketed to newborns and infants. *Pediatr Dermatol.* 2018;35(2):225–229.

15. Kwapniewski R, Kozaczka S, Hauser R, Silva MJ, Calafat AM, Duty SM. Occupational exposure to dibutyl phthalate among manicurists. *Journal of Occupational and Environmental Medicine / American College of Occupational and Environmental Medicine.* 2008;50(6):705–711.

16. Vuong AM, Webster GM, Romano ME, et al. Maternal polybrominated diphenyl ether (PBDE) exposure and thyroid hormones in maternal and cord sera: the HOME study, Cincinnati, USA. *Environ Health Perspect*. 2015;123(10):1079–1085.

17. Sathyanarayana S, Calafat AM, Liu F, Swan SH. Maternal and infant urinary phthalate metabolite concentrations: are they related? *Environ Res*. 2008;108(3):413–418.

18. Wolff MS, Engel SM, Berkowitz GS, et al. Prenatal phenol and phthalate exposures and birth outcomes. *Environ Health Perspect*. 2008;116(8):1092–1097.

19. Watkins DJ, Sanchez BN, Téllez-Rojo MM, et al. Impact of phthalate and BPA exposure during in utero windows of susceptibility on reproductive hormones and sexual maturation in peripubertal males. *Environmental Health*. 2017;16(69).

20. Rudel RA, Camann DE, Spengler JD, Korn LR, Brody JG. Phthalates, alkylphenols, pesticides, polybrominated diphenyl ethers, and other endocrine-disrupting compounds in indoor air and dust. *Environmental Science & Technology*. 2003;37(20):4543–4553.

21. EWG. Teen girls' body burden of hormone-altering cosmetics chemicals. http://www.ewg.org/research/teen-girls-body-burden-hormone-altering-cosmetics-chemicals. Published 2008. Accessed December 11, 2016.

22. Giudice LC. Environmental toxicants: hidden players on the reproductive stage. *Fertility and Sterility*. 2016;106(4):791–794.

23. Centers for Disease Control and Prevention (CDC). Fourth National Report on Human Exposure to Environmental Chemicals. 2013 (March).

24. Houten SM, Chen J, Belpoggi F, et al. Changes in the metabolome in response to low-dose exposure to environmental chemicals used in personal care products during different windows of susceptibility. *PLoS One*. 2016;11(7):e0159919.

25. Buttke DE, Sircar K, Martin C. Exposures to endocrine-disrupting chemicals and age of menarche in adolescent girls in NHANES (2003–2008). *Environ Health Perspect* 2012;120(11):1613–1618.

26. Harley KG, Kogut K, Madrigal DS, et al. Reducing phthalate, paraben, and phenol exposure from personal care products in adolescent girls: findings from the HERMOSA Intervention Study. *Environ Health Perspect*. 2016.

27. Pestana D, Teixeira D, Faria A, Domingues V, Monteiro R, Calhau C. Effects of environmental organochlorine pesticides on human breast cancer: putative involvement on invasive cell ability. *Environmental Toxicology*. 2015;30(2):168–176.

28. Golubnitschaja O, Debald M, Yeghiazaryan K, et al. Breast cancer epidemic in the early twenty-first century: evaluation of risk factors, cumulative questionnaires and recommendations for preventive measures. *Tumour*

Biology: The Journal of the International Society for Oncodevelopmental Biology and Medicine. 2016.

29. Ingber SZ, Buser MC, Pohl HR, Abadin HG, Murray HE, Scinicariello F. DDT/DDE and breast cancer: a meta-analysis. *Regul Toxicol Pharmacol.* 2013;67(3):421–433.

30. Thongprakaisang S, Thiantanawat A, Rangkadilok N, Suriyo T, Satayavivad J. Glyphosate induces human breast cancer cells growth via estrogen receptors. *Food Chem Toxicol.* 2013;59:129–136.

31. Gray JM, Rasanayagam S, Engel C, Rizzo J. State of the evidence 2017: an update on the connection between breast cancer and the environment. *Environmental Health: A Global Access Science Source.* 2017;16(1):94.

32. Ociepa-Zawal M, Rubis B, Wawrzynczak D, Wachowiak R, Trzeciak WH. Accumulation of environmental estrogens in adipose tissue of breast cancer patients. *Journal of Environmental Science and Health Part A, Toxic/Hazardous Substances & Environmental Engineering.* 2010;45(3):305–312.

33. Johnson RH, Chien FL, Bleyer A. Incidence of breast cancer with distant involvement among women in the United States, 1976 to 2009. *JAMA.* 2013;309(8):800–805.

34. Myers SL, Yang CZ, Bittner GD, Witt KL, Tice RR, Baird DD. Estrogenic and anti-estrogenic activity of off-the-shelf hair and skin care products. *Journal of Exposure Science & Environmental Epidemiology.* 2015;25(3):271–277.

35. Sauer SJ, Tarpley M, Shah I, Save AV, Lyerly HK, Patierno SR, et al. Bisphenol A activates EGFR and ERK promoting proliferation, tumor spheroid formation and resistance to EGFR pathway inhibition in estrogen receptor-negative inflammatory breast cancer cells. *Carcinogenesis.* 2017;38(3):252–260.

36. EWG. Big market for black cosmetics, but less-hazardous choices limited. http://www.ewg.org/research/big-market-black-cosmetics-less-hazardous-choices-limited#ref1. Published 2016. Accessed December 11, 2016.

37. Helm JS, Nishioka M, Brody JG, Rudel RA, Dodson RE. Measurement of endocrine disrupting and asthma-associated chemicals in hair products used by Black women. *Environ Res.* 2018.

38. Wise LA, Palmer JR, Reich D, Cozier YC, Rosenberg L. Hair relaxer use and risk of uterine leiomyomata in African-American women. *American Journal of Epidemiology.* 2012;175(5):432–440.

39. Donovan M, Tiwary CM, Axelrod D, et al. Personal care products that contain estrogens or xenoestrogens may increase breast cancer risk. *Medical Hypotheses.* 2007;68(4):756–766.

40. Stiel L, Adkins-Jackson PB, Clark P, Mitchell E, Montgomery S. A review of hair product use on breast cancer risk in African American women. *Cancer Medicine.* 2016;5(3):597–604.

41. Wolff MS, Britton JA, Wilson VP. Environmental risk factors for breast cancer among African-American women. *Cancer.* 2003;97(1 Suppl):289–310.

42. Nourbese NF, Teiope A. Black women for wellness: a five year study of the black beauty industry. 2016. http://www.bwwla.org/wp-content/uploads/2016/03/One-Hair-Story-Final-small-file-size-3142016.pdf. Accessed April 24, 2020.

43. Eberle CE, Sandler DP, Taylor KW, White AJ. Hair dye and chemical straightener use and breast cancer risk in a large US population of black and white women. *International Journal of Cancer.* 2019.

44. Kanaan YM, Sampey BP, Beyene D, et al. Metabolic profile of triple-negative breast cancer in African-American women reveals potential biomarkers of aggressive disease. *Cancer Genomics & Proteomics.* 2014;11(6):279–294.

45. Department of Labor. All About OSHA. OSHA 3302–08R.

46. Nohynek GJ, Fautz R, Benech-Kieffer F, Toutain H. Toxicity and human health risk of hair dyes. *Food Chem Toxicol.* 2004;42(4):517–543.

47. Bolt HM, Golka K. The debate on carcinogenicity of permanent hair dyes: new insights. *Critical Reviews in Toxicology.* 2007;37(6):521–536.

48. La Vecchia C, Tavani A. Epidemiological evidence on hair dyes and the risk of cancer in humans. *European Journal of Cancer Prevention: The Official Journal of the European Cancer Prevention Organisation (ECP).* 1995;4(1):31–43.

49. Liu S, Hammond SK, Rojas-Cheatham A. Concentrations and potential health risks of metals in lip products. *Environ Health Perspect.* 2013;121(6):705–710.

50. Hepp NM. Determination of total lead in 400 lipsticks on the U.S. market using a validated microwave-assisted digestion, inductively coupled plasma-mass spectrometric method. *Journal of Cosmetic Science.* 2012;63(3):159–176.

51. Hepp NM, Mindak WR, Cheng J. Determination of total lead in lipstick: development and validation of a microwave-assisted digestion, inductively coupled plasma-mass spectrometric method. *Journal of Cosmetic Science.* 2009;60(4):405–414.

52. Farage MA, Lennon L, Ajayi F. Products used on female genital mucosa. *Current Problems in Dermatology.* 2011;40:90–100.

53. Farage MA, Miller KW, Ledger WJ. Can the behind-the-knee clinical test be used to evaluate the mechanical and chemical irritation potential for products intended for contact with mucous membranes? *Current Problems in Dermatology.* 2011;40:125–132.

54. Farage MA, Scheffler H. Assessing the dermal safety of products intended for genital mucosal exposure. *Current Problems in Dermatology.* 2011;40:116–124.

55. Farage MA, Warren R. Emollients on the genital area. *Current Problems in Dermatology.* 2011;40:101–106.

56. Lang C, Fisher M, Neisa A, et al. Personal care product use in pregnancy and the postpartum period: implications for exposure assessment. *Int J Environ Res Public Health.* 2016;13(1).

57. Rigg LA, Hermann H, Yen SS. Absorption of estrogens from vaginal creams. *The New England Journal of Medicine.* 1978;298(4):195–197.

58. Santen RJ. Vaginal administration of estradiol: effects of dose, preparation and timing on plasma estradiol levels. *Climacteric: The Journal of the International Menopause Society.* 2015;18(2):121–134.

59. van der Bijl P, van Eyk AD. Comparative in vitro permeability of human vaginal, small intestinal and colonic mucosa. *International Journal of Pharmaceutics.* 2003;261(1–2):147–152.

60. Branch F, Woodruff TJ, Mitro SD, Zota AR. Vaginal douching and racial/ethnic disparities in phthalates exposures among reproductive-aged women: National Health and Nutrition Examination Survey 2001-2004. *Environmental Health: A Global Access Science Source.* 2015;14:57.

61. Kim KH, Kabir E, Jahan SA. The use of personal hair dye and its implications for human health. *Environ Int.* 2016;89–90:222–227.

62. Nohynek GJ, Antignac E, Re T, Toutain H. Safety assessment of personal care products/cosmetics and their ingredients. *Toxicol Appl Pharmacol.* 2010;243(2):239–259.

63. Skov T, Lynge E. Cancer risk and exposures to carcinogens in hairdressers. *Skin Pharmacology: The Official Journal of the Skin Pharmacology Society.* 1994;7(1–2):94–100.

64. Freni-Titulaer LW, Kelley DB, Grow AG, McKinley TW, Arnett FC, Hochberg MC. Connective tissue disease in southeastern Georgia: a case-control study of etiologic factors. *American Journal of Epidemiology.* 1989;130(2):404–409.

65. Cooper GS, Dooley MA, Treadwell EL, St Clair EW, Gilkeson GS. Smoking and use of hair treatments in relation to risk of developing systemic lupus erythematosus. *The Journal of Rheumatology.* 2001;28(12):2653–2656.

66. Darbre PD. Aluminium and the human breast. *Morphologie: bulletin de l'Association des anatomistes.* 2016;100(329):65–74.

67. Johnson RH, Chien FL, Bleyer A. Incidence of breast cancer with distant involvement among women in the United States, 1976 to 2009. *JAMA.* 2013;309(8):800–805.

9

Squeaky Clean
How to Stay Clean without Toxins!

In every aspect of life, purity and holiness, cleanliness and re-
finement, exalt the human condition . . . even in the physical
realm, cleanliness will conduce to spirituality.

—Abdu'l-Baha (1844–1921)

We each have our own perspective on cleanliness, whether it is the way we dress or the way we keep our home, including the odor of the house. Some of us are raised with beliefs, either traditional or cultural, that the degree to which one is clean on the outside, translates to the cleanliness of our mind. But the degree to which many in modern society seek to be "hyperclean" is, in fact, creating both short-term and long-term health problems due to excessive use of cleaning products, most of which contain toxic chemicals. Here we present approaches to maintaining a safe and clean lifestyle as alternatives to the approaches presented in TV and magazine advertisements intended to entice you to purchase products.

Since the 19th century, when French microbiologist Louis Pasteur elucidated the "germ theory of disease," humans have been trying to reduce and eradicate the microscopic bugs responsible for infectious diseases. Cleanliness took on a new meaning, which involved ridding our environment, homes, and bodies of microscopic invaders that were believed to take down whole cities if left unattended. Soon, the pharmaceutical industry began spending billions of dollars on antibiotic research. The consumer product industry soon followed, tasked with creating and marketing bacterial annihilation, not just to hospitals, which house the infected, but to consumers for use in our homes, schools, daycares, and on natural and synthetic-turf fields.

We now know that the balance between eradicating disease and eradicating *all* bacteria from our surroundings has gone unchecked; the idea that humans can be safe and even thrive *from* a variety of bacteria and other microorganisms living in and around their bodies is not obvious to the general public. As such, over the last 60 years, a multibillion dollar industry has emerged based more on the fear of bacteria than on harnessing a sound scientific understanding with which to manage health risks. Both short-term (acute poisoning, respiratory issues, asthma, skin burns) and long-term (developmental risks to newborns, preterm delivery, hormone changes, and cancer) health risks have been identified from exposure to toxic cleaning chemicals found in food, drinking water, and products that touch human skin. The discovery of beneficial microbes that have lived symbiotically on, as well as inside, human bodies for millions of years (i.e., the human microbiome), makes the indiscriminate eradication of bacteria through antibiotic chemicals in common household products not only unwise, but dangerous. Today, the overuse of antibiotics in medicine and in farm animals used for food has resulted in growing antibiotic resistance, accompanied by a lack of replacement antibiotics, creating a looming health crisis.

The Problem with Being Squeaky Clean

Oven cleaners, air fresheners, toilet bowl liquid, laundry detergent and softeners, chemical wipes, and mildew sprays—the effort to make our homes sparkling clean has become a billion dollar industry.[1]

Cleaning products are among the most toxic products you will find in homes today. In fact, because of their high toxicity, they are the only household products regulated by the Consumer Product Safety Commission under the 1966 Federal Hazardous Substances Act. Household cleaning products that have *known* hazardous ingredients will have one of three warning signs:

- **Danger** (skull and crossbones): could kill an adult if just a pinch is ingested
- **Warning**: could kill an adult if a teaspoon is ingested
- **Caution**: will not kill unless an amount greater than 2 tablespoons is ingested

This method of assigning poison risk is outdated, since products with these warnings can kill you and are particularly dangerous to have around children for whom the ingested amounts do not apply due to their small size and greater sensitivity to toxic chemicals.

When it comes to cleaning products, one of the first things to decide is *how aggressively* one needs to clean that area or object, because *that* will determine the degree of cleaning chemical risk you will be managing!

For example, cleaning refers to the *removal* of dirt and germs from surfaces, but does not *kill* germs. BUT, by removing them, it lowers their numbers and the risk of spreading infection. Removal of germs, the vast majority of which cause *no harm* to human health, can be done with products that are a lot less harmful to the human body than stronger chemicals used to remove infectious bacteria and viruses. For simple cleaning, we can use safe, effective cleaners such as simple bar and liquid soap made *without* fragrance, coloring, preservative, and anti-bacterial chemicals; all of these are not necessary to remove dirt, and the safe cleaners do a great job!

Disinfecting, on the other hand, refers to using chemicals to *kill* germs on surfaces, and can potentially use chemicals with stronger ingredients; this may involve the use of chemicals that can affect human health with both short- and long-term use. Bleach is one example of a strong disinfecting chemical that can cause short-term health issues like cough (bronchospasm), shortness of breath, and even trigger an asthma attack. Long-term use may cause risk to the thyroid gland and other endocrine disorders, if protection for skin contact, inhalation, and ventilation of the space, are not managed properly.

Disinfectants and COVID-19

With the new coronavirus that causes COVID-19, as well with other viral diseases such as the seasonal flu, disinfection is critical to reduce spread of the virus, especially on door handles, light switches, table and counter surfaces, and arms of chairs, so both a *diluted* household bleach solution or an alcohol solution with at least 70% alcohol should be effective.

- Diluted household bleach solutions can be inappropriate for the surface you want to clean, so follow manufacturer's instructions for application as well as for proper ventilation. Check to ensure the product is not past its expiration date. Never mix household bleach with ammonia or any other cleanser. Unexpired household bleach will be effective against coronaviruses when properly diluted (see below).
- Avoid handling bleach if you have a history of asthma, COPD, emphysema or other lung condition. Use skin protection (rubber gloves), eye protection (clear mask, eye glasses, sunglasses, or swim goggles) when handling bleach, and make sure the room is well ventilated and/or windows are open, and no children or pets are present. When working with bleach avoid touching your face.
- Accidental poisonings from cleaners and disinfectant has increased by 20% in the first quarter of 2020 as compared to rates from 2018 and 2019, according to one CDC report. Researchers believe the increase coincides with stay-at-home orders and guidelines to clean hands and surfaces to prevent COVID-19 infection.

Note: Take special care to store and /or lock all cleaning chemicals away from pets and children, and use them only when children, people with respiratory illness, and pets are at a reasonable distance.[2]

- The Center for Disease Control (CDC) in the US recommends this bleach solution mixture:
  - 5 tablespoons (1/3 cup) bleach per gallon of water *or*
  - 4 teaspoons bleach per quart of water

Resources for Effective COVID Disinfection Cleaning Products:

- https://www.cdc.gov/coronavirus/2019-ncov/prepare/cleaning-disinfection.html
- https://www.epa.gov/pesticide-registration/list-n-disinfectants-use-against-sars-cov-2

Cleaning Products and the Endocrine System

Many cleaning ingredients are categorized as endocrine-disrupting chemicals (EDCs) because they can disrupt and alter hormones in humans and wildlife at doses measured in parts per billion to parts per trillion, the equivalent of 1 drop in 20 Olympic-sized swimming pools. These incredibly small doses negatively impact the endocrine system, which manages hormones that are critical for thousands of biological functions. Effects of EDC exposure include disruption of normal fetal brain development; fertility and reproduction; and cancers of the breast, prostate, and thyroid gland. However, despite it being known that exposure to these chemical ingredients results in elevated health risks, they are not listed on product labels.

The reality is that in the United States, with the exception of products with older known hazardous ingredients, manufacturers of cleaning products are NOT required to list the full ingredient content of their products, nor are they responsible for supplying information about any testing or toxicity findings for the products that they create. Each product must have what is called a material safety data sheet (MSDS) or a more simplified Safety Data Sheet (SDS), listing known toxic ingredients, which can be found online from a number of non-profit and government web sites (for example, CDC, NIOSH, OSHA, IARC, WHO). But much like the ingredients for Coca Cola, some of the ingredients can be considered to be "trade secrets." Thus, some ingredients in cleaning products may not be listed on the ingredients list at all (coloring, preservatives, and other additives), because they are "proprietary," and under the current law are exempted from inclusion on the MSDS or SDS. In the event of an accidental poisoning, even poison control centers do not know the full ingredient details of the product ingested. While industries argue that protecting profits by keeping ingredients secret is essential, not informing consumers about the presence of chemicals in these products that have been shown to cause harm is unacceptable.

Labeling

Applying the words "organic" or "natural" to a cleaning product has no legal value unless the product carries the USDA Organic label. "Organic" implies that the ingredients are made from plants grown without use of synthetic fertilizers or pesticides, but only products bearing the USDA certified organic logo are legally obligated to comply with this claim. According to the dictionary, "natural" means that the substance or product is 'based on the state

Table 9.1 Criteria for Organic Product Labeling, Depending on the Amount of Organic Ingredients They Contain.

		ORGANIC INCREMENTS
100% ORGANIC All ingredients and processing aids must be certified organic. These foods may use the USDA organic seal as well as 100% organic claim.	USDA ORGANIC	**100%**
ORGANIC All agricultural ingredients must be certified organic, but product can contain up to 5% non-organic content. These foods may use the USDA organic seal.	USDA ORGANIC	AT LEAST **95%**
MADE WITH ORGANIC INGREDIENTS Contains at least 70% certified organic ingredients; remaining 30% not required to be certified organic, but may not be produced using excluded methods. These foods may not use the USDA organic seal.		AT LEAST **70%**
SPECIFIC ORGANIC INGREDIENTS Contains less than 70% certified organic ingredients. May list certified organic ingredients as organic in the ingredient list. These foods may not use the USDA organic seal.		LESS THAN **70%**

of things in nature,' which is meaningless under US product safety laws. Thus, the use of the term "natural" on a product has no legal or regulatory meaning.

The placement of this label also matters; products that have 100% organic ingredients are allowed to put the organic label on the front packaging. Products made with less than 70% organically grown ingredients may not use the USDA organic seal, but may list organic ingredients in the ingredients for the product. A "Made with Organic Ingredients" label may be used for products with at least 70% organic ingredients (see Table 9.1).[3]

Cleaning Chemicals to Avoid

Parabens

Parabens are synthetic chemicals first used in the 1920s as preservatives in medications, but later added to thousands of cleaning and other consumer products. The most recognizable parabens on an ingredient label are methylparaben, ethylparaben, isobutylparaben, and n-propylparaben. They are all water soluble, inexpensive to manufacture, and do not break down easily (i.e., they are persistent environmental pollutants), which makes them particularly problematic for the ecosystems that they make their way into. Parabens also have antibiotic capabilities, primarily against gram-positive species such as staphylococcus. They can kill most yeasts and molds, but they are not capable of killing viruses. Parabens are considered EDCs because of their ability to bind to both testosterone and thyroid hormone receptors (disrupting their normal activity), and they also stimulate estrogenic responses at low concentrations.

Fragrance

Before the 1900s, fragrances and perfumes were made from natural substances, such as flowers, berries, fragrant barks, and roots. Today, according to the National Academy of Sciences, up to 95% of the chemicals used to make fragrances are synthetic compounds derived from petroleum. Fragrances are infused into fabrics, added to cosmetics and cleaning products, and air fresheners are sprayed outside of teen clothing stores to entice customers to come inside to shop. Because the United States has no laws in place to require individual ingredients to be listed, the word "fragrance" or "perfume" on a label may mean up to 300+ chemicals have been added but are not listed as ingredients.

And what about products that claim to be "fragrance-free" or "unscented"? Many cleaning products (like detergents and fabric softeners) may say they have no fragrance, but what they actually mean is that the product contains no *perceptible* odor because the manufacturer added neutralizing chemicals to mask the fragrance, but the harmful chemicals remain! Clearly, you cannot rely on unregulated statements on product labels to assess the safety of these products.

How do you buy a non-toxic cleaning product? You can lessen your risk of exposure to harmful chemicals by eliminating cleaning products that you know contain added synthetic fragrance. The "less is more approach" is always best. Buy and use fewer products. Dispense with fabric softener, dryer sheets, and air fresheners. This is only the first step in eliminating hundreds, if not thousands, of undisclosed chemicals that may be harmful to your health.

Triclosan and Other Antibacterial Chemicals

Did you know that the cleaning products you lather, spray, and pour onto household surfaces may actually have antibiotics in them? That's right, everyday cleaners often contain chemicals similar to the medications doctors prescribe for an infection. But that's not all. These antibiotic chemicals are often added to makeup and shampoo and infused into the matrix of plastic products, and are actually designed to release the chemical for extended periods of time. They are listed as an "active" ingredient, as "antimicrobial," "germ fighting," or "antibacterial," and are designed to remove all bacteria that they come into contact with. Triclosan is perhaps the most widely known antimicrobial; it is registered with the EPA as a pesticide, and it is marketed under more than a dozen different names including Microban, Irgasan, Biofresh, Lexol-300, Ster-Zac, Bactroban, and Cloxifenolum. Other products containing triclosan include deodorant, cosmetics, clothing, cutting boards and kitchen utensils, tile sealant, and fitness mats.

Triclosan is also used as a preservative in adhesives, fabrics, vinyl, plastics, and sealants; in total, over 2100 products include triclosan. And, antibiotic chemicals, such as triclosan, are *readily absorbed through human skin* and are often detected in blood. In fact, 75% of urine samples[4] and 97% of breast milk samples in the United States and Sweden were found to include triclosan. After only one shower using a body wash containing triclosan, researchers found blood levels of triclosan immediately increased![5-9]

Why are these antibiotic chemicals a problem for the health of humans and wildlife? They create bacterial resistance in humans; that is, antibiotics that were once effective at treating infections are effective no longer. Worse, although all of the bacteria are supposed to be eradicated, some bacteria survive and multiply as bacteria strains that are now resistant to that particular antibiotic. The result is that people who are regularly exposed to bacteria-killing chemicals like triclosan, who then undergo routine elective procedures such as hip or knee replacements, give birth, or get treated for a bacterial cold, may no longer be protected from infection. And the truth is that antibiotic-resistant strains of bacteria, not manageable by current available antibiotics, develop much more quickly relative to the long time required to develop and get approval for new, effective antibiotics.

What happens when cleaning/antimicrobial chemicals go down the drain? They end up in waterways around the globe, and because they don't break down for years, they affect the normal ecosystems of plants and wildlife.[9-14] Triclosan is among the top 10 most frequently encountered contaminants in US rivers and streams.[15,16]

Fortunately, the FDA ruled on September 2, 2016, that 19 "antibacterial" chemicals would be banned from liquid soap, including triclosan, triclocarban, and methylbenzethonium chloride (Hyamine). This ruling applies only to consumer products intended to be used with water and subsequently washed off. The ban does NOT include products where the chemicals are left on the skin, such as hand sanitizers, wet wipes, first aid antiseptics, and other products, such as cosmetics, yoga mats, cooking utensils (where the chemical is infused into the material), and thousands of other products (see Figure 9.1). Note that hospitals and medical clinics are among the few locations where

(a)

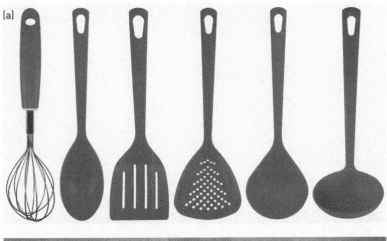

(b)

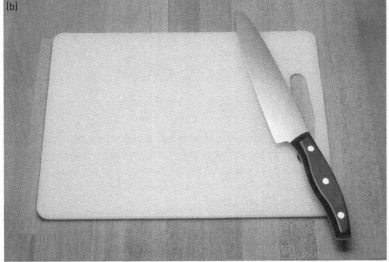

FIGURE 9.1 Continued

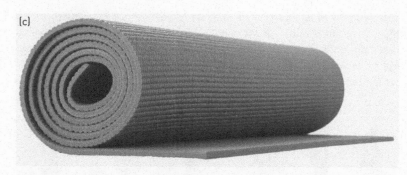

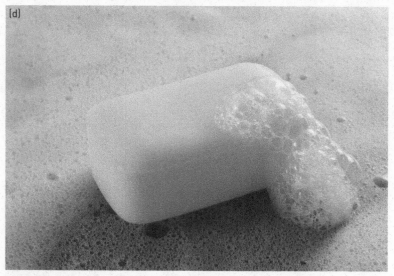

Figure 9.1 Common household items with triclosan bactroban, microban, and triclocarban (e.g., bar soap).

antibacterial soaps are still used due to increased exposure to patients of resistant bacteria. As illogical as it may seem, antibacterial soaps, which perpetuate the growth of antibiotic resistant strains of bacteria, are often used in the very locations where resistant strains of bacteria would be most worrisome, a "catch-22" scenario.

It turns out that using soap containing triclosan is *no more effective* in preventing infectious illness than washing with plain soap.[17] Chemicals that were deferred for later judgment by the FDA include benzalkonium chloride, benzethonium chloride, and chloroxylenol, also known as para-chloro-meta-xylenol or PCMX.

Health Issues from Cleaning Products

There are many "active" ingredients in common household cleaning products that kill bacteria, viruses, or mold (e.g., triclosan, bactroban, triclocarban, microban), which are associated with bacterial resistance. Cleaning products may also have chemicals that release 1-4 dioxane and formaldehyde, which are associated with increased risk for some cancers and acute respiratory issues. Often, these chemicals infiltrate households, daycare centers, and work spaces, wafting through the air and landing on other surfaces far from the surfaces where they were originally applied. These chemicals irritate the lungs when inhaled and cause a throat tickle, coughing, shortness of breath, burning eyes, or an allergic reaction from airborne exposure. They can also cause life-threatening exacerbation of asthma and COPD. Other cleaning chemicals, such as cresol, ammonia, and chlorine bleach, may cause irritation and even burns when they come into contact with skin.

Prenatal exposure to many chemicals is of great concern because many disclosed *and* undisclosed chemicals can easily cross from the mother through the placenta into a developing fetus, causing a whole host of health effects. Many popular cleaners contain chemicals that act as endocrine disruptors (e.g., parabens, triclosan, triclocarban), increasing the risk for later infertility[18] and hormone-sensitive cancers[19,20] (breast, prostate, ovarian, endometrial), as well as affecting normal thyroid function. Triclosan exposure during fetal development has been found to have neurodevelopmental effects in infants,[21,22] effects on sex hormones (testosterone, progesterone) in adolescent boys,[23] immune system dysfunction,[24-29] and increased risk for obesity[22] later in life. Most of these chemicals can be found at measurable levels in human blood, urine, tissues, and breast milk.

Passive exposure to these chemicals through breathing and skin contact are bad enough, but what about acute poisoning? Many of today's cleaning chemicals are highly toxic if ingested by infants or toddlers[30,31]—who find dishwashing detergent packets with bright swirling colors, in small clear packages, very enticing to eat. In 2016, US poison-control centers received reports of 162,791 human exposures to household cleaning products, with another 20,000+ pet exposures. The top two poison exposures in children five years of age or younger were cosmetics/personal care products (13.3%) and household cleaning substances (11.1%).[32] Never underestimate the curiosity and draw of a toddler to brightly colored objects!

How to Clean Safely

Cleaning safely involves old-fashioned elbow grease (physical effort!), a little extra work to find ready-made non-toxic products, and/or a trip to the store to create DIY products. The benefit of reduced toxin exposure in your and your family's life will be well worth it.

Using safe products is certainly important, but certain cleaning tools can offset the need for toxic chemicals as well. A steam cleaner, for instance, can do wonders; hot water can literally melt away caked-on dirt, grime, grease, soap scum, mold, mildew, and calcium and lime deposits, without chemicals or scrubbing. Microfiber dust cloths and mops, an abrasive brush or sponge, and a squeegee for showers and windows all support the non-toxic battle against dirt.

It turns out that many ecofriendly brands found in stores across the United States are as effective for cleaning common household surfaces as products containing toxic chemicals. In 2015, researchers looked at the effectiveness of products used in cleaning and disinfection against two types of bacteria, *Staphylococcus aureus* and *Escherichia coli*, on home surfaces. The researchers compared products such as conventional bleach, environmentally preferable (EP) products (Seventh Generation brand), do-it-yourself (distilled white vinegar, club soda, tea tree oil), DIY products that are 24 hours old, and individual DIY ingredients in water. The results showed that environmentally preferable (EP) products, were an effective alternative to bleach. DIY products were found to be effective in cleaning areas not required to be sterile—but they must be freshly prepared in order to work as well as the EP products.[33]

Cleaning Product Recommendations

- In general, it's wise to avoid products that contain ammonia, chlorine bleach, or nonchlorine bleach substitutes such as oxygen bleach, which are corrosive and irritating to skin.
- Avoid using air fresheners, carpet powders, cleaning products with lung irritants (such as bleach), and products containing fragrance or perfume. Limonene and other citrus fragrances are often added to cleaning products and should be avoided because of their ability to form formaldehyde when mixed with ozone in the air.
- Drain cleaners typically contain lye (sodium hydroxide), an extremely corrosive chemical that can cause severe skin burns and irritation.

Non-Toxic

Ingestion of lye can cause severe illness and death. Lye is often mixed with volatile liquid chemicals such as ammonia and petroleum chemicals that can cause severe respiratory reactions.

- Use a plunger or flexible metal snake for major drain clogs, and use a drain strainer to prevent food from going down the drain in the first place. It is important to discard grease into the garbage instead of down the drain where it can stick to debris and cause foul odors as well as clogging the drain. Make a safe DIY drain cleaner from the recipes below.
- Disinfection from salmonella and *E. coli* in kitchens (not hospital settings) that handle meat and poultry can be accomplished through the use of hot water and active scrubbing of exposed surfaces. Contrary to instinct, *DO NOT* wash off meat or poultry in the kitchen sink when preparing meals, because it can cause splashing that will disperse harmful bacteria onto other surfaces and make contact with other foods. Use separate, color-coded cutting boards for cooked versus uncooked food to reduce exposure to pathogens present in the uncooked food. Avoid placing uncooked meat or fish on a plate that will then be used for a meal unless the plate is thoroughly washed before being reused—this is a common source of transmission of harmful bacteria to the cooked food from the unwashed plate, particularly problematic with outdoor grilling.
- Look for USDA Certified Organic labeling: Again, the words "natural" or "organic" do not mean anything, only the USDA Organic seal has any legitimate value when it comes to safe cleaning products (Figure 9.2).

(a)   (b)

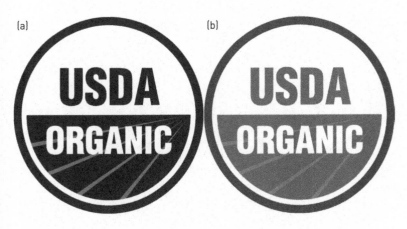

Figure 9.2 USDA certified organic labels can be black and white or green and white.

- Look for third-party-tested products. Organizations such as Green Seal or EcoLogo, provide such independent certification of environmentally friendly cleaning products. They evaluate cleaning products for the presence of toxic ingredients and require manufacturers to submit ongoing data showing that their products are both effective and continue to maintain green standards. Their seals of approval remain the best standard that is currently available in the US market (Figure 9.3).

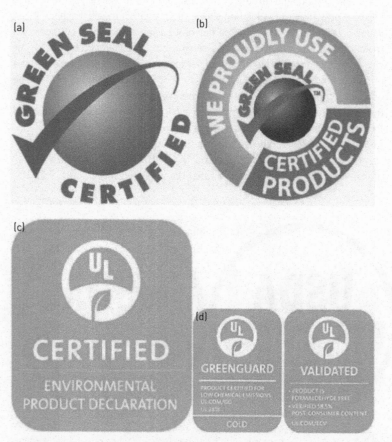

Figure 9.3 Seals found on cleaning product packaging indicating less toxic ingredients.

- Find safe cleaning products at EWG's Guide to Healthy Cleaning:
The EWG (Environmental Working Group) is a nonprofit, consumer product advocacy group that participates in research and testing of consumer products to evaluate their chemical ingredients and potential health risks. Their database of cleaning products ranks over 2,000 household cleaning products currently available in the US market and in big-box stores. You can also download their mobile app, Healthy Living, to check products in stores and on the go.

http://www.ewg.org/guides/cleaners/

Making Your Own Cleaning Products

The best way to know what's in your cleaning products is to make them yourself. These DIY cleaning recipes require only the time to purchase the ingredients and mix. Keep in mind that the shelf-life of these home-made cleaning products is limited because they contain no synthetic chemicals that act as preservatives. Essential oils used for fragrance will wear off over time because phthalate chemicals are not in the ingredients, but these recipes will result in fewer toxic chemicals lingering on countertops, filling indoor air, and touching the skin of pregnant women, kids, and pets. Of courses these chemicals also impact adults and the elderly.

In general, opposites attract. An acidic substance, such as white vinegar, will do a good job of cleaning alkaline stains, such as rust, grass stains, and hard water stains. Baking soda, which is alkaline, will do a good job of cleaning acidic stains caused by urine, tomato sauce, and coffee.

Ingredients for Do-It-Yourself Household Cleaning Products

- Water, a universal solvent (can dissolve other added ingredients)

- Course salt (large grain) can be used as an abrasive to clean caked-on food stuck to pots, pans, and the inside of an oven.
- White vinegar removes soap scum, breaks up grease and mineral deposits, and acts as a deodorizer. (Note: apple cider vinegar and wine vinegar can stain!)
- Baking soda (sodium bicarbonate) absorbs odor and is a mild abrasive.
- Lemon juice cuts grease and mineral buildup, and is a natural whitener.
- Organic or pure essential oils (e.g., peppermint, lavender) can be used for fragrance.
- Castile soap, made from plant oils that are natural degreasers
- Borax (sodium borate) is similar to baking soda but stronger; it removes odors and has antifungal, antimold, and antibacterial activity.
  (Note: toxic if ingested, so keep out of reach of children.)
- Fragrance-free and color-free liquid soap (not antibacterial soap) may be used.
- Club soda (with sodium citrate) loosens dirt and fabric stains, dries without water spots.
- Washing soda (i.e., sodium carbonate) cuts grease but may scratch waxed floors, aluminum pots, or fiberglass (wear gloves when using this ingredient).
- Sodium percarbonate is a bleach alternative that works well to whiten a tub, a sink, or even clothes without bleach (wear gloves to avoid skin irritation).

DIY Non-toxic Cleaning Product Recipes

All-Purpose Spray Cleaner

Empty spray bottle
2 cups of very hot water
1 teaspoon of liquid castile soap (not antibacterial and without added fragrance or perfume)
1/2 teaspoon of washing soda

Or

Empty spray bottle
1 cup of white vinegar
1 cup warm, water
1 tablespoon of organic liquid soap
1 teaspoon baking soda

Combine all ingredients in the bottle and shake to dissolve the powders.

Dishwashing Soap

Empty bottle or large jar
2 cups of water
2 tablespoons of liquid castile soap (not antibacterial and without added fragrance or perfume)
1 teaspoon vegetable glycerin

Combine the castile soap and water in the empty container. Add the glycerin, stir, and apply to sponge with warm water.

Squeaky Clean

Dishwasher Detergent

Most automatic dishwasher detergents contain harmful chemicals and phosphate that can harm the environment. Use DIY dishwashing soap (see above) and fill only half of the soap reservoir to avoid excessive sudsing.

Oven Cleaner

Empty spray bottle
2 tablespoons castile or non-toxic liquid soap (not detergent)
2 teaspoons borax (inhibits mold growth)
Warm water to fill bottle

Combine ingredients in bottle. Spray closely to the oven surface to avoid inhaling or getting into your eyes. Leave solution for 20 minutes, then scrub with coarse sea salt and damp cloth, steel wool, or pumice stone (found at hardware store) for really baked-on spots.

   *Also try using baking soda on oven stains. Moisten with water and let stand overnight, wipe, and rinse.

Mold/Mildew Cleaner

First, try to limit sources of moisture, where molds thrive—no high moisture, no mold. Keep windows open or bathroom dehumidifier on for an hour after showering
Empty spray bottle
1 cup borax or vinegar
Fill with water (4 parts water to one part vinegar)

Air Freshener (air mist)

Empty spray bottle
5 drops of orange, lemon, or lime nonsynthetic essential oil
2 cups clean, warm water

Carpet and Clothing Stain Remover

Buy machine washable rugs when possible. Use non–flame-retardant carpet padding when possible.
1 spray bottle

¼ cup baking soda or ¼ club soda
2 cups warm water

Combine ingredients in the bottle and spray on the stain, allow 15 minutes and then dab with a moist towel to lift the stain. This recipe also works well with sweat stains on clothing.

Window Cleaner

Empty spray bottle
3 cups water
¼ cup white vinegar
1½ tablespoons real lemon juice

Wood Polish

1 medium size squirt bottle
2 parts vegetable or olive oil
1 part lemon juice

Combine all ingredients, gently squirt onto a cloth and then apply to wood surface, and keep refrigerated.

Toilet Bowl Cleaner

Use a solution made with 1 part borax powder to 3 parts warm water for the inside of the bowl

Use equal parts white vinegar and water to clean the toilet seat and rim (where children come in contact with the toilet)

Drain Cleaner

½ cup baking soda
½ cup white vinegar

Combine and pour mixture down drain and wait 15 minutes. Pour a full pot of boiling water (careful!) down the drain to dissolve caked-on food and grease.

Stainless Steel Polisher

¼ cup baking soda
2 cups water

Mix, then apply using a soft sponge, allow 15 minutes, and then remove with a moist cloth or sponge.

Laundry Detergent (powdered)

1 bar castile soap (grated)
2 cups borax
2 cups washing soda
1 cup baking soda
30 drops of essential oil
Mix all of the ingredients together and put into an air-tight jar.
Use 1 tablespoon per load.

Fabric Softener

Commercial fabric softeners leave a chemical residue on the fabric
to control static cling, as well as strong fragrance that can cause
allergic symptoms, and skin irritation.
Add ½ cup white vinegar *or* ¼ cup baking soda to the rinse cycle
Vinegar helps prevent static cling, brightens and softens fabrics, and
reduces strong odors.

Sources for More Household Cleaner Recipes:

The Smart Human: http://thesmarthuman.com/educational-resources/
Healthy Child Healthy World: http://www.healthychild.org/easy-
steps/green-spring-cleaning-9-diy-recipes-for-natural-cleaners/
Clean Mama's household cleaner recipes (printable PDF): http://www
.cleanmama.net/wp-content/uploads/2013/04/cleaningrecipepic2
.png
The Healthy Home: Vanguard Press

Dry Cleaning

Conventional dry cleaning is somewhat of a mystery to most people. The actual process is not actually "dry," but involves many harmful "wet" chemicals
that are not soluble in water. Dry cleaning is popular because it helps keep
fabric from being stretched, matted, or torn, and dyes do not fade or run. But
research now shows that the risks of dry cleaning may outweigh the benefits.

There are over 30,000 dry cleaners in the United States, and roughly 80% of them routinely use toxic chemicals.[34] Despite the fact that in 1991 the Air Resources Board of California identified perchloroethylene (Perc) as a "toxic air contaminant," this chemical continues to be the most pervasively used chemical in dry cleaning in the United States. Perc is a solvent and a volatile organic compound (VOC) with a pungent odor and the appearance of water, but the consistency of oil. Perc has both short- and long-term health effects for humans and was classified by the International Agency for Research on Cancer (IARC), part of the World Health Organization (WHO), as a Group 2A carcinogen. In other words, Perc is "probably" a cancer-causing agent for humans.[35] Short-term exposure, perhaps breathing in Perc while hanging clothes that were recently dry cleaned, can cause headache, skin irritation, rapid heart rate, nausea, and dizziness. Long-term inhalation can cause kidney and liver damage in humans, and Perc has been shown to cause cancer in lab animals. It is a known central nervous system neurotoxin and "depressant" and tends to collect over time in fat cells, being slowly released over weeks into the bloodstream after heavy exposure.[36] One study looked at the air quality in New Jersey homes where dry-cleaned clothes were brought inside. The study found that the exposed residents had 2- to 6-fold higher levels of Perc than people who had not been directly exposed to dry-cleaned clothes, and Perc lingered in the air for up to 48 hours after clothes were brought inside the home.[37] Exposure of pregnant women to Perc may in turn cause exposure to growing fetuses—Perc, along with many other toxic airborne chemicals, was found in the urine of pregnant women tested through the National Children's Study, which collected data on 488 pregnant women in their third trimester of pregnancy.[38] California has pledged to phase out the use of Perc by 2023 and awards grants to incentivize business owners to adopt safe replacement chemicals. California often leads by example on environmental chemical restrictions and labeling, so other states will likely follow this example.

See the following box for suggested alternatives to dry cleaning.

Alternatives to Dry Cleaning

- Buy clothing that does not require dry cleaning.
- Use an iron or inexpensive steam machine to remove wrinkles.

- Spot-clean garments with a non-toxic fabric cleaner (see EWG.org for recommendations).
- Use a half-cup of white vinegar in place of fabric softener in the wash to reduce static cling, soften clothes, and remove stains

If You Do Dry Clean:
- Carefully unwrap and air out clothing for 2–3 days in an outdoor space (covered deck, garage, porch) away from open windows or doors or in a well-ventilated room.
- Keep fresh dry cleaning away from children's bedrooms and play areas.
- Wear undershirts or tank tops under perc-treated clothing to prevent skin exposure.
- Look for less toxic alternatives:
  - "wet cleaning" technology combines spot cleaning, steaming, and hand-washing techniques, using water along with mild, biodegradable detergents and specialized humidity- controlled drying machines
  - Liquid CO_2 (carbon dioxide) is effective, non-toxic, and is a closed-loop system that has no effects on the environment or global warming. The EPA and Natural Resources Defense Fund (NRDC) recognize CO_2 dry cleaning as a truly green dry-cleaning method, and in 2003, it was rated #1 by Consumer Reports for effectiveness. For more information on non-toxic dry cleaning: https://www.arb.ca.gov/toxics/dryclean/grant_faqs.htm
  Use these websites to locate wet or CO2 dry cleaners: http://www.nodryclean.com
  http://wetcleanersusa.com/wcu/find-a-certified-store/

Carpet Cleaning

If you are interested in cleaning your carpeted areas beyond what a HEPA vacuum can accomplish, steam cleaners are readily available for rent at local grocery stores or can be purchased online or at retail stores. Steam cleaners or vapor cleaners are very effective at eliminating dirt, dust mites, and mold, which can be very important to residents who suffer from allergies and asthma. When purchasing a steam cleaner, the trick is to avoid any chemical cleaners designed to be sold with it. Often these cleaners contain as many harmful chemicals as handheld spray. Avoid commercial carpet sprays or powders, and use only non-toxic spot cleaner for tough stains (see recipe above).

Commercial carpet cleaning companies are wildly popular, and they clean carpets, rugs, and upholstered furniture very well, but be sure to specifically ask for steamed water *only* to be used, without any added chemicals. Steam cleaning companies may advertise certification by the Asthma and Allergy Association of America, and their employees will often claim that the chemicals used are "safe," but this is often not the case! Most commercial spot cleaners use Perc, the same toxic solvent used in dry cleaning.

And, chemicals are almost always *unnecessary* for routine cleaning with a heavy-duty steamer because of the high temperature and heavy pressure used. If necessary, you can provide a non-toxic (store-bought or DIY) spot cleaner for specific areas that need more aggressive cleaning.

Bottom line

Cleaning products in the United States are under minimal regulatory oversight and often contain chemicals known to cause many health issues. Avoid buying harmful cleaning products, use reliable sources to find recommended products, or make your own cleaners with basic, inexpensive natural ingredients. Open windows to air out odors, spot-clean spills and messes at the source, and throw in some old fashioned elbow grease instead of relying on a toxic chemical fix. And finally, do not try to mask odors with air fresheners that release toxic chemicals into the air you breath in your home and at work.

References

1. Wire B. ACI Report: Cleaning products industry has $59 billion direct impact on U.S. economy. Businesswire.com. https://www.businesswire.com/news/home/20181001005781/en/ACI-Report-Cleaning-Products-Industry-59-Billion. Published 2018. Accessed November 22, 2019.

2. Stobbe M. US lockdowns coincide with rise in poisonings from cleaners. Associeated Press; 2020. https://apnews.com/5621611ac1e1c04de36d5b6dfb0b6422. Accessed April 24, 2020.

3. US Department of Agriculture (USDA). USDA organic labeling standards. https://www.ams.usda.gov/grades-standards/organic-labeling-standards. Published 2018. Accessed October 11, 2018.

4. Calafat AM, Ye X, Wong LY, Reidy JA, Needham LL. Urinary concentrations of triclosan in the U.S. population: 2003-2004. *Environ Health Perspect.* 2008;116(3):303–307.

5. Dayan AD. Risk assessment of triclosan [Irgasan] in human breast milk. *Food Chem Toxicol.* 2007;45(1):125–129.

6. Allmyr M, Adolfsson-Erici M, McLachlan MS, Sandborgh-Englund G. Triclosan in plasma and milk from Swedish nursing mothers and their exposure via personal care products. *The Science of the Total Environment.* 2006;372(1):87–93.

7. Allmyr M, McLachlan MS, Sandborgh-Englund G, Adolfsson-Erici M. Determination of triclosan as its pentafluorobenzoyl ester in human plasma and milk using electron capture negative ionization mass spectrometry. *Analytical Chemistry.* 2006;78(18):6542–6546.

8. Adolfsson-Erici M, Pettersson M, Parkkonen J, Sturve J. Triclosan, a commonly used bactericide found in human milk and in the aquatic environment in Sweden. *Chemosphere.* 2002;46(9–10):1485–1489.

9. Toms LM, Allmyr M, Mueller JF, et al. Triclosan in individual human milk samples from Australia. *Chemosphere.* 2011;85(11):1682–1686.

10. Li X, Brownawell BJ. Quaternary ammonium compounds in urban estuarine sediment environments—a class of contaminants in need of increased attention? *Environmental Science & Technology.* 2010;44(19):7561–7568.

11. Li X, Luo X, Mai B, Liu J, Chen L, Lin S. Occurrence of quaternary ammonium compounds (QACs) and their application as a tracer for sewage derived pollution in urban estuarine sediments. *Environmental Pollution (Barking, Essex: 1987).* 2014;185:127–133.

12. Reiss R, Lewis G, Griffin J. An ecological risk assessment for triclosan in the terrestrial environment. *Environmental Toxicology and Chemistry.* 2009;28(7):1546–1556.

13. Reiss R, Mackay N, Habig C, Griffin J. An ecological risk assessment for triclosan in lotic systems following discharge from wastewater treatment plants in the United States. *Environmental Toxicology and Chemistry.* 2002;21(11):2483–2492.

14. Lindesjoo E, Adolfsson-Erici M, Ericson G, Forlin L. Biomarker responses and resin acids in fish chronically exposed to effluents from a total chlorine-free pulp mill during regular production. *Ecotoxicology and Environmental Safety.* 2002;53(2):238–247.

15. Kolpin DW, Thurman EM, Lee EA, Meyer MT, Furlong ET, Glassmeyer ST. Urban contributions of glyphosate and its degradate AMPA to streams in the United States. *The Science of the total environment.* 2006;354(2–3):191–197.

16. Worral F, Besien T, Kolpin DW. Groundwater vulnerability: interactions of chemical and site properties. *The Science of the Total Environment.* 2002;299(1–3):131–143.

17. Kuehn BM. FDA pushes makers of antimicrobial soap to prove safety and effectiveness. *JAMA.* 2014;311(3):234.

18. Kumar V, Chakraborty A, Kural MR, Roy P. Alteration of testicular steroidogenesis and histopathology of reproductive system in male rats treated with triclosan. *Reproductive Toxicology (Elmsford, NY).* 2009;27(2):177–185.

19. Rutkowska AZ, Szybiak A, Serkies K, Rachon D. Endocrine disrupting chemicals as potential risk factor for estrogen-dependent cancers. *Polskie Archiwum Medycyny Wewnetrznej.* 2016;126(7–8):562–570.

20. Rachon D. Endocrine disrupting chemicals (EDCs) and female cancer: informing the patients. *Reviews in Endocrine & Metabolic Disorders.* 2015;16(4):359–364.

21. Braun JM, Bellinger DC, Hauser R, et al. Prenatal phthalate, triclosan, and bisphenol A exposures and child visual-spatial abilities. *Neurotoxicology.* 2016;58:75–83.

22. Braun JM. Early-life exposure to EDCs: role in childhood obesity and neurodevelopment. *Nature Reviews Endocrinology.* 2016.

23. Eskenazi B, Rauch SA, Tenerelli R, et al. In utero and childhood DDT, DDE, PBDE and PCBs exposure and sex hormones in adolescent boys: the CHAMACOS study. *Int J Hyg Environ Health.* 2016.

24. Anderson SE, Meade BJ, Long CM, Lukomska E, Marshall NB. Investigations of immunotoxicity and allergic potential induced by topical application of triclosan in mice. *Journal of Immunotoxicology.* 2016;13(2):165–172.

25. Ashley-Martin J, Dodds L, Arbuckle TE, Marshall J. Prenatal triclosan exposure and cord blood immune system biomarkers. *Int J Hyg Environ Health.* 2016;219(4–5):454–457.

26. Clayton EM, Todd M, Dowd JB, Aiello AE. The impact of bisphenol A and triclosan on immune parameters in the U.S. population, NHANES 2003–2006. *Environ Health Perspect.* 2011;119(3):390–396.

27. Hurd-Brown T, Udoji F, Martin T, Whalen MM. Effects of DDT and triclosan on tumor-cell binding capacity and cell-surface protein expression of human natural killer cells. *Journal of Applied Toxicology.* 2013;33(6):495–502.

28. Marshall NB, Lukomska E, Long CM, et al. Triclosan induces thymic stromal lymphopoietin in skin pomoting Th2 allergic responses. *Toxicological Sciences: An Official Journal of the Society of Toxicology.* 2015;147(1):127–139.

29. Palmer RK, Hutchinson LM, Burpee BT, et al. Antibacterial agent triclosan suppresses RBL-2H3 mast cell function. *Toxicol Appl Pharmacol.* 2012;258(1):99–108.

30. Calafat AM, Ye X, Valentin-Blasini L, Li Z, Mortensen ME, Wong LY. Co-exposure to non-persistent organic chemicals among American pre-school aged children: A pilot study. *Int J Hyg Environ Health.* 2016.

31. Garcia-Hidalgo E, von Goetz N, Siegrist M, Hungerbuhler K. Use-patterns of personal care and household cleaning products in Switzerland. *Food Chem Toxicol.* 2016;99:24–39.

32. Gummin DD MJ, Spyker DA, Brooks DE, et al. 2016 Annual Report of the American Association of Poison Control Centers' National Poison Data System (NPDS): 34th Annual Report. *Clin Toxicol.* 2017;55(10):1072–1252.

33. Goodyear N, Brouillette N, et al. The effectiveness of three home products in cleaning and disinfection of *Staphylococcus aureus* and *Escherichia coli* on home environmental surfaces. *J Applied Microbiology.* 2015;119(5):1245–1252.

34. Bounds G. Finding an eco-friendly dry cleaner. *The Wall Street Journal* https://www.wsj.com/articles/SB122834783552077505. Published 2008. Accessed October 12, 2018.

35. Caldwell J, Lunn R, Ruder A. Tetrachloroethylene (perc, tetra, PCE). *International Agency for Research on Cancer, IARC Monographs.* 1995;63:145–158.

36. California Air Resources Board (CARB). Dry Cleaning Program. https://www.arb.ca.gov/toxics/dryclean/dryclean.htm. Published 2017. Accessed October 11, 2018.

37. Thomas KW, Pellizzari ED, Perritt RL, Nelson WC. Effect of dry-cleaned clothes on tetrachloroethylene levels in indoor air, personal air, and breath for residents of several New Jersey homes. *Journal of Exposure Analysis and Environmetal Epidemiology.* 1991;1(4):475–490.

38. Boyle EB, Viet SM, Wright DJ, et al. Assessment of Exposure to VOCs among Pregnant Women in the National Children's Study. *Int J Environ Res Public Health.* 2016;13(4):376.

10

Insecticides, Herbicides, and Other Pesticides
Chemicals Designed to Kill

-cide definition: from Latin meaning "killer," "act of killing," used in the formation of compound words: pesticide, homicide.
—www.merriam-webster.com

A Brief History of Pesticides

A pesticide is a chemical or biological agent that deters, incapacitates, kills, or otherwise discourages pests. Since before 2000 BCE, humans have used pesticides to preserve their crops. The first-known pesticide was elemental sulfur dusting, used about 4,500 years ago in the Sumer region in ancient Mesopotamia. Since that time, heavy metals (e.g., lead arsenate, mercury compounds, copper sulfate, and calcium arsenate) and tobacco leaf derivatives, such as nicotine sulfate, have been used to ward off insects and other pests.[1] By the beginning of the 1930s, usage of other, newer pesticide chemicals was well underway, however, the types of chemicals used as active ingredients in pesticides have changed greatly since the 1930s. In general, inorganic chemicals (such as the metals listed above) have declined in use, and synthetic organic chemicals have taken over, particularly since the 1940s. By the start of WWII, herbicide usage had increased dramatically with the advent of the synthetic organic pesticide industry.[2] Pesticides, such as dichloro-diphenyl-trichloroethane (DDT), BHC, aldrin, dieldrin, endrin, and 2,4-D were designed to be inexpensive and effective, and they soon became enormously popular. By the early 1950s, pesticide use had increased by more than 50%, and pesticides were being used in hundreds of applications and products.

"Inert" additives—supposedly chemically inactive—are commonly added to pesticides. These chemicals are used to enhance absorption and help spread the "active" ingredients. However, they are often not actually inert, and in some cases have been found to add greater toxicity than the "active" ingredients. As we shall discuss later on in the chapter, it is important to note that these "inert" additives are proprietary (i.e., trade secrets) and are not disclosed on labels. As of 2002, the EPA reported that, "In the US, more than 18,000 products are licensed for use . . . each year approximately 2 billion pounds of pesticides are applied to crops, homes, schools, parks and forests. US expenditures at the user level for conventional and other pesticides totaled $11.8 billion in 2006 and $12.5 billion in 2007."[3]

Regulation of Pesticides

The regulation of pesticides was given very little attention until around the turn of the 20th century. In 1910, as the usage of pesticides became more widespread, Congress passed the Federal Insecticide Act, primarily aimed at protecting farmers against fraud as they purchased insecticides, often by mail or from traveling dealers. The Insecticide Act of 1910 was the beginning of pesticide regulation in the United States.[2] It was later replaced by the Federal Insecticide, Fungicide and Rodenticide Act (FIFRA) in 1947, which expanded coverage to all pesticides (not just insecticides) and required that all pesticide active ingredients be registered with the US Department of Agriculture; any ingredient not considered by the manufacturer to be an active ingredient was exempt from disclosure. It was primarily a labeling act, providing no sanctions for misuse, no authority for immediate stop-sale orders against dangerous pesticides, and limited penalties for companies selling such products.

The Miller Bill, passed in 1954, gave the FDA responsibility for monitoring food for pesticide residues (the amount that remains on food) and provided a new mechanism for setting "tolerances" (known in other countries as a "maximum residue limit" or MRL) of pesticide residues in foods. Tolerances are not the same as safe daily level of exposure, which the EPA refers to as the "reference dose" or RfD, and the FDA refers to as the "acceptable daily intake" dose or ADI. Tolerances are based on the sensitivity of the chemical-detection method. Pesticide levels in water, supposedly not to be exceeded, are referred to as maximum contaminant levels (MCLs). These different terms are clearly confusing to the public. In 1958, the Delaney clause was passed by Congress to prohibit any pesticide additives "found to induce cancer when ingested by man or animal."[2] It wasn't until the early 1960s, with the publication of biologist Rachel Carson's groundbreaking book *Silent Spring*, in which she revealed the detrimental effects of pesticide exposure, especially DDT, on animal life and ecosystems, that serious attention was paid to their likely health effects on human health. The book ignited a social movement that resulted in congressional hearings in 1963, and the formation of the EPA in 1970. DDT was withdrawn from use in the United States in 1972 (but production of DDT was still allowed if it was sold outside of the US). DDT's pervasive use and its persistence in the environment is evident in that, even decades later, it still is detectable as a contaminant in soil and water and in people's blood throughout the United States. DDT is still being used around the world to fight malaria and other insect-borne diseases.[4]

However, it has been determined from the Legacy Tobacco Documents Library (created as part of the multibillion-dollar tobacco industry settlement) that funding for the antimalaria pesticide program, Africa Fighting Malaria, was proposed for funding to the tobacco company Philip Morris. This was done in order to keep the focus of the World Health Organization in Africa off of tobacco, and create an issue that would promote conflict between public health officials focusing only on malaria, and environmental scientists concerned about the impact of DDT on the development of cancer and impaired fertility. DDT can kill malaria-carrying mosquitos, but (a) this eventually results in resistance of mosquitos to DDT, and (b) DDT is a persistent and very harmful endocrine-disrupting chemical. The reason for proposing that Philip Morris should provide funding to support this sham was that their tobacco grown in Africa was highly contaminated with DDT. The tobacco industry strategy has been to make false claims with the help of paid experts, a strategy that has been adopted by chemical and petroleum corporations because it worked so well for tobacco companies for decades. Even the World Health Organization was duped into thinking Africa Fighting Malaria was a legitimate organization.[5]

Classification of Pesticides

Pest-control chemicals are classified by the target pests for which they are to be used. Most commonly known are fungicides, herbicides, algicides, insecticides, and rodenticides. Other classes include termiticides, molluscicides, piscicides (i.e., fish), avicides (i.e., birds), and predacides (e.g., wolves, coyotes, red foxes). There is overlap because some pesticides control more than one type of pest. The mechanism of action also may vary. As mentioned above, "inert" additives, which are proprietary and thus *not* disclosed on labels, are used to enhance absorption and spread of the "active" ingredient, and may be more toxic than the "active" ingredients that *are* reported on labels. For example, the additives in Roundup confer greater toxicity than is due to the active ingredient of glyphosate alone.[6] The EPA report from 2004 has identified almost 3,000 substances, with widely varying toxicity, that are used as "inert" ingredients in the United States.[7–9]

Health Effects from Pesticides

Pesticides, which are widely applied in the environment, are intended to kill living organisms through mechanisms that can make them toxic to humans. For example, many herbicides designed to have a specific mode of action to kill plants actually have multiple other, endocrine-disrupting, actions in animals, including humans; examples include atrazine and glyphosate (found in Roundup), which both have estrogenic activity. Since insecticides are often designed to be neurotoxins, it is not surprising that epidemiologic evidence suggests that exposure to a variety of insecticides increases the risk of many health disorders, including ADHD,[10] decreased cognitive development,[9,11,12] autism[13] in children, and dementia in adults.[14,15] Pesticide exposure is also associated with increased risk for cancers in children[16,17] and adults (multiple myeloma and other lymphohematopoietic cancers,[18,19] breast,[20] prostate[21]) and neurodegenerative diseases (Parkinson's,[22,23] ALS,[24-28] and Alzheimer's[15,29,30]). Pesticides are also linked to birth defects (neural tube defects, gastroschisis), reproductive problems,[31] delayed or premature onset of menopause, and thyroid disorders.[32] Studies also suggest that residential and workplace insecticide exposure is associated with risk of developing autoimmune rheumatic diseases (ARD) in postmenopausal women.[33] Clearly the vast majority of synthetic pesticides have now been discovered to cause much greater harm to human health, with these diseases occurring at a higher frequency than in the decades prior to their use.[34] Yet, the US pesticide industry continues to grow, protected by the illusion of science-based regulation by the EPA. There is no end in sight to their creation, production, or distribution!

Parkinson's Disease

Evidence from animal and human studies, as well as from animal and human cell culture models, suggests that pesticides are one cause of the neurodegenerative process leading to Parkinson's disease.[35-37] Parkinson's disease is the second-most-prevalent neurodegenerative disorder (prevalence of 500/100,000, with an annual incidence of 20/100,000); it affects as many as 1.5 million individuals in the United States, with about 70,000 new cases diagnosed annually.[29] Exposure to pesticides such as Paraquat, one of the most commonly used herbicides in the world, and Maneb (a common fungicide), has been linked to increased risk for developing Parkinson's disease. A study showed human exposure to both of these pesticides was associated with an even greater risk for Parkinson's disease, especially if the exposure occurred at an early age—the possibility of pesticide interactions resulting in adverse outcomes, which is a big concern with drugs, is not considered by the EPA in assessing the risks of pesticides.[38] Multiple epidemiologic studies have linked farmers, field workers, rural living, and drinking (unfiltered) well water with increased risk for Parkinson's disease.[39,40]

Although studies are ongoing, research in both animals and humans shows possible mechanisms of action for pesticide exposure contributing to neurodegenerative diseases. Some people who carry variants of specific genes associated with Parkinson's disease, such as the dopamine transporter (DAT) gene, may be more sensitive to the neurotoxic effects of exposure to certain pesticides and thus be at increased risk for developing Parkinson's disease.[36] For example, a study showed that people with a specific genetic variant may be at increased risk if they are exposed to organophosphates, diazinon, chlorpyrifos, and parathion pesticides.[35] One variant of the PON gene has also been implicated in an increased risk for Alzheimer's disease.[41,42] Mitochondria, microscopic components of the human cell responsible for generating the molecule (ATP) that provides the energy for cells to function, may also be responsible for increased risk when humans are exposed to pesticides that can destabilize the normal function of the mitochondria. This can lead to "oxidative stress," which involves the generation of molecules that can damage many critical cell functions, leading to a wide range of diseases.[43] Parkinson's disease risk clearly exemplifies the potential toxic interplay between our genes and our environment, typically referred to as nature (our genetic makeup) and nurture (effects due to the environment we live in). A focus only on genes as the source of disease involves looking at only one-half of the cause, yet the (largely futile) search for genes that cause diseases has been the primary focus of medical research funded by the National Institutes of Health (NIH).

Glyphosate and Other Endocrine Disruptors

Some pesticides may cause adverse health effects in humans because of their ability to act as endocrine disruptors. Take glyphosate, the active ingredient in the most widely used weed killer (herbicide) Roundup, which is now marketed by many corporations under different names and is used on 70 crops as of 2020 (see Table 10.1).[44,45]

Several studies show that low concentrations of glyphosate possess the ability to disrupt the normal workings of estrogen via estrogenic receptors (ERs) through which natural and synthetic estrogens control estrogen-regulated genes. Estrogenic endocrine disruptors such as glyphosate alter the estrogen receptor's ability to control gene activity.[46,47] Glyphosate was first sold to farmers in 1974, but since then, the volume of glyphosate-based herbicides (GBHs) applied to crops worldwide has increased approximately 100-fold (see Figure 10.1). Now, GBHs are the most heavily applied herbicide in the world, and usage continues to rise. Glyphosate-*resistant* weeds have now developed, requiring even more GBH spraying. Extremely worrisome is that glyphosate is now also being applied *just prior* to harvest as a drying or desiccating agent to promote "dry down" so that farmers can rapidly harvest the crops; thus glyphosate will not only be absorbed into the produce during crop growth, unable to washed off, but will also remain on the surface of the produce (such as wheat) immediately after harvest.[48] Glyphosate doesn't break down and become less toxic as fast as researchers once thought.

Table 10.1 Type of produce and amount of glyphosate pesticide sprayed on these crops annually.

| | | Date: October 5,2015 | | |
| | | Annual Average | Percent Crop Treated | |
	Crop	Lbs. A.I.	Average	Maximum
1	Alfalfa	400,000	<2.5	5
2	Almonds	2,100,000	85	95
3	Apples	400,000	55	70
4	Apricots	10,000	55	80
5	Artichokes	1,000	10	15
6	Asparagus	30,000	55	70
7	Avocados	80,000	45	65
8	Barley	600,000	25	40
9	Beans, Green	70,000	15	25
10	Blueberries	10,000	20	25
11	Broccoli	3,000	<2.5	<2.5
12	Brussels Sprouts*	<500	<1	<2.5
13	Cabbage	20,000	10	25
14	Caneberries	4,000	10	25
15	Canola	500,000	65	80
16	Cantaloupes	20,000	10	25
17	Carrots	3,000	5	10
18	Cauliflower	1,000	<2.5	5
19	Celery	1,000	<2.5	10
20	Cherries	200,000	65	85
21	Chicory*	<500	<2.5	<2.5
22	Corn	63,500,000	65	85
23	Cotton	18,400,000	85	95
24	Cucumbers	30,000	20	35
25	Dates	8,000	65	25
26	Dry Beans/Peas	600,000	30	45
27	Fallow	8,800,000	55	70
28	Figs	10,000	85	100
29	Garlic	4,000	10	25
30	Grapefruit	400,000	85	100
31	Grapes	1,500,000	70	80
32	Hazelnuts	30,000	65	90
33	Kiwifruit	5,000	70	95
34	Lemons	200,000	75	90
35	Lettuce	10,000	5	10

(Continued)

Table 10.1 Continued

36	Nectarines	20,000	45	70
37	Oats	100,000	5	10
38	Olives	40,000	60	75
39	Onions	40,000	30	40
40	Oranges	3,200,000	90	95
41	Pasture	600,000	<2.5	<2.5
42	Peaches	100,000	55	70
43	Peanuts	300,000	25	35
44	Pears	100,000	65	90
45	Peas, Green	20,000	10	20
46	Pecans	400,000	35	45
47	Peppers	30,000	20	35
48	Pistachios	500,000	85	95
49	Plums/Prunes	200,000	70	85
50	Pluots*	1,000	65	90
51	Pomegranates*	40,000	70	90
52	Potatoes	90,000	10	20
53	Pumpkins	20,000	20	25
54	Rice	800,000	30	50
55	Sorghum	3,000,000	40	60
56	Soybeans	101,200,000	105	100
57	Spinach	1,000	<2.5	10
58	Squash	10,000	20	40
59	Strawberries	10,000	10	20
60	Sugar Beets	1300,000	60	100
61	Sugarcane	300,000	45	60
62	Sunflowers	1,100,000	60	75
63	Sweet Corn	100,000	15	25
64	Tangelos	9,000	55	80
65	Tangerines	60,000	65	80
66	Tobacco	10,000	5	10
67	Tomatoes	100,000	35	45
68	Walnuts	600,000	75	90
69	Watermelon*	30,000	15	25
70	Wheat	8,600,000	25	70

All numbers are rounded
  <500: less than 500 pounds of active ingredients.
  <2.5: less than 2.5 percent of crop is treated.
  < I: less than 1 percent of crop is treated.

*Based on CA DPR data only (80% or more of U.S. acres grown are in California).

SLUA data sources include:
  USDA-NASS (United States Department of Agriculture's National Agricultural Statistics Service)
  Private Pesticide Market Research
  California DPR (Department of Pesticide Regulation)
These results reflect amalgamated data developed by the Agency and are releasable to the public.

In the United States, at the time of this publication, soy beans and corn are among the 12 allowable genetically modified (GMO) crops which have been modified to resist the destructive effects of GBHs. (For a full list of allowable GMO crops in the United States, see chapter 4.) Human exposure to GBHs is rising, despite the fact that the World Health Organization's International Agency for Research on Cancer (IARC) recently concluded that glyphosate is "probably carcinogenic to humans."[49,50]

GBHs are implicated in heightened risk of developing non-Hodgkin's lymphoma among populations exposed to glyphosate either occupationally or by virtue of living in an area routinely treated with GBHs.[51] GBHs have also been linked to increased rates of autism spectrum disorder,[52,53] neurodevelopmental delay,[53] chronic kidney disease,[54] celiac disease and gluten sensitivity,[55] and infertility.[56] There is no doubt this toxic pesticide will leave lasting devastation, similar to the effects of DDT. Have we not learned our lesson?

Since 2018, juries in several high-profile glyphosate-exposure cases have awarded hundreds of millions of dollars in reparations to people who developed cancer from ongoing exposure to glyphosate. There are thousands of pending glyphosate suits. Once again the American public's only hope for removing toxic chemicals has been through litigation, where internal documents obtained through the process of discovery show Monsanto's executives were well aware of the toxicity of glyphosate, which accounts for the large sums of money awarded to plaintifs. The EPA, however, is still defending the safety of formulations containing glyphosate.

Epigenetic Changes

Epigenetics, as discussed in chapter 2, also occur with pesticide exposures. Researchers have found changes in gene expression that occur without a corresponding change in the sequence of bases in DNA (i.e., there was no change in the genetic code) with some pesticide exposures, and those changes occur through still-undetermined mechanisms that are transmitted to subsequent generations. For example, studies using pregnant mice exposed to the biocide tributyltin produced generations of offspring that became obese.[57,58] Exposures to pesticides may cause a variety of epigenetic changes, and these epigenetic changes may correlate with the development of diseases in generations beyond those initially exposed, known as transgenerational effects.[43,59]

How We Get Exposed

Human exposure to pesticides can occur both inside and outside of the home. Exposure may be unintentional, through food and water ingestion; exposure to household dust (many pesticides stick to dust); or inhalation via agricultural spraying and drift; it may also occur intentionally, through deliberate spraying in the home or workplace (a very bad idea, particularly if there are pregnant women, infants, or children in the home). Pesticides end up in waterways and eventually in drinking water (Figures 10.2), and only a handful are monitored and regulated under the 1974 Safe Drinking Water Act (SDWA) (see chapter 5).[60] Pesticides often contaminate drinking water sources, such as lakes, streams, and rivers, as well as compromising the air quality in agricultural regions. Because of their structure, halogenated pesticides that have bromine, fluorine, or chlorine atoms attached to their molecular core, can persist in the environment for decades or centuries.

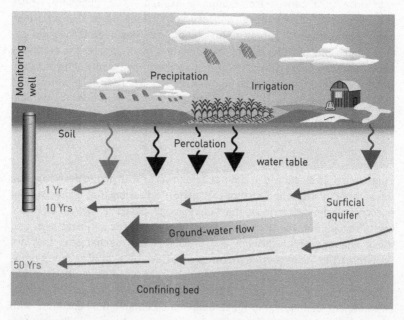

Figure 10.2 Graphic showing a variety of ways that chemicals make their way into ground water that will often become drinking water.

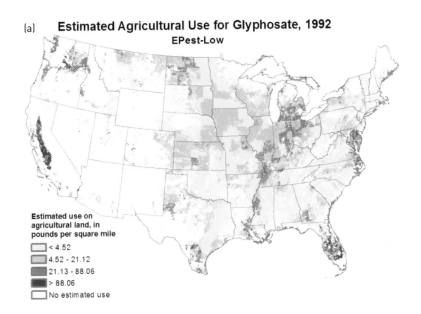

(a)

Estimated Agricultural Use for Glyphosate, 1992
EPest-Low

Estimated use on
agricultural land, in
pounds per square mile

< 4.52
4.52 - 21.12
21.13 - 88.06
> 88.06
No estimated use

FIGURE 10.1 Glyphosate usage in the United States in 1992 and 2016. Courtesy of the USGS and the Pesticide National Synthesis Project.

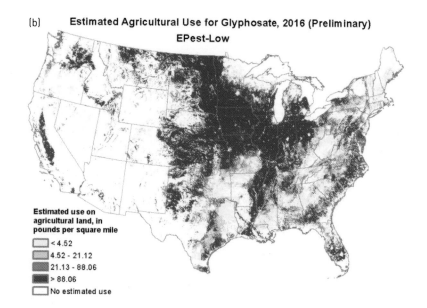

(b) **Estimated Agricultural Use for Glyphosate, 2016 (Preliminary)**
EPest-Low

Estimated use on
agricultural land, in
pounds per square mile
- < 4.52
- 4.52 - 21.12
- 21.13 - 88.06
- > 88.06
- No estimated use

FIGURE 10.1 Continued

How Pesticides Are Transported throughout the Environment

Pesticides and Household Dust Levels

According to a recent survey, 75% of US households used at least one pesticide product indoors during the past year—most often insecticides and disinfectants. Another study suggests that 80% of most people's exposure (excluding farm workers) to pesticides occurs indoors, and that measurable levels of up to a dozen pesticides have been found in the air inside homes.[62] Dust can accumulate pesticides as well.[63] Results from a large meta-analysis indicated that children exposed to insecticides indoors, but not to outdoor residential insecticides, showed a significant increase in risk for childhood leukemia.[16]

In addition to pesticides, household air and dust have been shown to harbor hundreds of chemicals from indoor products and materials, including alkylphenols, parabens, phthalates, and flame-retardant chemicals.[64,65] It is extremely important to note that, due to their hand-to-mouth behaviors and smaller size relative to adults, children will absorb greater amounts of toxic chemicals from dust, exposing them to greater health risks.[17,66] As parents know, toddlers spend a great deal of time on the floor, where dust collects and gets stuck to toys, teethers, pacifiers, and hands, as well as to the paws of pets living in the home.

Pesticides in Food

We consume an enormous amount of pesticides from both food and municipal drinking water; these pesticides inadvertently kill off the good bacteria in the gut as well as the potentially harmful bacteria. (See chapters 4 and 5 on pesticides in food and drinking water.)

Practical Methods for Reducing Pesticide Exposure from Food

- Buy organic produce whenever possible. Frozen organics are often more accessible and maintain the same nutrients as fresh produce, but without the abundance of pesticides that conventional produce has.
- Wash all produce with clean, warm water and white vinegar; although rinsing of produce reduces pesticides levels, it does not eliminate them

entirely. White vinegar can be added to clean warm water, using a ratio of 1 part vinegar to 4 parts water. Soak and mildly agitate produce for 5 minutes, then rinse with clean water. Peeling off the outer layer of produce also can reduce pesticide ingestion, but many of the best nutritional assets of the produce will likely be wasted with this approach.

- If choosing non-organic produce, check the "Dirty Dozen & Clean Fifteen" lists from the Environmental Working Group (EWG) (https://www.ewg.org/foodnews/dirty_dozen_list.php), which is updated yearly (see Table 4.2.) EWG research has found that people who eat five fruits and vegetables a day from the Dirty Dozen list consume an average of 10 pesticides a day. Those who eat from the "Clean Fifteen" (i.e., the 15 least-contaminated conventionally grown fruits and vegetables) ingest fewer than 2 pesticides daily.
- Limit foods with high animal fat content, where persistent pesticides (e.g., DDT) can accumulate.
- Limit intake of the skin of fish, which contains fat that absorbs pesticides.
- Drink and cook with water that is filtered to remove chlorinated chemicals that kill off healthy gut bacteria. Choose a water filter from the Water Filter Buying Guide found on EWG.org (https://www.ewg.org/tapwater/water-filter-guide.php). Water filters, in general, are inexpensive and provide significant protection from many of the toxins in water.
- Avoid spraying pesticides (rodenticides, insecticides, etc.) either inside the home or outside (which is particularly dangerous for children and pets). Ask about pesticide use in your workplace and your children's school. Mechanical traps, chemical baits and gels are placed in specific locations and thus less likely to contaminate the entire home environment; make sure that these are placed outside of the reach of children and pets.
- Avoid whole house fumigation, which leaves pesticide residues behind.
- Avoid cleaners and personal care products that claim to be antimicrobial, germ fighting, or antibacterial. One popular antimicrobial ingredient, triclosan, is marketed under more than a dozen different names, including Bactroban, Microban, Irgasan, Biofresh, Lexol-300, Ster-Zac, and Clonifexenolum; triclosan affects the heart and other muscles and the endocrine system (it interferes with thyroid hormone and with estrogen), and its use contributes to bacterial resistance.
- Remove contaminated shoes and boots before entering the home or workplace to avoid tracking chemicals inside; if clothes are exposed due to personal use or occupational exposure, remove them prior to entering your home.
- Be aware of agricultural spraying near home, work, and schools and advocate for change.

- Avoid using pesticides (flea and tick collars, shampoos and dips) on pets whenever possible, since the pet will spread these in your home.
- Vacuum with a high-efficiency particulate air (HEPA) filter, and dust regularly with a wet cloth (using water only). Household dust is not benign.
- When using pesticides, wear personal protective equipment (PPE), including gloves, long sleeves, eye protection, closed shoes, hats, and masks. Wash (PPE) in hot water and soap after use.
- When gardening/farming, use Integrated Pest Management (IPM) alternatives, which apply safe techniques without the use of synthetic pesticides.

Resources

- US Geological Survey: https://www.usgs.gov/science-explorer-results?es=pesticides
- National Pesticide Information Center (http:// www.npic.orst.edu) is a cooperative venture between the EPA and Oregon State University. Information on pesticides is available as downloadable handouts.
- Bugs (www.livingwithbugs.com) is a great resource for information and advice on DIY pest management.
- University of California Statewide IPM Program (http:// www.ipm.ucdavis.edu/ PDF/ PESTNOTES/ index.html) is an extensive library of information on IPM for the home. Downloadable PDFs are also effective as patient handouts.
- "Rachel Carson" video on YouTube: https://youtu.be/Ipbc-6IvMQI
- "From DDT to Glyphosate: Rachel Carson, We Need You Again" on YouTube: https://youtu.be/mF2iS5vlamg
- Beyond Pesticides offers the latest information on the hazards of pesticides and least-toxic alternatives, as well as ongoing projects including children's health, pollinators and pesticides, organic food and agriculture, mosquito control and lawn care. www.BeyondPesticides.org
- Environmental Working Group "Dirty Dozen" and "Clean Fifteen" (https://www.ewg.org/foodnews/dirty_dozen_list.php)

References

1. Ranga Rao, CV, et al. The role of biopesticides in crop protection: present status and future prospects. *Indian Journal of Plant Protection*. 2007;35(1):1–9.

2. USDA National Institute of Food and Agriculture. Pesticide usage in the United States: Trends during the 20th century. CIPM Technical Bulletin 105. https://nifa.usda.gov/sites/default/files/resources/Pesticide%20Trends.pdf Published 2003. Accessed April 24, 2020.

3. Environmental Protection Agency (EPA). Pesticides industry sales and usage: 2006 and 2007 market estimates. https://www.epa.gov/sites/production/files/2015-10/documents/market_estimates2007.pdf. Published 2007. Accessed January 16, 2017.

4. EPA. DDT—a brief history and status. https://www.epa.gov/ingredients-used-pesticide-products/ddt-brief-history-and-status. Published 2016. Accessed January 16, 2017.

5. Sarvana A. *Bate and switch: How a free-market magician manipulated two decades of environmental science.* Natural Resources News Services, 2019.

6. Martinez A, Reyes I, Reyes N. [Cytotoxicity of the herbicide glyphosate in human peripheral blood mononuclear cells]. *Biomedica.* 2007;27(4):594–604.

7. Cox C, Surgan M. Unidentified inert ingredients in pesticides: implications for human and environmental health. *Environ Health Perspect.* 2006;114(12):1803–1806.

8. Androutsopoulos VP, Hernandez AF, Liesivuori J, Tsatsakis AM. A mechanistic overview of health associated effects of low levels of organochlorine and organophosphorous pesticides. *Toxicology.* 2013;307:89–94.

9. Hernandez AF, Parron T, Tsatsakis AM, Requena M, Alarcon R, Lopez-Guarnido O. Toxic effects of pesticide mixtures at a molecular level: their relevance to human health. *Toxicology.* 2013;307:136–145.

10. Bouchard MF, Bellinger DC, Wright RO, Weisskopf MG. Attention-deficit/hyperactivity disorder and urinary metabolites of organophosphate pesticides. *Pediatrics.* 2010;125(6):e1270–1277.

11. Butler-Dawson J, Galvin K, Thorne PS, Rohlman DS. Organophosphorus pesticide exposure and neurobehavioral performance in Latino children living in an orchard community. *Neurotoxicology.* 2016;53:165–172.

12. Eskenazi B, Huen K, Marks A, et al. PON1 and neurodevelopment in children from the CHAMACOS study exposed to organophosphate pesticides in utero. *Environ Health Perspect.* 2010;118(12):1775–1781.

13. De Felice A, Greco A, Calamandrei G, Minghetti L. Prenatal exposure to the organophosphate insecticide chlorpyrifos enhances brain oxidative stress and prostaglandin E2 synthesis in a mouse model of idiopathic autism. *Journal of Neuroinflammation.* 2016;13(1):149.

14. Baldi I, Gruber A, Rondeau V, Lebailly P, Brochard P, Fabrigoule C. Neurobehavioral effects of long-term exposure to pesticides: results from

the 4-year follow-up of the PHYTONER study. *Occupational and Environmental Medicine.* 2011;68(2):108–115.

15. Bosma H, van Boxtel MP, Ponds RW, Houx PJ, Jolles J. Pesticide exposure and risk of mild cognitive dysfunction. *Lancet (London, England).* 2000;356(9233):912–913.

16. Chen M, Chang CH, Tao L, Lu C. Residential exposure to pesticide during childhood and childhood cancers: a meta-analysis. *Pediatrics.* 2015;136(4):719–729.

17. Roberts JR, Karr, C.J. Pesticide exposure in children. *Pediatrics.* 2012;130(6): e1757–1763.

18. Presutti R, Harris SA, Kachuri L, et al. Pesticide exposures and the risk of multiple myeloma in men: an analysis of the North American Pooled Project. *International Journal of Cancer Journal International du Cancer.* 2016;139(8):1703–1714.

19. Chang ET, Delzell E. Systematic review and meta-analysis of glyphosate exposure and risk of lymphohematopoietic cancers. *Journal of Environmental Science and Health Part B, Pesticides, Food Contaminants, and Agricultural Wastes.* 2016;51(6):402–434.

20. Eldakroory SA, Morsi DE, Abdel-Rahman RH, Roshdy S, Gouida MS, Khashaba EO. Correlation between toxic organochlorine pesticides and breast cancer. *Human & Experimental Toxicology.* 2016:960327116685887.

21. Koutros S, Berndt SI, Hughes Barry K, et al. Genetic susceptibility loci, pesticide exposure and prostate cancer risk. *PLoS One.* 2013;8(4):e58195.

22. Caudle WM, Guillot TS, Lazo CR, Miller GW. Industrial toxicants and Parkinson's disease. *Neurotoxicology.* 2012;33(2):178–188.

23. Tanner CM, Kamel F, Ross GW, et al. Rotenone, paraquat, and Parkinson's disease. *Environ Health Perspect.* 2011;119(6):866–872.

24. Malek AM, Barchowsky A, Bowser R, et al. Exposure to hazardous air pollutants and the risk of amyotrophic lateral sclerosis. *Environmental Pollution (Barking, Essex: 1987).* 2015;197:181–186.

25. Malek AM, Barchowsky A, Bowser R, et al. Environmental and occupational risk factors for amyotrophic lateral sclerosis: a case-control study. *Neurodegenerative Diseases.* 2014;14(1):31–38.

26. Malek AM, Barchowsky A, Bowser R, Youk A, Talbott EO. Pesticide exposure as a risk factor for amyotrophic lateral sclerosis: a meta-analysis of epidemiological studies: pesticide exposure as a risk factor for ALS. *Environ Res.* 2012;117:112–119.

27. Kamel F, Umbach DM, Bedlack RS, et al. Pesticide exposure and amyotrophic lateral sclerosis. *Neurotoxicology.* 2012;33(3):457–462.

28. Ingre C, Roos PM, Piehl F, Kamel F, Fang F. Risk factors for amyotrophic lateral sclerosis. *Clinical Epidemiology.* 2015;7:181–193.

29. Tanner CM, Goldman SM, Ross GW, Grate SJ. The disease intersection of susceptibility and exposure: chemical exposures and neurodegenerative disease risk. *Alzheimer's & Dementia: the Journal of the Alzheimer's Association.* 2014;10(3 Suppl):S213–225.

30. Baldi I, Lebailly P, Mohammed-Brahim B, Letenneur L, Dartigues JF, Brochard P. Neurodegenerative diseases and exposure to pesticides in the elderly. *American Journal of Epidemiology.* 2003;157(5):409–414.

31. Hu JX, Li YF, Li J, et al. Toxic effects of cypermethrin on the male reproductive system: with emphasis on the androgen receptor. *Journal of Applied Toxicology.* 2013;33(7):576–585.

32. American College of Obstetricians and Gynecologists. Exposure to toxic environmental agents. *Fertility and Sterility.* 2013;100(4):931–934.

33. Parks CG, Walitt BT, Pettinger M, et al. Insecticide use and risk of rheumatoid arthritis and systemic lupus erythematosus in the Women's Health Initiative Observational Study. *Arthritis Care & Research.* 2011;63(2):184–194.

34. Mostafalou S, Abdollahi M. Pesticides and human chronic diseases: evidences, mechanisms, and perspectives. *Toxicol Appl Pharmacol.* 2013;268(2):157–177.

35. Manthripragada AD, Costello S, Cockburn MG, Bronstein JM, Ritz B. Paraoxonase 1, agricultural organophosphate exposure, and Parkinson disease. *Epidemiology (Cambridge, Mass).* 2010;21(1):87–94.

36. Ritz BR, Manthripragada AD, Costello S, et al. Dopamine transporter genetic variants and pesticides in Parkinson's disease. *Environ Health Perspect.* 2009;117(6):964–969.

37. Rohlman DS, Lasarev M, Anger WK, Scherer J, Stupfel J, McCauley L. Neurobehavioral performance of adult and adolescent agricultural workers. *Neurotoxicology.* 2007;28(2):374–380.

38. Costello S, Cockburn M, Bronstein J, Zhang X, Ritz B. Parkinson's disease and residential exposure to maneb and paraquat from agricultural applications in the central valley of California. *American Journal of Epidemiology.* 2009;169(8):919–926.

39. de Lau LM, Breteler MM. Epidemiology of Parkinson's disease. *The Lancet Neurology.* 2006;5(6):525–535.

40. Wan N, Lin G. Parkinson's disease and pesticides exposure: new findings from a comprehensive study in Nebraska, USA. *The Journal of Rural Health: Official Journal of the American Rural Health Association and the National Rural Health Care Association.* 2016;32(3):303–313.

41. Erlich PM, Lunetta KL, Cupples LA, et al. Serum paraoxonase activity is associated with variants in the PON gene cluster and risk of Alzheimer disease. *Neurobiology of Aging.* 2012;33(5):1015.e1017–1023.

42. Erlich PM, Lunetta KL, Cupples LA, et al. Polymorphisms in the PON gene cluster are associated with Alzheimer disease. *Human Molecular Genetics.* 2006;15(1):77–85.

43. Mostafalou S, Abdollahi M. Pesticides and human chronic diseases: evidences, mechanisms, and perspectives. *Toxicol Appl Pharmacol.* 2013; 268(2):157–177.

44. Fraser C. What crops are sprayed with glyphosate? Over 70 of them to be exact. livelovefruit.com. https://livelovefruit.com/what-crops-are-sprayed-with-glyphosate/. Published Sept 10, 2018. Updated January 7, 2020. Accessed April 24, 2020.

45. Weedbusters. Herbicides & Trade Names. https://www.weedbusters.org.nz/weed-information/herbicides-trade-names/ Accessed January 10, 2020.

46. Thongprakaisang S, Thiantanawat A, Rangkadilok N, Suriyo T, Satayavivad J. Glyphosate induces human breast cancer cells growth via estrogen receptors. *Food Chem Toxicol.* 2013;59:129–136.

47. Hokanson R, Fudge R, Chowdhary R, Busbee D. Alteration of estrogen-regulated gene expression in human cells induced by the agricultural and horticultural herbicide glyphosate. *Human & Experimental Toxicology.* 2007;26(9):747–752.

48. Pope S. Roundup sprayed on dozens of crops pre-harvest. https://www.thehealthyhomeeconomist.com/pre-harvest-roundup-crops-not-just-wheat. Published 2019. Updated October 21, 2019. Accessed January 10, 2020.

49. Myers JP, Antoniou MN, Blumberg B, et al. Concerns over use of glyphosate-based herbicides and risks associated with exposures: a consensus statement. *Environmental Health: A Global Access Science Source.* 2016;15:19.

50. Vandenberg LN, Blumberg B, Antoniou MN, et al. Is it time to reassess current safety standards for glyphosate-based herbicides? *Journal of Epidemiology and Community Health.* 2017;71(6):613–618.

51. Schinasi L, Leon ME. Non-Hodgkin lymphoma and occupational exposure to agricultural pesticide chemical groups and active ingredients: a systematic review and meta-analysis. *Int J Environ Res Public Health.* 2014;11(4):4449–4527.

52. Sealey LA, Hughes BW, Sriskanda AN, et al. Environmental factors in the development of autism spectrum disorders. *Environ Int.* 2016;88:288–298.

53. Nevison CD. A comparison of temporal trends in United States autism prevalence to trends in suspected environmental factors. *Environmental Health: A Global Access Science Source.* 2014;13:73.

54. Jayasumana C, Paranagama P, Agampodi S, Wijewardane C, Gunatilake S, Siribaddana S. Drinking well water and occupational exposure to Herbicides

is associated with chronic kidney disease, in Padavi-Sripura, Sri Lanka. *Environmental Health: A Global Access Science Source.* 2015;14:6.

55. Samsel A, Seneff S. Glyphosate, pathways to modern diseases II: Celiac sprue and gluten intolerance. *Interdisciplinary Toxicology.* 2013;6(4):159–184.

56. Sanin LH, Carrasquilla G, Solomon KR, Cole DC, Marshall EJ. Regional differences in time to pregnancy among fertile women from five Colombian regions with different use of glyphosate. *Journal of Toxicology and Environmental Health Part A.* 2009;72(15–16):949–960.

57. Kirchner S, Kieu T, Chow C, Casey S, Blumberg B. Prenatal exposure to the environmental obesogen tributyltin predisposes multipotent stem cells to become adipocytes. *Mol Endocrinol.* 2010;24(3):526–539.

58. Chamorro-Garcia R, Sahu M, Abbey RJ, Laude J, Pham N, Blumberg B. Transgenerational inheritance of increased fat depot size, stem cell reprogramming, and hepatic steatosis elicited by prenatal exposure to the obesogen tributyltin in mice. *Environ Health Perspect.* 2013;121(3):359–366.

59. Collotta M, Bertazzi PA, Bollati V. Epigenetics and pesticides. *Toxicology.* 2013;307:35–41.

60. EPA. Table of regulated drinking contaminants. http://www.epa.gov/your-drinking-water/table-regulated-drinking-water-contaminants. Published 2016. Accessed February 2016.

61. United States Geological Survey (USGS). Pesticides are transported throught the environment. https://www.usgs.gov/media/images/pesticides-are-transported-throughout-environment. Published 1995. Accessed November 25, 2019.

62. EPA. Pesticides' Impact on Indoor Air Quality. https://www.epa.gov/indoor-air-quality-iaq/pesticides-impact-indoor-air-quality. Published 2016. Accessed January 14, 2017.

63. Mitro SD, Dodson RE, Singla V, et al. Consumer product chemicals in indoor dust: a quantitative meta-analysis of US studies. *Environmental Science & Technology.* 2016.

64. Rudel RA, Camann DE, Spengler JD, Korn LR, Brody JG. Phthalates, alkylphenols, pesticides, polybrominated diphenyl ethers, and other endocrine-disrupting compounds in indoor air and dust. *Environmental Science & Technology.* 2003;37(20):4543–4553.

65. Rudel RA, Perovich LJ. Endocrine disrupting chemicals in indoor and outdoor air. *Atmospheric Environment (Oxford, England: 1994).* 2009;43(1):170–181.

66. Payne-Sturges D, Cohen J, Castorina R, Axelrad DA, Woodruff TJ. Evaluating cumulative organophosphorus pesticide body burden of children: a national case study. *Environmental Science & Technology.* 2009;43(20):7924–7930.

11

Home Furnishings
How to Avoid Flame Retardants and Other Toxic Chemicals

Every accident is a notice that something is wrong with men, methods, or materials—investigate—then act.
—Safety saying, circa early 1900s

What Are Flame Retardants?

Currently used flame-retardant chemicals are a group of industrial chemicals that were developed during the late 1970s after PCB (polychlorinated biphenyl) flame retardants were banned due to their neurotoxic effects. These chemicals resist burning and breaking down under high heat and fire, so they have been added into the materials of various products with the intention to reduce deaths from household fires. Household fires are a real issue in the United States, despite the use of fire alarms; approximately 386,000 residential fires were reported in 2011, with 3,005 deaths and 17,500 injuries.[1] Flame-retardant chemicals were designed to allow residents more time (12 seconds) to get out of the home safely in the case of an accidental fire, often caused by an unextinguished cigarette (one of the main causes of house fires), burning candles or the stove.

Unfortunately, these chemicals have become an ongoing environmental and human health debacle that has plagued us for over 40 years, just as PCBs did between the 1920s until they were banned in 1979. As discussed in chapter 1, a California law called TB-117 that was passed in 1975 to promote the use of flame retardants in clothes and household products, was uncovered by a team of investigative reporters to be based on fraudulent information. The law was based on information that distorted the actual ability of these chemicals to suppress fires (see "The Real Story" box below). Most residential fires are started by unextinguished cigarettes, and tobacco corporations, not surprisingly, were involved in this fraud, that was revealed in a stunning series of investigative newspaper articles in the *Chicago Tribune* in 2012.[2] Confirmation of this fraudulent behavior led California to eventually reverse the 1975 law, which went into effect at the beginning of 2015, undoing the mandate requiring the use of flame retardants in household products. The exposé by the *Chicago Tribune* also led to numerous lawsuits against the manufacturers of these chemicals, such as Dupont and 3M.

The Real Story: California's 1975 Flame Retardant Law

In 1975, California legislators decided to enact a law intended to protect residents from home fires started by small open flames such as cigarettes, candles, matches, and lighters. California's legislature passed Technical Bulletin 117 (TB-117), which required that furniture and other materials used in the home be infused with flame-retardant chemicals that allow for a 12-second "burn time" or time for the material to ignite. This extra time would allow inhabitants to get out safely in the event of a fire. This turned out to be a false claim, since the amounts of flame retardants used were not adequate to suppress fires—but were high enough to be toxic to humans.

In reality, this law was promoted by the tobacco industry, which for cost and other factors, was not willing to change the formulation of cigarettes to include self-extinguishing features that would automatically burn out if dropped on the floor, couch, or other household material. They devised a legal "fix" that put the onus of fire safety onto product manufacturers instead of reworking the cigarette design.

Manufacturers found it costly to produce flame-retardant products only for California, so they began infusing flame-retardant chemicals into all of their products (e.g., household furniture, pillows, rugs, carpet padding, draperies, children's clothes) sold throughout the United States. TB-117 became a major driver of toxic chemicals used in residential furniture in the US. After studies showed high blood levels of flame retardants in adults and children and its associated health risks, the tide began to turn. In January 2015, the law mandating flame-retardant chemicals in home furnishings was rescinded, and manufacturers were allowed to voluntarily remove fire-retardant chemicals from their products. Manufacturers who have removed chemical flame retardants in their couches, pillows, and other furnishings use the tag, "TB-117-2013," instead of "TB-117" or "Technical Bulletin 117" (see Figures 11.3 and 11.4).

Where Are Flame-Retardant Chemicals Found?

Today, flame retardants are used in clothes, couches, mattresses, electronics, carpeting and carpet backing, blankets, and other housewares (see Box11.1).[3] They are used at amounts equivalent to about 1– 30% of the weight of foam or plastic found in products such as baby products, building insulation, and wire and cable.[4-7] Commonly used flame retardants include TCEP (tris (2-chloroethyl) phosphate) and BEHTBP (a tetrabromophthalate). Bromine-based flame-retardants (BFRs) are applied to 2.5 million tons of product materials (polymers) annually. Between 2001 and 2008, the volume of BFRs worldwide doubled from approximately 200,000 to 410,000 metric tons annually.

> **Box 11.1 Flame-Retardant Chemicals Are Found In:**
>
> - The plastic casing of electronics, such as televisions, stereos, computers
> - Electronic cables, plugs
> - Textiles, including upholstered couches, pillows, padded (with polyurethane foam) furniture
> - Infant car seats
> - Carpeting and foam carpet backing
> - Insulation
> - Firefighting foam and fire emergency equipment
> - Uniforms for occupations at risk for burns, including firefighting, members of the military, and other occupations

Exposure to Flame Retardants

We are exposed to an enormous amount of flame-retardant chemicals in daily life, since they continue to migrate out of products over time, showing up in humans as well as pets and wildlife.[8-11] Polybrominated diphenyl ethers (PBDEs) are a class of organohalogen flame-retardant chemicals that have emerged as a major environmental pollutant. PBDEs are added to thousands of products and textiles to reduce flammability in order to comply with the prior safety regulations. This is a sad example of what is referred to as a "regrettable substitution," since chlorinated chemicals (PCBs) were banned and quickly replaced with another halogen, bromine; bromine is used to manufacture PBDEs, which are as neurotoxic as the PCBs they replaced.

Organohalogen and organophosphorous flame retardants are considered persistent organic pollutants (POPs) and do not break down into safer chemicals in the environment because of the extremely strong bond formed between the carbon atoms that are bonded to bromine or chlorine molecules. POPs are also able to travel in air far from the source of release and become distributed worldwide. POPs are able to bioaccumulate and build up in people and animals with levels becoming more concentrated further up the food chain. POPs are such an environmental concern worldwide that of all POPs banned globally under the Stockholm Convention, 22 are organohalogens, with three of them being brominated flame retardants.[12] The Stockholm Convention on Persistent Organic Pollutants is an international environmental treaty, signed in 2001, that aims to eliminate or restrict the production and use of persistent organic pollutants. The United States signed the treaty in 2001, but has yet to ratify it because in the United States, we currently lack the regulatory authority to implement all of its provisions.

How Do Humans Get Exposed?

Household Dust

Flame-retardant chemicals are additives and usually are mixed with, rather than chemically bound to, a product. As a result, flame-retardant chemicals can easily leach out of products and into the air, sticking to particles of dust, dirt, and sediment (see Figure 11.1). One study showed that exposures to PBDE flame retardants in house dust accounted for 82% of all exposure in the United States.[13] A recent quantitative meta-analysis of other US studies on consumer product chemicals present in indoor dust, showed US indoor dust consistently contains chemicals from multiple classes of chemicals, and that many chemicals in dust share hazardous traits such as reproductive and endocrine toxicity.[3,14,15]

Dust is estimated to account for 80–93% of flame-retardant exposure in toddlers, and their small bodies and developing brains and other organs compound the effects of their exposures. Toddlers are on the floor more than other age groups, often putting objects in their mouths, and pound-for-pound, tend to have higher amounts of exposure to chemicals than adults. Reducing the amount of dust in the home is a critical factor in

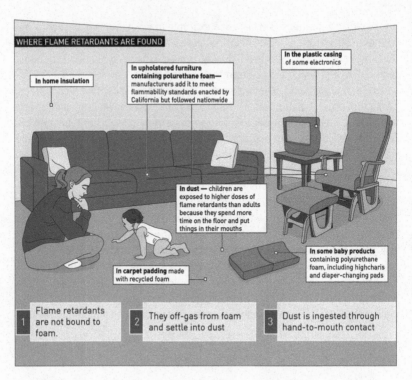

FIGURE 11.1 Where flame retardants are found and how they spread into the air and dust.

reducing exposure to toxic chemicals that attach to dust and accumulate in our bodies, contributing to multiple diseases.

In 2011, 80% of tested products containing foam designed for infants, toddlers, and children were found to contain chemical flame retardants considered toxic to children (e.g., car seat covers, nursing pillows, and changing pads).[4] Strollers, baby carriers, nursing pillows, and many more baby products were exempt from California's EPA 1975 law, TB-117, that required flame-retardant chemicals be added to these products. Currently, *infant car seats still contain flame-retardant chemicals*; infant car seat regulations are mandated by the Federal Transportation Laws, not the EPA.

The Textile and Fashion Industries

Most fabrics are not required to have an "ingredients" label; so even though they are infused with many (undisclosed) chemicals, trying to decipher *which* chemicals are in fabrics is almost impossible. However, the nature of the marketing used for many types of clothing and furniture will hint at the chemical contaminants they contain. "Stain-Guard" chemicals, for instance, are often marketed to consumers as a beneficial feature, despite the adverse health effects associated with exposure to these chemicals. Lawsuits have been initiated against manufacturers such as Dupont and 3M. In 2018 3M settled for $850 million from a lawsuit initiated by the attorney general of Minnesota regarding the hazards of its product Scotchgard, a fabric and carpet protector. Antibacterial chemicals and "silver-nano" beads are marketed to sell sportswear to ward off odor caused by bacteria from sweating.

Despite savvy marketing, chemicals used in fabrics can cause health issues. Colored fabrics used for clothing, couches, pillows, and chairs may use harmful dyes that can irritate skin with repeated contact.[16] Recently, airline attendants from a major US airline raised concern over the health issues that many experienced shortly after their uniforms were redesigned. Complaints ranging from cough, asthma exacerbation, rash, memory loss, fatigue, and change in mental function made headlines and alerted airline officials to remediate the problem.[17]

Many uniforms are manufactured with stain-guard and waterproofing chemicals to add longevity and minimize wear-and-tear. Other uniforms may contain flame-retardant chemicals and pesticides, particularly for soldiers who may be serving in countries where mosquitoes and other insects pose a threat for malaria and other infections (at one time military uniforms were soaked in DDT). Firefighter uniforms are infused with flame retardants to ward off occupational burns when putting out fires. As is true with other clothing, most uniforms containing toxic chemicals will eventually end up in landfills; this poses further environmental issues. Unbelievably, the average American disposes of approximately 70 pounds of clothing per year, and 85% of clothing in the US eventually ends up in landfills.[18]

Flame Retardants and Body Burden

The CDC has found PBDEs in the bodies of 97% of adult Americans sampled in the nationally representative NHANES report.[19] PBDEs are found in 95% of US homes, and because they are not bound to the materials (matrix) they are found in, they migrate out of products over time.[20] Despite the ban on PentaBDE and OctaBDE brominated flame retardants, studies in North America show concentrations of flame-retardant chemicals in humans have been doubling every 4–6 years since the late 1970s. For example, a recent study showed elevated halogenated flame-retardant concentrations in settled dust at gymnastics-training facilities and in the homes of gymnasts.

These facilities have large quantities of polyurethane foam that releases fine particulate matter that is easily inhaled.[21] United States residents have 20 times the blood levels of PBDEs than Europeans.[13,22] California residents experience the highest exposures due to lingering effects of the 1975 California state law mandating the use of flame retardants, which was finally reversed in 2013 after the *Chicago Tribune's* exposé in 2012.[23]

Flame-retardant chemicals have been detected in human adipose (fat) tissue, serum, and breast milk samples collected from populations in Asia, Europe, North America, Indonesia, Australia, and the Arctic.[20] The concentration of these chemicals in human serum and breast milk has exponentially increased in the last three decades.[24] As previously mentioned, toddlers have levels of flame retardants in their bodies three-times higher than adults due to their hand-to-mouth behavior and extensive time spent on the floor.[23,25] In one recent study looking at 22 mothers and 26 children, the children exhibited on average nearly five times the level of a biomarker for the popular fire-retardant TDCIPP compared to their mothers. In the most extreme case, a child had 23 times the level measured in the mother. According to findings from one study, children in California, who have some of the highest measured serum PBDE levels, showed deficits in attention, fine motor skills, and cognition. Another study showed prenatal PBDE concentration was inversely associated with reading skills at 8 years of age.[26]

Flame Retardants and Human Health

Organohalogen flame retardants are often toxic and resistant to breakdown, leading to persistence and bioaccumulation both in our bodies and in the environment. Many also are semivolatile, enabling them to continuously migrate out of products into air where they attach to dust particles and are inhaled by humans (particularly toddlers) and pets.

Brominated flame-retardant chemicals carry the element bromine in their molecular structure. The number and carbon position of the bromines designates its chemical name; PentaPBDE has 4-6 bromines, OctaPBDE has 6-8 bromines, and DecaPBDE has 10 bromines in its structure (see Figure 11.2). The bromine flame-retardant molecule is very similar to the iodine molecule in thyroxine, an important hormone that is produced by the thyroid gland. PentaPBDE has a similar structure to PCBs, dioxins, and furans, other toxic chemicals found in the environment. Dioxins are carcinogenic, persistent chlorine-containing compounds, produced when

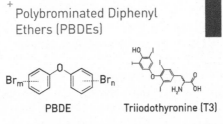

Polybrominated Diphenyl
Ethers (PBDEs)

PBDE   Triiodothyronine (T3)

Two halogenated phenolic chemicals

Figure 11.2 Molecular structure of a brominated flame-retardant chemical and the similar structure of the human thyroid hormone, triiodothyronine (T3), which contains 3 iodine molecules. Iodine and bromine are both halogens.

consumer products containing organochlorine compounds are incinerated. PBDEs that replaced the chlorine-containing PCBs have been found to be neurotoxins and affect neurodevelopment in newborns exposed through the mother's exposure. Children exposed to PBDEs are prone to subtle but measurable developmental problems. PBDEs also have been shown to have endocrine-disrupting effects in humans and wildlife.[13,27]

Many current flame retardants, such as tris (1,3-dichloro-isopropyl) phosphate (TDCPP) and Firemaster 550 (FM 550), as well as older persistent flame retardants, act as endocrine disruptors, disrupting the human body's own thyroid hormone actions, resulting in changes in biological functions.[28] Specifically, health effects from flame-retardant chemicals include endocrine system effects such as thyroid dysfunction, early onset of menstruation, lowered sperm counts, brain development disruption in young children, infertility, and breast and testicular cancers.[29–39]

Brominated flame retardants are particularly persistent, with estimated half-lives ranging between 2 and 12 years in humans. One study showed that, despite discontinuing the use of pentaBDE in 2004, human PBDE serum concentrations did not fall even after 10 years.[20]

Firefighters are among the most vulnerable to the effects of these chemicals because they are regularly exposed to burning home furnishings, with these volatile chemicals making up to 30% of the total weight of these objects.[40] Firefighters have been found to have elevated rates of cancer, such as multiple myeloma, non-Hodgkin's lymphoma, prostate cancer, and testicular cancer.[41]

Home Furnishings

Humans are not the only living creatures whose health is affected by flame-retardant chemicals. Over the past several decades, veterinarians have seen a noticeable increase in feline hyperthyroidism (overactive thyroid hormone) among indoor cats. The condition presents with chronic weight loss, hair loss, and heart issues, and would eventually be called the "Wasting Cat Syndrome." Studies were undertaken to see what factors may be playing a role, and researchers found elevated blood levels of flame-retardant chemicals in indoor cats overall, and also found associations between cats diagnosed with hyperthyroidism and elevated levels of several flame retardants compared to healthy indoor cats.[42,43] Much like toddlers who spend lots of time on the floor, cats are continuously exposed to household dust that collects flame-retardant chemicals, phthalates, and many other hormone-disrupting chemicals. These chemicals are then ingested through "paw/fur-to-mouth" behavior due to their constant grooming. (Dogs have also shown elevated levels of these chemicals but no strong association with hyperthyroidism.) Word of this phenomenon spread among veterinarians and pet owners alike and even became a feature article in the Health Issue section of the *New York Times* in 2017.[44]

Legislation: A Clever Spin

There is a history of unfortunate substitutions of one flame retardant for another. Brominated tris was used in children's sleepwear in the 1970s until it was banned as a mutagen;[26] it was then replaced by chlorinated tris, a known carcinogen.[45] Although several classes of brominated flame retardants have been taken off of the market, including OctaPBDE (2005) and PentaPBDE (2004), studies show that other PBDEs continue to leach out of aging household products.[46] PBDEs resist breakdown in the environment and may persist for decades.[47] One flame retardant, DecaPBDE, is still used commercially and has been found to break down into Octa and PentaPBDEs. Replacement brominated flame retardants are thus still on the market and are raising similar health concerns.[46] Moreover, it has been discovered that these chemicals add no fire-safety benefit, because fires in home furnishings start in the exterior fabric, not the filling.

One-third of flame-retardant products currently contain TCEP, TDCIPP, or bromine, all of which are linked to thyroid and reproductive disorders, cancers, neurodevelopmental effects, and fertility disruption in animal and human models.

Flame-Retardant Legislation Now

In 2012, tobacco lobbyists began their battle against the repeal of California's TB-117, which finally went into full effect in January 2015 based on research showing the harmful effects of flame-retardant chemicals.[31,48-52] After many years of legislative battling by California congressional leaders, environmental and health advocates, researchers, and the public, California's TB-117 mandating the use of flame retardants in many products was repealed in 2013. The use of flame retardants was not actually banned under this new law, but the reality is that manufacturers throughout the United States made changes in the use of flame retardants to be in compliance with this California law and also due to increasing awareness by consumers of the health risks of flame-retardant chemicals.

Other Toxins of Concern: Stain-Proofing/ Water-Resistant Chemicals

Perfluoroalkyls (PFAS) are a class of fluorine-containing halogenated chemicals used to make materials grease and water resistant. They have been used for decades in cookware, grease-proof paper, fabrics, and firefighting foam. Textile uses of PFAS include carpeting, home and office furniture, rain gear, duffle bags, Gortex, and other outerwear. Fluorine containing chemicals poses a threat to human health due to its abundant presence and inability to break down in the environment, similar to environmentally persistent chlorine- and bromine-containing compounds. Health effects linked to exposure to this class of chemicals include endocrine disruption, immune system changes, decreased birth weight, preeclampsia, developmental effects in fetuses, testicular and kidney cancer, cardiovascular disease, and blunted immune response to vaccinations.[53-55] PFAS have contaminated hundreds of waterways and water treatment plants across the United States due to their hydrophilic (water loving) nature, affecting millions of people (PFAS chemicals are actually amphiphilic, which means that they are both hydrophobic and hydrophilic, which is a characteristic of surfactants.). State regulators are currently working to set safety standards for human exposure.[56]

What You Can Do

Clothing and Textiles

- Avoid all clothing and pillows with stain-guard chemicals.
- Swap non-chemical containing clothing with friends.
- Before use, wash all newly purchased stuffed toys, pet beds, bedding, and clothing well, especially children's clothing.
- Avoid "wrinkle-free" clothing, bedding, and other fabrics; it is often infused with formaldehyde and other chemicals.
- Avoid buying clothing that requires dry-cleaning; harmful chemicals such as perchloroethylene (Perc) are often used and can cause a variety of respiratory issues such as cough asthma and long-term risks for cancers (see chapter 9).
- If you use dry-cleaning services, air out your dry cleaning for 24 to 48 hours to reduce chemical fumes.

Home Cleaning

- Vacuum homes regularly to remove house dust.
- Use a vacuum equipped with a HEPA filter, which traps dust in the bag.
- Use a mop dampened with *water*, not with cleaning chemicals.

Carpeting and Rugs

- Choose carpeting and rugs with woven instead of rubberized backing.
- Avoid stain-guard and antimicrobial chemicals.
- Use wool and organic cotton that are naturally flame retardant.
  If you use a synthetic-fiber carpet or rug, choose 100% nylon, which is the safest synthetic material.
- Air out (outside, if possible) before installation to allow for offgassing of common volatile toxins:
  o benzene, formaldehyde, xylene, toluene, butadiene, styrene, and 4-phenylcycloghexene (4PC)
- Avoid padding containing styrene-butadiene rubber.
- Clean regularly to avoid mold, bacteria, dust, and pesticide build-up.
- Use a HEPA filter vacuum to remove mold spores, dust mites, mite feces, and chemicals; ask comercial carpet cleaning services to use steam cleaning with water and no chemicals.
- Establish a "no-shoes in the house" policy.

- Avoid wall-to-wall carpeting in bathrooms, kitchens, laundry rooms, or mechanical rooms due to the potential for water exposure and dampness.

Furniture

- Buy couches and furniture made with naturally flame-resistant materials such as wool or polyester fill, which are unlikely to contain synthetic flame-retardant chemicals.
- Look for products and furniture labeled as free of flame-retardant chemicals, such as couches with labels stating: TB-117-2013.
- Use glass and metal home goods and decor.
- Furniture imported from tropical countries is often sprayed with pesticides while in transit.
- Look for furniture made in Europe, which will meet EU emission standards and is often constructed with low-emission materials.
- Avoid buying furniture with stain-guard chemicals.
- Look for furniture that meets Green Guard emission standards (www.greenguard.org), which must achieve formaldehyde emission rates of <0.05 ppm.
- Look for certification from ECOLOG (www.ul.com), which certifies that furniture has low emissions and was produced sustainably.
- Look for certification from the Global Organic Textile Standard (GOTS) (www.global-standard.org). The GOTS seal shows that a product does not contain toxin-emitting polyurethane foam or other hazardous chemicals.
- Look for certification from Green Seal (https://www.greenseal.org), a nonprofit environmental-standard development and certification organization that certifies products, services, restaurants, and hotels based on Green Seal standards, which contain performance, health, and sustainability criteria.

As of January 2015, manufacturers are *voluntarily allowed* to remove fire-retardant chemicals from their products, *but* they are required to label products if these chemicals are added! Read labels on home furnishings: if a label says TB-117, it likely has flame-retardant chemicals in the materials. If the label lists TB-117-2013, then there is a strong likelihood that the materials DO NOT contain flame-retardant chemicals (see Figures 11.3 and 11.4).

You will still need to contact the manufacturer to see if flame retardants were used or not. And be careful—manufacturers are still allowed to sell off old chemical-laced stock before *voluntarily* switching to safer practices.

Here are a few companies that are voluntarily going flame-retardant free in their furnishings:

- Ethan Allen has been using the CertiPUR-US furniture designation since 2013. CertiPUR-US is a certification that ensures that products are made with low-volatile-emission materials for reduced indoor air pollution, and made without formaldehyde, mercury, lead, heavy metals, PBDEs, ozone depleters, or prohibited phthalates.
- La-Z-Boy
- Crate and Barrel
- IKEA
- The Futon Shop

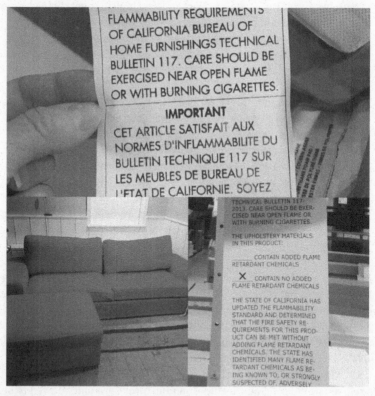

FIGURE 11.3 Author's old couch with label showing old legislation "technical bulletin 117" (top figure). Couches without chemical flame retardants are now labeled "TB-117-2013" (bottom figure).

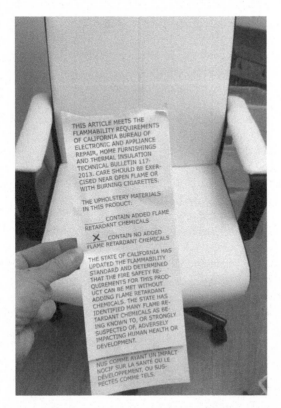

Figure 11.4 Author's new office chair with new flame retardant label. Technical Bulletin 117-2013, stating no flame-retardant chemicals were added.

Additional Product Resources

For survey results of recently tested furniture and a much more extensive list of manufacturers who supply flame-retardant-free furniture, visit:

Center for Environmental Health: http://www.ceh.org/residential-furniture/

Green Science Policy: http://greensciencepolicy.org/wp-content/uploads/2015/03/Buying_FR-free_furniture.pdf

http://greensciencepolicy.org/topics/furniture/

Centers for Disease Control and Prevention: https://www.cdc.gov/biomonitoring/PBDEs_FactSheet.html

EPA: https://www.epa.gov/assessing-and-managing-chemicals-under-tsca/fact-sheet-assessing-risks-flame-retardants

National Resources Defense Council (NRDC): https://www.nrdc.org/stories/fight-against-flame-retardants

Chicago Tribune Watchdog: http://media.apps.chicagotribune.com/flames/index.html

Chicago Tribune Pulitzer Prize-winning reporting on flame-retardant chemicals "Playing With Fire": https://www.pulitzer.org/files/finalists/2013/chictrib2013/chictrib01.pdf

How to buy flame-retardant-free furniture: http://greensciencepolicy.org/wp-content/uploads/2015/03/Buying_FR-free_furniture.pdf

Rate It Green: https://www.rateitgreen.com/green-building-directory/sustainable-building-products/appliances

California Office of Environmental Health Hazard Assessment: https://oehha.ca.gov

California's Proposition 65 list: https://oehha.ca.gov/proposition-65/proposition-65-list

For a list of PFAS-Free Products . . . outdoor gear, shoes, apparel, car seats, dental floss, carpet, furniture, nonstick cookware: https://pfascentral.org/pfas-basics/pfas-free-products/

Mind the Store (see Table 11.1): https://saferchemicals.org/mind-the-store/ A non-profit group that ranks retailers on use of toxic chemicals and creates a report card on retailer actions to eliminate toxic chemicals in their products (published by the "Mind the Store Campaign" of the national non-profit Safer Chemicals, Healthy Families).

Leading Retailers

Retailer	Grade	Points
Apple	A+	109.75
Target	A	102.5
Walmart	A	98.25
Ikea	A−	89
Rite Aid	B+	85.5
Whole Foods Market	B+	81.75
Sephora	B+	81
Home Depot	B+	80.5
CVS Health	B	71
Lowe's	B−	66
Walgreens	B−	65.25

References

1. National Fire Protection Association (NFPA). NFPA Report: Fire loss in the United States during 2011. http://www.nfpa.org/news-and-research/publications/nfpa-journal/2012/september-october-2012/features/fire-loss-in-the-united-states-during-2011. Accessed December 1, 2016.

2. *The Chicago Tribune*. Tribune Watchdog: Playing With Fire. TheChicagoTribune.com: The Chicago Tribune; 2012 [updated 2014]. Available from: http://media.apps.chicagotribune.com/flames/index.html.

3. Schecter A, Papke O, Joseph JE, Tung KC. Polybrominated diphenyl ethers (PBDEs) in U.S. computers and domestic carpet vacuuming: possible sources of human exposure. *Journal of Toxicology and Environmental Health Part A*. 2005;68(7):501–513.

4. Stapleton HM, Klosterhaus S, Keller A, et al. Identification of flame retardants in polyurethane foam collected from baby products. *Environmental Science & Technology*. 2011;45(12):5323–5331.

5. Stapleton HM, Klosterhaus S, Eagle S, et al. Detection of organophosphate flame retardants in furniture foam and U.S. house dust. *Environmental Science & Technology*. 2009;43(19):7490–7495.

6. Hale RC, La Guardia MJ, Harvey E, Mainor TM. Potential role of fire retardant-treated polyurethane foam as a source of brominated diphenyl ethers to the US environment. *Chemosphere*. 2002;46(5):729–735.

7. Allen JG, McClean MD, Stapleton HM, Webster TF. Linking PBDEs in house dust to consumer products using X-ray fluorescence. *Environmental Science & Technology*. 2008;42(11):4222–4228.

8. de Wit CA, Herzke D, Vorkamp K. Brominated flame retardants in the Arctic environment—trends and new candidates. *The Science of the Total Environment*. 2010;408(15):2885–2918.

9. Shaw SD, Berger ML, Brenner D, et al. Polybrominated diphenyl ethers (PBDEs) in farmed and wild salmon marketed in the Northeastern United States. *Chemosphere*. 2008;71(8):1422–1431.

10. Shaw SD, Berger ML, Weijs L, Papke O, Covaci A. Polychlorinated biphenyls still pose significant health risks to northwest Atlantic harbor seals. *The Science of the Total Environment*. 2014;490:477–487.

11. Annamalai J, Namasivayam V. Endocrine disrupting chemicals in the atmosphere: Their effects on humans and wildlife. *Environ Int*. 2015;76:78–97.

12. United Nations Environment Programme. Listing of POPs in the Stockholm Convention. http://chm.pops.int/TheConvention/ThePOPs/ListingofPOPs. Accessed December 1, 2016.

13. Lorber M. Exposure of Americans to polybrominated diphenyl ethers. *Journal of Exposure Science & Environmental Epidemiology.* 2008;18(1):2–19.

14. Mitro SD, Dodson RE, Singla V, et al. Consumer product chemicals in indoor dust: a quantitative meta-analysis of U.S. studies. *Environmental Science & Technology.* 2016.

15. Natural Resources Defense Council (NRDC). Not just dirt: toxic chemicals in indoor dust. https://www.nrdc.org/resources/not-just-dirt-toxic-chemicals-indoor-dust. Published 2016. Accessed April 14, 2019.

16. Chung KT. Azo dyes and human health: A review. *Journal of Environmental science and health Part C, Environmental Carcinogenesis & Ecotoxicology Reviews.* 2016;34(4):233–261.

17. The Guardian. "Chemical burns": Delta flight attendants say new uniforms cause rashes. https://www.theguardian.com/business/2019/apr/03/delta-flight-attendants-uniforms-rash-claims. Published 2019. Accessed April 4, 2019.

18. Tasha Lewis PhD. What makes us human [Internet]; 2019. Podcast. Available from: https://soundcloud.com/cornellcas/future-fashion.

19. Hendryx M, Luo J. Children's environmental chemical exposures in the USA, NHANES 2003–2012. *Environmental Science and Pollution Research International.* 2018;25(6):5336–5343.

20. Sjodin A, Jones RS, Caudill SP, Wong LY, Turner WE, Calafat AM. Polybrominated diphenyl ethers, polychlorinated biphenyls, and persistent pesticides in serum from the national health and nutrition examination survey: 2003-2008. *Environmental Science & Technology.* 2014;48(1):753–760.

21. La Guardia MJ, Hale RC. Halogenated flame-retardant concentrations in settled dust, respirable and inhalable particulates and polyurethane foam at gymnastic training facilities and residences. *Environ Int.* 2015;79:106–114.

22. Hites RA. Polybrominated diphenyl ethers in the environment and in people: a meta-analysis of concentrations. *Environmental Science & Technology.* 2004;38(4):945–956.

23. Fischer D, Hooper K, Athanasiadou M, Athanassiadis I, Bergman A. Children show highest levels of polybrominated diphenyl ethers in a California family of four: a case study. *Environ Health Perspect.* 2006;114(10):1581–1584.

24. Schecter A, Papke O, Tung KC, Joseph J, Harris TR, Dahlgren J. Polybrominated diphenyl ether flame retardants in the U.S. population: current levels, temporal trends, and comparison with dioxins, dibenzofurans, and polychlorinated biphenyls. *Journal of Occupational and Environmental Medicine / American College of Occupational and Environmental Medicine.* 2005;47(3):199–211.

25. Wu XM, Bennett DH, Moran RE, et al. Polybrominated diphenyl ether serum concentrations in a Californian population of children, their parents, and older adults: an exposure assessment study. *Environmental Health: A Global Access Science Source.* 2015;14:23.

26. Zhang H, Yolton K, Webster GM, Sjodin A, Calafat AM, Dietrich KN, et al. Prenatal PBDE and PCB exposures and reading, cognition, and externalizing behavior in children. *Environ Health Perspect.* 2017;125(4):746–752.

27. Blum A, Ames BN. Flame-retardant additives as possible cancer hazards. *Science (New York, NY).* 1977;195(4273):17–23.

28. Dishaw LV, Macaulay LJ, Roberts SC, Stapleton HM. Exposures, mechanisms, and impacts of endocrine-active flame retardants. *Curr Opin Pharmacol.* 2014;19:125–133.

29. Johnson PI, Stapleton HM, Mukherjee B, Hauser R, Meeker JD. Associations between brominated flame retardants in house dust and hormone levels in men. *The Science of the Total Environment.* 2013;445–446:177–184.

30. Chevrier J, Harley KG, Bradman A, Gharbi M, Sjodin A, Eskenazi B. Polybrominated diphenyl ether (PBDE) flame retardants and thyroid hormone during pregnancy. *Environ Health Perspect.* 2010;118(10):1444–1449.

31. Eskenazi B, Chevrier J, Rauch SA, et al. In utero and childhood polybrominated diphenyl ether (PBDE) exposures and neurodevelopment in the CHAMACOS study. *Environ Health Perspect.* 2013;121(2):257–262.

32. Meeker JD, Stapleton HM. House dust concentrations of organophosphate flame retardants in relation to hormone levels and semen quality parameters. *Environ Health Perspect.* 2010;118(3):318–323.

33. Caserta D, Mantovani A, Marci R, et al. Environment and women's reproductive health. *Human Reproduction Update.* 2011;17(3):418–433.

34. Small CM, Murray D, Terrell ML, Marcus M. Reproductive outcomes among women exposed to a brominated flame retardant in utero. *Archives of Environmental & Occupational Health.* 2011;66(4):201–208.

35. Terrell ML, Rosenblatt KA, Wirth J, Cameron LL, Marcus M. Breast cancer among women in Michigan following exposure to brominated flame retardants. *Occupational and Environmental Medicine.* 2016;73(8):564–567.

36. Reers AR, Eng ML, Williams TD, Elliott JE, Cox ME, Beischlag TV. The Flame-retardant tris(1,3-dichloro-2-propyl) phosphate represses androgen signaling in human prostate cancer cell lines. *Journal of Biochemical and Molecular Toxicology.* 2016;30(5):249–257.

37. Pi N, Chia SE, Ong CN, Kelly BC. Associations of serum organohalogen levels and prostate cancer risk: Results from a case-control study in Singapore. *Chemosphere.* 2016;144:1505–1512.

38. Allen JG, Gale S, Zoeller RT, Spengler JD, Birnbaum L, McNeely E. PBDE flame retardants, thyroid disease, and menopausal status in U.S. women. *Environmental Health: A Global Access Science Source.* 2016;15(1):60.

39. Hoffman K, Sosa JA, Stapleton HM. Do flame retardant chemicals increase the risk for thyroid dysregulation and cancer? *Current Opinion in Oncology.* 2016.

40. Shaw SD, Berger ML, Harris JH, et al. Persistent organic pollutants including polychlorinated and polybrominated dibenzo-p-dioxins and dibenzofurans in firefighters from Northern California. *Chemosphere.* 2013;91(10):1386–1394.

41. LeMasters GK, Genaidy AM, Succop P, et al. Cancer risk among firefighters: a review and meta-analysis of 32 studies. *Journal of Occupational and Environmental medicine / American College of Occupational and Environmental Medicine.* 2006;48(11):1189–1202.

42. Affairs C. Study finds indoor cats have high levels of flame retardants. https://www.consumeraffairs.com/news/study-finds-indoor-cats-have-high-levels-of-flame-retardants-022717.html. Published 2017. Accessed April 17, 2020.

43. J. Norrgran Engdahl, A. Bignert et al. Cats' internal exposure to selected brominated flame retardants and organochlorines correlated to house dust and cat food. *Environmental Science & Technology.* 2017;51:3012–3020.

44. Anthes E. The mystery of the wasting house-cats. Health Issue website. https://www.nytimes.com/2017/05/16/magazine/the-mystery-of-the-wasting-house-cats.html. Published 2017. Accessed June 18, 2019.

45. Gold MD, Blum A, Ames BN. Another flame retardant, tris-(1,3-dichloro-2-propyl)-phosphate, and its expected metabolites are mutagens. *Science (New York, NY).* 1978;200(4343):785–787.

46. Stapleton HM, Sharma S, Getzinger G, et al. Novel and high volume use flame retardants in US couches reflective of the 2005 PentaBDE phase out. *Environmental Science & Technology.* 2012;46(24):13432–13439.

47. Lin W, Li X, Yang M, Lee K, Chen B, Zhang BH. Brominated Flame Retardants, Microplastics, and Biocides in the Marine Environment: Recent Updates of Occurrence, Analysis, and Impacts. *Advances in Marine Biology.* 2018;81:167–211.

48. Chen A, Yolton K, Rauch SA, et al. Prenatal polybrominated diphenyl ether exposures and neurodevelopment in U.S. children through 5 years of age: the HOME study. *Environ Health Perspect.* 2014;122(8):856–862.

49. Collaborative on Health and the Environment. Chemical contaminants and human disease: a summary of the evidence. March 18, 2004. https://www.healthandenvironment.org/partnership_calls/60. Accessed April 24, 2020.

50. Vuong AM, Yolton K, Webster GM, et al. Prenatal polybrominated diphenyl ether and perfluoroalkyl substance exposures and executive function in school-age children. *Environ Res.* 2016.

51. Sagiv SK, Kogut K, Gaspar FW, et al. Prenatal and childhood polybrominated diphenyl ether (PBDE) exposure and attention and executive function at 9-12 years of age. *Neurotoxicology and Teratology.* 2015;52(Pt B):151–161.

52. Braun JM, Kalkbrenner AE, Just AC, et al. Gestational exposure to endocrine-disrupting chemicals and reciprocal social, repetitive, and stereotypic behaviors in 4- and 5-year-old children: the HOME study. *Environ Health Perspect.* 2014;122(5):513–520.

53. Huang M, Jiao J, Zhuang P, Chen X, Wang J, Zhang Y. Serum polyfluoroalkyl chemicals are associated with risk of cardiovascular diseases in national US population. *Environ Int.* 2018;119:37–46.

54. Coperchini F, Awwad O, Rotondi M, Santini F, Imbriani M, Chiovato L. Thyroid disruption by perfluorooctane sulfonate (PFOS) and perfluorooctanoate (PFOA). *Journal of Endocrinological Investigation.* 2017;40(2):105–121.

55. Rappazzo KM, Coffman E, Hines EP. Exposure to perfluorinated alkyl substances and health outcomes in children: a systematic review of the epidemiologic literature. *Int J Environ Res Public Health.* 2017;14(7).

56. Guelfo JL, Marlow T, Klein DM, et al. Evaluation and management strategies for per- and polyfluoroalkyl substances (PFASs) in drinking water aquifers: perspectives from impacted U.S. northeast communities. *Environ Health Perspect.* 2018;126(6):065001.

12

Radiation: Safer Use of Cell Phones, Tech Toys, and Gadgets

One cannot escape the feeling that these mathematical formulas have an independent existence and an intelligence of their own, that they are wiser than we are, wiser even than their discoverers.

—Heinrich Hertz (1857–1894), who proved the existence of electromagnetic waves

Much like plastic products today, which are cheap, available, and convenient, so too are cellular gadgets, making their use irresistible and addictive to consumers. According to mobile industry analysis groups, there are over 5 billion cell phones in use around the globe, and two-thirds of the world's population is now connected by mobile devices.[1] Add to this countless number of tablets, laptops, Bluetooth, and other wireless technologies worldwide, the number of radiofrequencies used and towers needed to power them, and the number of people surrounded by ANY type of radiation at any given time, and the picture begins to look alarming. Younger users, a wider variety of wireless transmitting devices, rapid advances in cellular technology, lack of public health monitoring, regulation, and precautionary recommendations contribute to the confusion about safety. There continues to be tremendous product excitement surrounding these "magical" objects that we have come to love and depend on so much.

Statistics

According to Pew Research Center, the vast majority of Americans—95%—now own a cell phone of some kind. The share of Americans that own smartphones is now 77%, up from just 35% in Pew Research Center's first survey of smartphone ownership conducted in 2011. As of January 2018, 100% of people aged 18–29 owned a cell phone, 94% of which were smartphones. Owners span all age groups, household incomes, education levels, locations (suburban vs. urban vs. rural), religions, ethnicities, and cultures.[2]

In 2005, only 5% of American adults used at least one social media platform. By 2011 that share had risen to half of all Americans. In the age 18–29 demographic, 88% use social media regularly as compared to 37% of those aged 65+.[3] As of 2019, 69% of the US public used some type of social media (e.g., Facebook, Pinterest, Instagram, LinkedIn, WhatsApp, Twitter).

Radiation Basics

Our cell phones, tablets, computers, microwaves, fitness trackers, transistor radios, x-ray machines, cordless phones, baby monitors, and WiFi water/electric meters all emit electromagnetic frequency radiation—also known as microwave/radiofrequency radiation (MW/RF), which is made up of invisible waves of electric and magnetic energy moving through space. There are generally two types of radiation, *ionizing* radiation and *non-ionizing* radiation; these are used for different functions, based on their speed of movement and ability to penetrate through materials such as air, water, and skin. Ionizing radiation, the type of radiation used by x-ray machines, consists of higher-energy and shorter-wavelength, high-frequency radiation (wave frequency is measured in Hertz (Hz) or cycles per second). In contrast, non-ionizing radiation, used in microwave ovens, cell phones, tablets, visible light, and radio waves from transistor and car radios, consists of lower-energy, longer-wavelength, low-frequency radiation (Figure 12.1). Extremely low frequency radiation (ELF) is non-ionizing and is used for household appliances, with varying cycles depending on the country. In the United States, ELF operates at 50 or 60 Hz. Devices that

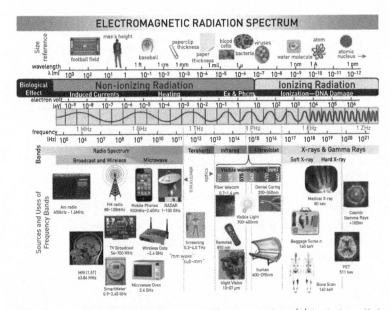

FIGURE 12.1 Electromagnetic spectrum. Wireless devices (*) include cellular and cordless phones; computers, laptops, tablets, and peripheral equipment; antennae, WiFi, access points, and drones; monitors (e.g., security, medical, for babies); toys and entertainment systems; smart utility meters and appliances; control systems (e.g., indoor climate or lighting); "wearables"; and power transfer/battery charging stations.

emit microwave radiation, such as cell phones, baby monitors, tablets, fitness trackers, virtual reality (VR) systems, and the so-called internet of things (e.g., smart refrigerators, utility meters, alarm systems) operate at between 900 million and 5 billion Hz. Although ionizing radiation has the capacity for greater disruption and harm to cells of the body than nonionizing, the frequencies of radiation used in the "microwave zone" (see Figure 12.1.) are now under greater scrutiny as health risks.

Unlike a microwave oven, which is an enclosed system and heats up with 1000 watts (W) of continuous radiation when you push "Start," cell phones and other microwave-emitting gadgets are NOT enclosed in a radiation-blocking box. Instead, these devices release radiation to their surroundings as they communicate with nearby cell towers using pulsed, irregular signals, with rapid changes in their electric and magnetic fields. These wireless devices thus act as a two-way microwave radio that sends and receives silent, invisible signals from towers at a rate of around 900 times per minute.

Regulatory Standards and Safety Testing

Safety testing for cellular devices was originally designed to measure heat, or "thermal" changes, as an endpoint for radiation harm, since radiation increases the movement of molecules in human cells, which in turn, generates heat that can disrupt cellular functions. The specific energy absorption rate (SAR) is a measure commonly used to calculate the RF energy absorbed by the body during mobile phone use. The Federal Communications Commission (FCC) certification process requires cellular phone testing—but still uses an old testing model—a Specific Anthropomorphic Mannequin (SAM), a human head and body made from plastic (polycarbonate) that is filled with liquids that simulate the RF absorption characteristics of different human tissues. The size and weight of the SAM was chosen to represent the top 10% of US military recruits in 1989 (220-pound man with an 11-pound head).[4] Radiofrequency radiation (RFR) exposure limits adopted by the FCC in the late 1990s were based upon behavioral change in rats exposed to microwave radiation and were designed to protect us from short-term heating risks due to RFR exposure. Clearly, there are problems with this outdated testing model: It does not take into account the size and make up of a woman's or child's skull and brain, the varying signal power that occurs during cell phone use, or the health risks from continual usage over time. The American Association of

Pediatrics wrote to the FCC urging that new standards be developed, noting that "Current FCC standards do not account for the unique vulnerability and use patterns specific to pregnant women and children."[5] How ironic that our most technologically advanced inventions are using decades-old science for safety regulations!

Over two decades ago, regulatory bodies, including the US Institute of Electrical and Electronic Engineers (IEEE), the US National Council on Radiation Protection (NCRP), and the European International Commission for Non-Ionizing Radiation Protection (ICNIRP), reviewed standards for the use and safety of electronic devices, and found that technologies in use at the time complied.[6] But much has changed in the intervening years: faster signals, broader use of radiofrequencies, pulsing versus continuous signaling from cell towers, product materials that mask heat, use of multiple devices at once and proximity to multiple cell towers, and younger users of microwave technology whose physical immaturity puts them at greater risk for harm. So too have the data changed. It is now well established that, in addition to thermal changes, weak MW/RF can cause all sorts of dramatic *non-thermal* effects in the body's cells, tissues, and organs. As with many of the products sold on the US market, safety standards have not kept up with rapid changes in technology. Pressure by technology and telecommunications companies, lobbyists, and politicians to paralyze and block balanced, scientifically based review of safety standards makes it nearly impossible to slow down "progress" to make time for appropriate, well-funded safety testing.

Checking RF Exposure from your Smart Phone

What does the maker of your cell phone say about its safety and recommendations for safe use? Often, this information is quietly located in the fine print of your phone.

If you have an iPhone, for example, go to "Settings," "General," "Legal & Regulatory" (it's toward the bottom), and, finally, "RF Exposure."

What Are 2G, 3G, 4G, and 5G Technology?

The "G" stands for "generation," and these labels refer to the 2nd, 3rd, 4th and 5th generations of wireless technology. The newer generation is designed to be faster, more secure, with more reliable signal strength. Each generation tends to use higher-frequency, lower-power signals than previous generations. So, when cellular carriers boast about their technology running on 2G, 3G, 4G, and 5G technology, you would think that what they are marketing to customers is a good thing, right? For convenience and usability, this may be true; but from a human health perspective, a wider spectrum of frequencies and faster rates of data movement may have health implications that have not been fully examined, especially as cellular companies begin to roll out 5G in the United States and around the globe. The newest cellular technology, 5G, will employ millimeter waves for the first time, in addition to the microwaves used in 2G–4G technologies. Because millimeter waves have a more limited reach, 5G requires cell antennas every 100 to 200 meters (each emitting radiation), with an additional 800,000 new antennas required to be built across the United States, close to where we live, work, and play.[7] The regulatory agencies have avoided discussing the implications of having people literally surrounded by radiation-producing antennas.

Health Issues

Are all of the tech gadgets that have infiltrated our lives harmful? A growing body of evidence shows that cell phone and wireless radiation—at even very low levels—could harm our health in a number of different ways. There are now over 500 peer-reviewed studies from around the world showing biologic or health effects from exposure to radiofrequency radiation at intensities too low to cause significant heating, which is one of the endpoints adopted by the FCC in the late 1990s to indicate harm. WHO listed cell phones as a "Class 2B Carcinogen" in 2011, a category that indicates it is "possibly carcinogenic to humans"—the same category as lead, engine exhaust, DDT, and jet fuel.[8,9] In their report, the International Agency for Research on Cancer (IARC) working group, which is part of the WHO, stated, "The average MW/RF radiation energy deposition for children exposed to mobile phone MW/RF is two times higher in the brain and 10 times higher in the bone marrow of the skull compared with mobile phone use by adults."[10] Clearly, safety standards based only on large adults are not protective of children.

The millimeter waves used in 5G technology are mostly absorbed within a few millimeters of human skin and in the surface layers of the cornea, potentially posing health risks to the skin (e.g., melanoma), the eyes (e.g., ocular melanoma), and the testes (e.g., sterility). 5G will not replace 4G; it will accompany 4G for the near future and possibly over the long term, raising questions of synergistic effects, but as of the beginning of 2020, no safety testing has been undertaken to study health risks of 5G technologies.[7]

Despite the concern about 5G, US policymakers have been dragging their feet to enact precautionary changes, while technology-sophisticated nations, such as India, Belgium, and Israel, have already taken regulatory steps based on the growing body of data showing health risks. Even China and Russia have stronger regulations on the use of wireless radiation than the United States, which prompted unfounded claims that any concern about radiation was a Russian "hoax" to stop the supposedly wonderful new 5G technology from being advanced in the United States.[11]

Effects of MW/RF Radiation on Cells

Studies in the laboratory on human and animal body tissues show that microwave radiation can alter cells and tissues in several ways. MW/RF radiation can weaken electrical bonds, disrupt release of nitric oxide (which regulates cell functions) and other signaling and repair chemicals, cause structural and functional changes within membranes of cells, and create "free-radicals," substances known to cause damage to surrounding tissue and that are also a risk factor for cancer.[12-15] These types of effects have been ignored by regulatory agencies that have focused on measuring heat generated by MW/RF (the thermal standard).

Radiation Exposure in Children vs. Adults

As mentioned in previous chapters, children are generally more vulnerable to a number of harmful environmental exposures. So too are children more vulnerable to the effects of radiofrequency radiation.[16-18] Children have smaller heads and thinner skulls; their skulls contain a higher percentage of bone marrow, a fatty substance that allows radiation to pass through with greater ease. Children are still growing, so their brain tissue has greater water content and less fat (myelin) content, and therefore less

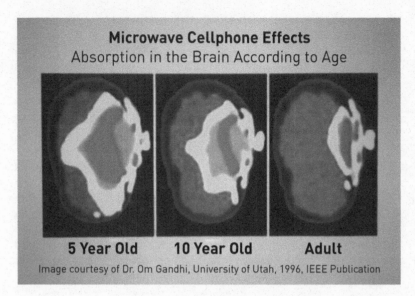

Microwave Cellphone Effects
Absorption in the Brain According to Age

| 5 Year Old | 10 Year Old | Adult |

Image courtesy of Dr. Om Gandhi, University of Utah, 1996, IEEE Publication

FIGURE 12.2 Image of cell phone radiation penetration of a child's vs. adult's head.

protective "coating," which allows higher doses and deeper penetration of cellphone radiation into the brain compared to an adult brain. The deeper structures in the brain include the cerebellum (controls movement, balance, coordination, speech) and the hippocampus (short-term, long-term, and spatial memory) (see Figure 12.2). In fact, because of the structural differences, a child's brain and skull can absorb up to ten times more radiation than the brain and skull of an adult![16,19,20]

MW/RF Radiation and Pregnancy

The developing embryo and fetus are much more vulnerable than adults to environmental toxins. Researchers are working to see if routine MW/RF exposure, at levels commonly experienced by pregnant women in industrialized communities, may have harmful effects. Some data have shown changes in fetal growth, while others show outcomes such as miscarriage. New studies find that mothers exposed to MW/RF radiation during routine exposure from WiFi in the home, buildings, and outdoor environments may have babies with worse birth outcomes, such as low birth weight. In one study, infant girls with higher exposure to electromagnetic radiation during pregnancy had a lower birth weight, compared with infant girls with lower prenatal electromagnetic radiation exposure.[21] As a precaution, it is strongly recommended that cell phones and tablets not be held near a pregnant belly, or computers held on the belly or lap of a pregnant woman. Radiation intensity decreases as a function of distance squared from the source, so the farther you are from any source of radiation, the lower your exposure will be.

***For more tips to reduce wireless radiation exposure during pregnancy: https://www.babysafeproject.org/

Brain Changes

Although data were sparse just a decade ago, a number of studies from research labs around the world are now demonstrating the health effects of MW/RF radiation to the brain, and the data continue to grow.[22] Several animal studies, which looked at health effects from MW radiation exposure, at the same level as cell phone users, have shown changes in decision making, while other studies have shown changes to heart rate, blood pressure, and EKG changes.[23,24] In humans, radiofrequency radiation has been found to affect sugar (glucose) metabolism in the brain. One study found that after a 50-minute cell phone exposure in healthy participants, there was increased brain glucose metabolism in the region closest to where the cell phone antennae was held against the head.[25]

One study looking at brain scans (MRIs) of children aged 3 to 5 years old, found that those children using screen technology (e.g., iPads, televisions, computers) greater than the recommended one hour a day by the American Academy of Pediatrics, had decreased development in their brain's white matter (the nerve fibers that transmit messages between brain cells), which is key to the development of literacy, language, and cognitive skills.[26]

Combining heavy metal exposure with cell phone use may make things even worse. One study showed children with very high blood lead levels experienced worsening of symptoms of ADHD when cell phones were held to their heads.[27]

Brain Tumors: Are the Data Real?

Several European studies have found a relationship between brain tumor (glioma) development and specifically ipsilateral (same side of the head as the tumor) cell phone use.[28-31] Acoustic neuroma, a type of tumor that affects the hearing centers of the brain, has also been implicated in some studies, but to a lesser degree than glioma.[32]

A major US government study on rats found a link between cell phones and cancer, an explosive finding in the long-running debate about whether mobile phones cause detrimental health effects. This multi-year, peer-reviewed study by the US National Toxicology Program (NTP) found "low incidences" of two types of tumors in male rats that were exposed to the type of radio frequencies commonly emitted by cell phones. The tumors discovered were gliomas in the brain as well as schwannomas, which are nerve sheath tumors located around the heart. The study also showed damaged DNA in rats and mice of both sexes. "Given the widespread global usage of mobile communications among people of all ages, even a very small increase in the incidence of disease resulting from exposure to [radio-frequency radiation] could have broad implications for public health," according to the study.[33]

A major criteria for the strength of scientific findings is the "reproducibility" of the results by other scientists. It is thus significant that the Ramazzini Institute in Italy was able to replicate the key finding of the NTP study using a different carrier frequency and much weaker exposure to cell phone radiation over the life of the rats.[34]

While not all biological effects observed in animals necessarily apply to humans, the majority do, and the NTP's $30 million study is one of the biggest and most comprehensive investigations into health effects of cell phones. The finding by the NTP that real-world MW/RF exposure caused a significant increase in tumors, contrasts with the lack of this finding in some smaller prior studies without appropriate unexposed controls. A major difference, however, was that the NTP shielded all animals from background radiation by building a giant Faraday cage around them, so that there was an actual unexposed (control) group; this had not previously been done. In the NTP study, the control animals did not get these tumors, while the MW/RF-exposed animals did.

Breast Cancer Risk

A series of case reports show an increase in the development of breast tumors, both benign and cancerous, in women who kept their cell phones in their bras. The four women ranged in age from 21 to 39, and all regularly carried their smartphones directly against their breasts in their bras for up to 10 hours a day for several years. All four women developed tumors in areas of their breasts immediately underlying the phones. These patients had no family history of breast cancer, tested negative for BRCA1 and

BRCA2 (genetic markers of high risk of breast cancer), and had no other known breast cancer risks.[35]

Sperm Quality and Quantity

Cell phone studies on animals that looked at changes to testicular tissue showed changes that were considered precancerous for testicular cancer. In the experiment, rats were exposed to 900 MHz (megahertz) of electromagnetic radiation for 0, 1, 2, or 4 hours per day for 30 consecutive days. Results indicated biochemical specific protein changes that can be extrapolated to radiation exposure in adult human males and that are related to cancer risk and reproductive damage.[36] Human studies also link cell phone and cordless telephone use to an increasing number of testicular cancers as well as cases of non-Hodgkin's lymphoma.[37,38] Testes, along with the brain, are particularly vulnerable to damage caused by MW/RF radiation. Given that in the United States and Europe, sperm count has been steadily decreasing, the impact of MW/RF radiation on sperm has to be of great concern.[39] Other studies show the harmful effects of radiation on sperm development, quality, and quantity, and therefore on fertility in men.[40]

Important Takeaway

There is a wide body of evidence available now along with the wisdom of the precautionary principle that underscores the importance of keeping cell phones *away from sensitive parts of the body*, including the testicles, ovaries, and breasts!

Cell phones should not be kept in front pockets close to male or female genitalia, and believe it or not, laptops should not sit on laps! Computers and tablet devices should be placed on a table or chair with reasonable distance, perhaps greater than 12 inches, from reproductive parts of both men AND women, and certainly not resting on the belly of a pregnant woman.

Sleep

Disrupted sleep from email and text pings, blue-light exposure, and social media addiction are among the obvious culprits when it comes to reduced sleep quantity and quality from cell phones, tablets, and computers. Light exposure, especially in the blue-light range of visible light, can cause melatonin levels (which normally increase at night) to drop, potentially contributing to poor sleep. Other important physiological changes that can occur with radiofrequency radiation include changes to melatonin levels and cortisol rhythms—two major hormone markers of the sleep-wake cycle (circadian system).[41] Melatonin levels can be affected even by low-level EMF given off by digital alarm clocks, stereos, computers, and other electrical appliances. Among other ways to improve both the quality and quantity of sleep (see chapter 13), would be to switch out your plug-in alarm clock for a battery operated one, and remove any other electrical appliances from the bedroom.

Other Health Problems

Use of cell phones and related technologies have been linked to headaches, migraines, tinnitus, poor concentration, mood changes, depression, fatigue, irritability, and vision changes in both children and adults.[42–45] Often, those who are sensitive to MW/RF radiation and experience electromagnetic hypersensitivity (EHS) will see a noticeable difference in their symptoms when they leave a space using WiFi and/or devices are turned off. Homes, hotels, the workplace, and schools can all be a source of electromagnetic radiation. And what about new WiFi technologies for managing home alarms, room temperature, refrigerator contents, and other conveniences? "Smart meters" are being required in many homes around the United States and the world to monitor electricity and water usage for utility companies. They are often set up in the basement of homes and apartment complexes and run continuously. Reports of health effects related to these meters have increased over the short period since they have been introduced. One Australian researcher reported cases of increased headaches, insomnia, cognitive dysfunction, irritability, and tinnitus in people with homes using smart meters.[46]

For the very young, reducing or eliminating WiFi technology in daycares is gaining popularity. On January 29, 2015, the French National Assembly made history by passing a new law to reduce exposures to wireless radiation electromagnetic fields by banning WiFi and wireless devices in nursery schools across the country. In September 2018, France's education minister announced a total ban on students using mobile phones in primary and secondary schools. Not only are cell phones now banned in classrooms, but students are barred from using them during breaks, at lunch time, and between lessons.[47] This is a clear example of Europeans using the principle of "precaution" rather than requiring "absolute proof" (that can never be achieved) prior to initiating regulations to protect children from plausible sources of harm.

Functional and anatomical effects from cellular technology include "texting thumb" and "texting neck," neck strain, muscle spasm, tingling hand, and carpal tunnel syndrome from overuse and poor posture. Despite millions of years of human evolution, use of modern-day tech toys is actually changing the anatomy and dynamics of our bodies in the span of just two generations since their invention!

Bluetooth and Ear Bud Safety

Is Bluetooth any safer for cell phone users? Although use of "hands-free kits" such as Bluetooth lowers exposure to the brain to below 10% of the exposure from use at the ear, an increase in exposure to other parts of the body may occur, and wireless hands-free kits still emit low dose but constant radiation.[48] Ear buds employ Bluetooth technology, but no long-term testing has yet been undertaken to evaluate their safety beyond that which complies with minimal FCC regulations. According to Dr. Devra Lee Davis, founder and president of the Environmental Health Trust, a nonprofit research and education organization focused on environmental health hazards: "The fact is that wireless ear buds still place a microwave transmitter next to the head, and as a result, these microwaves penetrate into your skull and brain. Yes, they are considered 'low level' microwaves as they do not cook your tissue, but these very low levels have been shown to cause biological effects."[49]

Cell Phone Cases and Protective Materials

Studies show that, paradoxically, "radiation-blocking" cell phone cases may increase rather than reduce radiation exposure. Consider how a phone case works: a signal must reach the cell phone antenna in order to pass data, so if a case is only partially surrounding the cell phone, the signal must work that much harder to reach the antenna. The only foolproof way to reduce radiation exposure to both incoming and outgoing signals is to place the phone on "airplane mode" to completely cut off the signal.

Another way to reduce MW/RF radiation is to place the cell phone in a Faraday bag, named after British scientist Michael Faraday (1791–1867). A Faraday bag, also known as a radiofrequency shielding bag, is a pouch consisting of layers of specially designed RF shielding material which *completely* surrounds the phone or tablet from signal transmission. The Faraday bag will block cell signals, WiFi, satellite, Bluetooth frequencies, and GPS.

Clothing made with silver or copper thread can also block MW/RF radiation. Several companies have developed products, such as baby blankets and maternity clothing, that act as a shield for infants and pregnant mothers. WiFi radiation can be reduced in the home simply by turning off the system when not in use (such as while sleeping), or adding special paints, foil, protective drapes, and metal sheeting for walls as a barrier to exposure from outside cell towers.

Social Media and Stress

Emotional highs and lows contributing to mood swings, interrupted sleep from personal and business texts, and anxiety resulting from NOT checking your phone for messages are just a few of the modern-day problems associated with social media and technology use.[50] And then there's FOMO (fear of missing out) the feelings of anxiety that arise from the realization that you may be missing out on a rewarding experience that others are having without you. Or "phubbing," a combination of "snubbing" and "phone." describing the practice of ignoring one's present company in order to pay attention to one's phone or other mobile device.[51,52]

No longer does one experience shame, bullying, or social pressure only at work or school—they are readily available now in the form of "cyberbullying" for those using any of the thousands of apps connecting humans through conversation. It is not surprising that depression and anxiety have increased over the past decade among both adults and children. Among teens surveyed, the number of teenagers experiencing depressed mood and feelings of anxiety on a daily basis has reached an all-time high, and cell phone use is likely contributing to these numbers.[53] Many people, in all age groups, are now looking to "unplug" from social media to reduce stress and anxiety and increase positive human-to-human interactions.

Distracted Driving and Walking

One of the most dramatic consequences of modern-day technologies is its effect on attention. You've seen these people, or been one; a driver passes you along a busy freeway, going 60+ miles per hour and looking down at a cell phone.[54,55] Not only does cell phone use while driving affect sensory function, such as visual fields and the ability to hear other drivers, but it also can disrupt basic driving skills, such as making lane changes, recognizing light signals, and stopping safely.[56] Teens who use cell phones while driving are a growing concern. Among young people aged 18–29, the number of car accidents and injuries have risen in the United States and abroad.[57] Studies continue to show that texting, calling, social media browsing, and taking "selfies," especially among young cell phone users, create distraction, redirecting both focus and attention. This also negatively affects social relationships, school work, and learning.[58–64] The number of injuries and fatal collisions from distracted walking, running, skiing, and taking selfies (victims have even fallen from cliffs) has skyrocketed; the irony is that these incidents are often captured on social media for all to see.[65,66] Generally, teens and young adults are not risk averse, which means they are more likely to engage in behaviors that later in life would be thought of as being "a really bad idea." The US educational system has not adapted to the rapid changes in technology that have occurred in just a decade, unlike the proactive steps being taken in France (as mentioned earlier), and so it is up to parents to deal with these issues in the United States and most other countries.

Policy and Funding

Currently, cell phones in the United States and many other countries are in compliance with standards set to prevent heating of skin that they are in contact with or when they are in the vicinity of microwave-emitting devices. Questions remain regarding whether the agencies that set the standards were influenced by tech manufacturers, lobbyists, and politicians to move technology forward as opposed to using the precautionary principle to protect the health of their citizens. In 2015, more than 252 scientists from 43 different countries, who have published a combined 2000 papers and letters on biologic and health effects of non-ionizing electromagnetic radiation, signed the International EMF [Electromagnetic Field] Scientist Appeal, which calls for stronger limits on exposure.[67] Collectively they request that:

1. children and pregnant women be protected;
2. guidelines and regulatory standards be strengthened;
3. manufacturers be encouraged to develop safer technology;
4. utilities responsible for the generation, transmission, distribution, and monitoring of electricity maintain adequate power quality and ensure proper electrical wiring to minimize harmful ground current;
5. the public be fully informed about the potential health risks from electromagnetic energy and taught harm reduction strategies;

6. medical professionals be educated about the biological effects of electromagnetic energy and be provided training on treatment of patients with electromagnetic sensitivity;

7. governments fund training and research on electromagnetic fields and health that is independent of industry and mandate industry cooperation with researchers;

8. media disclose experts' financial relationships with industry when citing their opinions regarding health and safety aspects of EMF-emitting technologies; and

9. white-zones (radiation-free areas) be established.

Where does the funding for radiofrequency radiation come from? One researcher looked into the available studies on cell phone radiation between 1996 and 2006 and where its funding came from. He found that 50% of the 326 studies showed some kind of biological effect from radiofrequency radiation, and 50% did not. But when he dug deeper, he found that studies independently conducted without corporate fundings were likely to find a biological effect (70% of these studies), as opposed to just 30% of the studies that were industry-funded (see Figure 12.3).[68] This is a common finding across issues relating to the struggle of corporate profits versus public health.[69]

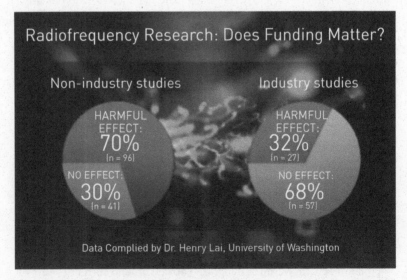

FIGURE 12.3 Slide showing funding-related biases for radiofrequency radiation safety studies; industry-funded studies show fewer results of biological harm than non-industry funded studies.

Non-Toxic

How Should We Handle Conflicting Data?

Once again, we need to utilize the precautionary principle to guide commonsense changes to improve health. "When an activity raises threats of harm to human health or the environment, precautionary measures should be taken, even if some cause and effect relationships are not fully established scientifically."[70] The data in Figure 12.3 also show that the industries involved in producing products that emit electromagnetic radiation have adopted the tobacco-industry strategy of funding fraudulent science (studies designed to fail), which is intended for use in future litigation and to result in increased industry profits at the expense of Use our health.

Therefore, with no expectation of help from US regulatory agencies, we should all harness the key tool for reducing harm caused by radiation: distance, distance, distance! The proximity to the body when we use cell phones, laptops, Bluetooth, and other technology, especially when children are using these MW/RF technologies, is key.[71] When you double the distance, the radiation level goes down by 4-fold. If you cut the distance between your body and the phone by half, it increases the radiation by 4-fold. Remember that radiation intensity decreases by a factor of distance squared. Distance is your friend! This is particulary true with regard to placement within the home of MW/RF devices in relation to where children sleep and play.

Key Safe Cell Phone, Tablet, and Computer Tips:

- Don't buy dumb stuff. The list of ridiculous tech toys that are now on the market or are set to launch is long. Take Bluetooth-controlled tampons, for instance, that let you know when they need to be changed, or Bluetooth-controlled pacifiers that will sound an alarm seconds before your baby does. Do we really need these products producing radiation from within the body? Avoidance is key to reducing any harmful exposure, and dumb tech products are no exception.
- Keep devices away from your body, particularly the head and reproductive organs (groin, breasts, abdomen). Choose landlines, wireless headphones (especially air tubes headsets), speakerphone, and texting options whenever possible, and keep calls short.
- Avoid wireless radiation exposure during pregnancy. Do not place your cell phone or computer on or near your pregnant belly.

- Do not attach your cell phone to your belt buckle, place in pants pockets, or carry it in your bra. The amount of radiation absorbed by the body drops dramatically even with a small amount of separation.
- Keep cell phones at least 8 inches from a cardiac pacemaker (don't carry your phone in your shirt chest pocket).
- Turn device onto "airplane mode" or "off" when carrying close to your body whenever possible and at night while sleeping.
- Text rather than talk. Phones emit less radiation when sending and receiving text messages than during voice calls, and texting keeps phones away from your head.
- Call only when the signal is strong (more signal bars on screen); fewer signal bars means the phone must try harder to broadcast its signal to/from the cell tower, which raises radiation levels. For the same reason, avoid calls in elevators and cars where the metal surroundings block the signal.
- Limit children's cell phone and tablet use whenever possible. Turn on "airplane mode" when children play games already downloaded to the phone or tablet.
- Avoid "radiation shields" such as phone cases, antennae caps, and keyboard covers, which reduce the connection quality and force the phone to transmit greater energy to connect with the device, generating more radiation.
- When looking at your phone, tablet, or computer screen for extended periods of time, use specialized glasses that block harmful blue light (blue blocker), to protect sensitive structures in the eyes (nerve cells in the retina).
- Adjust phone and computer screen using a "blue blocker" downloadable app that adjusts blue spectrum light emitted from digital devices, which can effect circadian rhythms and disrupts the human sleep/wake cycle.
- Take advantage of built-in screen time monitors that can track daily and weekly use of your phone, tablet, and other devices.
- Understand your tech radiation exposures beyond *personal* tech gadgets; for example, your WiFi use at work, in daycare centers and schools, hotels, and the required water and energy meters being implemented in homes to monitor usage. The hours of exposure may really add up!

Bottom Line

We all love our tech toys, but using them as infrequently as possible and using smart tools and behaviors to reduce exposure to radiation is the safest way to go.

Resources for Electromagnetic Field (EMF) Information

The Baby Safe Project: www.TheBabySafeProject.org
Environmental Heath Trust: www.EHTrust.org
Electronic Silent Spring www.electronicsilentspring.com
EUROPAEN EMF Guideline 2016 for the prevention, diagnosis, and treatment of
EMF-related health problems and illnesses (PDF): https://www.degruyter
.com/view/j/reveh.2016.31.issue-3/reveh-2016-0011/reveh-2016-0011.xml

EMF Scientist Appeal: https://emfscientist.org/index.php/emf-scientist- appeal
Electromagnetic Radiation Safety: https://www.saferemr.com

References

1. Hollander R. Two-thirds of the world's population are now connected by mobile
   devices. https://www.businessinsider.com/world-population-mobile-devices-
   2017-9. Published 2017. Accessed June 20, 2019.
2. Pew Research Center. Mobile fact sheet. Internet and technology web site.
   http://www.pewinternet.org/fact-sheet/mobile/. Published 2019. Updated June,
   2019. Accessed April 23, 2020.
3. Pew Research Center. Social media fact sheet. Internet and Technology web
   site. http://www.pewinternet.org/fact-sheet/social-media/. Published 2019.
   Accessed April 23, 2020.
4. Federal Communications Commission (FCC). Specific absorption rate (SAR)
   for cell phones: what it means for you. https://www.fcc.gov/consumers/guides/
   specific-absorption-rate-sar-cell-phones-what-it-means-you. Published 2017.
   Updated September 8, 2017. Accessed March 3, 2019.
5. McInerny T. Letter from the American Academy of Pediatrics to Commissioners
   of the US Federal Communications Commission regarding regulation of wireless technology. https://ecfsapi.fcc.gov/file/7520941318.pdf. Published 2013.
   Accessed April 23, 2020.
6. Morgan L, Miller AB, Davis DL. Why children absorb more microwave radiation than adults: the consequences. *Journal of Microscopy and Ultrastructure*.
   2014;2:197–204.
7. Joel Moskowitz. We have no reason to believe 5g is safe. https://blogs
   .scientificamerican.com/observations/we-have-no-reason-to-believe-5g-is-
   safe/. Published 2019. Accessed April 23, 2020.

8. International Agency for Research on Cancer (IARC). Press Release. http://www.iarc.fr/en/media-centre/pr/2011/pdfs/pr208_E.pdf. Published 2011. Accessed October 20, 2016.

9. Baan R, Grosse Y, Lauby-Secretan B, et al. Carcinogenicity of radiofrequency electromagnetic fields. *The Lancet Oncology.* 2011;12(7):624–626.

10. IARC. IARC Working group on the evaluation of carcinogenic risks to human, non-ionizing radiation, part 2: radiofrequency. http://monographs.iarc.fr/ENG/Monographs/vol102/mono102.pdf. Published 2013. Accessed April 24, 2020.

11. Davis D. 5G: The unreported global threat. Medium.com. 2019.

12. Kaszuba-Zwoinska J, Gremba J, Galdzinska-Calik B, Wojcik-Piotrowicz K, Thor PJ. Electromagnetic field induced biological effects in humans. *Przeglad lekarski.* 2015;72(11):636–641.

13. Van Huizen AV, Morton JM, Kinsey LJ, et al. Weak magnetic fields alter stem cell-mediated growth. *Science Advances.* 2019;5(1):eaau7201.

14. Yakymenko I, Tsybulin O, Sidorik E, Henshel D, Kyrylenko O, Kyrylenko S. Oxidative mechanisms of biological activity of low-intensity radiofrequency radiation. *Electromagnetic Biology and Medicine.* 2016;35(2):186–202.

15. Kostoff RN, Lau CGY. Combined biological and health effects of electromagnetic fields and other agents in the published literature. *Technol Forecast Soc Change.* 2013;80(7):1331–1349.

16. Gandhi OP, Morgan LL, de Salles AA, Han YY, Herberman RB, Davis DL. Exposure limits: the underestimation of absorbed cell phone radiation, especially in children. *Electromagnetic Biology and Medicine.* 2012;31(1):34–51.

17. Morgan RD. ML, Davis D. Children absorb higher doses of radio frequency Electtromagnetic radiation from mobile phones than adults. *IEEE.* 2015;3:2379–2387.

18. Fernandez-Rodriguez CE, Almeida De Salles AA, Davis DL. Dosimetric simulations of brain absorption of mobile phone radiation—the relationship between psSAR and age. *IEEE.* 2015;3:2425–2430.

19. Gandhi OMP, Lazzi G, Furse C. Electromagnetic absorption in the human head and neck for mobile telephones at 835 and 1900 MHz *IEEE.* 1996.

20. Christ A, Gosselin MC, Christopoulou M, Kuhn S, Kuster N. Age-dependent tissue-specific exposure of cell phone users. *Physics in Medicine and Biology.* 2010;55(7):1767–1783.

21. Ren Y, Chen J, Miao M, et al. Prenatal exposure to extremely low frequency magnetic field and its impact on fetal growth. *Environmental Health: A Global Access Science Source.* 2019;18(1):6.

22. Roosli M, Lagorio S, Schoemaker MJ, Schuz J, Feychting M. Brain and Salivary Gland tumors and mobile phone use: evaluating the evidence from various epidemiological study designs. *Annual Review of Public Health.* 2019.

23. Saili L, Hanini A, Smirani C, et al. Effects of acute exposure to WIFI signals (2.45GHz) on heart variability and blood pressure in Albinos rabbit. *Environ Toxicol Pharmacol.* 2015;40(2):600–605.

24. Deshmukh PS, Nasare N, Megha K, et al. Cognitive impairment and neurogenotoxic effects in rats exposed to low-intensity microwave radiation. *International Journal of Toxicology.* 2015;34(3):284–290.

25. Volkow ND, Tomasi D, Wang GJ, et al. Effects of cell phone radiofrequency signal exposure on brain glucose metabolism. *JAMA.* 2011;305(8):808–813.

26. Hutton JS, Dudley J, Horowitz-Kraus T, DeWitt T, Holland SK. Associations between screen-based media use and brain white matter integrity in preschool-aged children. *JAMA Pediatrics.* 2019:e193869.

27. Byun YH, Ha M, Kwon HJ, et al. Mobile phone use, blood lead levels, and attention deficit hyperactivity symptoms in children: a longitudinal study. *PLoS One.* 2013;8(3):e59742.

28. Hardell L, Carlberg M, Hansson Mild K. Use of mobile phones and cordless phones is associated with increased risk for glioma and acoustic neuroma. *Pathophysiology: The Official Journal of the International Society for Pathophysiology.* 2013;20(2):85–110.

29. Little MP, Rajaraman P, Curtis RE, et al. Mobile phone use and glioma risk: comparison of epidemiological study results with incidence trends in the United States. *BMJ (Clinical research ed).* 2012;344:e1147.

30. Hardell L, Carlberg M. Mobile phone and cordless phone use and the risk for glioma—Analysis of pooled case-control studies in Sweden, 1997-2003 and 2007-2009. *Pathophysiology: The Official Journal of the International Society for Pathophysiology.* 2015;22(1):1–13.

31. Hardell L, Carlberg M, Soderqvist F, Mild KH. Pooled analysis of case-control studies on acoustic neuroma diagnosed 1997-2003 and 2007-2009 and use of mobile and cordless phones. *International Journal of Oncology.* 2013;43(4):1036–1044.

32. Sato Y, Akiba S, Kubo O, Yamaguchi N. A case-case study of mobile phone use and acoustic neuroma risk in Japan. *Bioelectromagnetics.* 2011;32(2):85–93.

33. Smith-Roe SL WM, Stout MD, Winters JW. NTP Cell phone radiation study: final reports. https://www.saferemr.com/2018/11/NTP-final-reports31.html. Published 2019. Accessed April 23, 2020.

34. Moskowitz JM. Ramazzini Institute cell phone radiation study replicates NTP study. https://www.saferemr.com/2018/03/RI-study-on-cell-phone.html. Published 2018. Accessed April 23, 2020.

35. West JG, Kapoor NS, Liao SY, Chen JW, Bailey L, Nagourney RA. Multifocal breast cancer in young women with prolonged contact between their breasts and their cellular phones. *Case Rep Med.* 2013;2013:354682.

36. Sepehrimanesh M, Kazemipour N, Saeb M, Nazifi S, Davis DL. Proteomic analysis of continuous 900-MHz radiofrequency electromagnetic field exposure in testicular tissue: a rat model of human cell phone exposure. *Environmental Science and Pollution Research International*. 2017;24(15):13666–13673.

37. Hardell L, Carlberg M, Ohlson CG, Westberg H, Eriksson M, Hansson Mild K. Use of cellular and cordless telephones and risk of testicular cancer. *International Journal of Andrology*. 2007;30(2):115–122.

38. Hardell L, Eriksson M, Carlberg M, Sundstrom C, Hanson Mild K. Use of cellular or cordless telephones and the risk for non-Hodgkin's lymphoma. *International Archives of Occupational and Environmental Health*. 2005;78(8):625–632.

39. Levine H, Jorgensen N, Martino-Andrade A, et al. Temporal trends in sperm count: a systematic review and meta-regression analysis. *Human Reproduction Update*. 2017:1–14.

40. Adams JA, Galloway TS, Mondal D, Esteves SC, Mathews F. Effect of mobile telephones on sperm quality: a systematic review and meta-analysis. *Environ Int*. 2014;70:106–112.

41. Lewczuk B, Redlarski G, Zak A, Ziolkowska N, Przybylska-Gornowicz B, Krawczuk M. Influence of electric, magnetic, and electromagnetic fields on the circadian system: current stage of knowledge. *BioMed Research International*. 2014;2014:169459.

42. Divan HA, Kheifets L, Obel C, Olsen J. Cell phone use and behavioural problems in young children. *Journal of Epidemiology and Community Health*. 2012;66(6):524–529.

43. Sudan M, Kheifets L, Arah O, Olsen J, Zeltzer L. Prenatal and postnatal cell phone exposures and headaches in children. *The Open Pediatric Medicine Journal*. 2012;6(2012):46–52.

44. Pall ML. Microwave frequency electromagnetic fields (EMFs) produce widespread neuropsychiatric effects including depression. *Journal of Chemical Neuroanatomy*. 2016;75(Pt B):43–51.

45. Mohammadianinejad SE, Babaei M, Nazari P. The effects of exposure to low frequency electromagnetic fields in the treatment of migraine headache: a cohort study. *Electronic Physician*. 2016;8(12):3445–3449.

46. Lamech F. Self-reporting of symptom development from exposure to radiofrequency fields of wireless smart meters in Victoria, Australia: a case series. *Altern Ther Health Med*. 2014;20(6):28–39.

47. Samuel H. France to impose total ban on mobile phones in schools. https://www.telegraph.co.uk/news/2017/12/11/france-impose-total-ban-mobile-phones-schools/. Published 2017. Accessed March 4, 2019.

48. Kuhn S, Cabot E, Christ A, Capstick M, Kuster N. Assessment of the radio-frequency electromagnetic fields induced in the human body from

mobile phones used with hands-free kits. *Physics in Medicine and Biology.* 2009;54(18):5493–5508.

49. CIO. Opinion: Are truly wireless earbuds (like AirPods) safe? https://www.cio.com/article/3180345/are-truly-wireless-earbuds-like-airpods-safe.html. Published 2017. Accessed March 4, 2019.

50. Vannucci A, Flannery KM, Ohannessian CM. Social media use and anxiety in emerging adults. *Journal of Affective Disorders.* 2017;207:163–166.

51. Franchina V, Vanden Abeele M, van Rooij AJ, Lo Coco G, De Marez L. Fear of missing out as a predictor of problematic social media use and phubbing behavior among Flemish adolescents. *Int J Environ Res Public Health.* 2018;15(10).

52. Oxford Living Dictionaries. Phubbing. Oxford University Press. https://en.oxforddictionaries.com/definition/phubbing. Published 2019. Accessed March 1, 2019.

53. Hoge E, Bickham D, Cantor J. Digital media, anxiety, and depression in children. *Pediatrics.* 2017;140(Suppl 2):S76–s80.

54. Przybylski AK, Weinstein, N. Can you connect with me now? How the presence of mobile communication technology influences face-to-face conversation quality. *J Soc Pers Relat* 2013;30:237–246.

55. Huemer AK, Schumacher M, Mennecke M, Vollrath M. Systematic review of observational studies on secondary task engagement while driving. *Accident; Analysis and Prevention.* 2018;119:225–236.

56. Niu J, Wang X, Liu X, Wang D, Qin H, Zhang Y. Effects of mobile phone use on driving performance in a multiresource workload scenario. *Traffic Injury Prevention.* 2019:1–8.

57. McEvoy SP, Stevenson MR, McCartt AT, et al. Role of mobile phones in motor vehicle crashes resulting in hospital attendance: a case-crossover study. *BMJ (Clinical Research Ed).* 2005;331(7514):428.

58. Briskin JL, Bogg T, Haddad J. Lower trait stability, stronger normative beliefs, habitual phone use, and unimpeded phone access predict distracted college student messaging in social, academic, and driving contexts. *Frontiers in Psychology.* 2018;9:2633.

59. Linden PL, Endee LM, Flynn E, et al. High school student driving perceptions following participation in a distracted driving curriculum. *Health Promotion Practice.* 2019:1524839918824322.

60. Kim K, Ghimire J, Pant P, Yamashita E. Self-reported handheld device use while driving. *Accident; Analysis and Prevention.* 2019;125:106–115.

61. Gershon P, Sita KR, Zhu C, et al. Distracted driving, visual inattention, and crash risk among teenage drivers. *American Journal of Preventive Medicine.* 2019.

62. Wei FFY, Wang YK, Klausner M. Rethinking college students' self-regulation and sustained attention: does text messaging during class influence cognitive learning? *Commun Educ.* 2012(61):185–204.

63. Prabu D, Kim JH, Brickman JS, et al. Mobile phone distraction while studying. *New Media Soc* 2014;17:1661–1679.

64. Misra S, Cheng L, Genevie J, et al. The iPhone effect: the quality of in-person social interactions in the presence of mobile devices. *Environ Behav* 2014;48:275–298.

65. Courtemanche F, Labonte-LeMoyne E, Leger PM, et al. Texting while walking: an expensive switch cost. *Accident; Analysis and Prevention.* 2019;127:1–8.

66. Timmis MA, Bijl H, Turner K, Basevitch I, Taylor MJD, van Paridon KN. The impact of mobile phone use on where we look and how we walk when negotiating floor based obstacles. *PLoS One.* 2017;12(6):e0179802.

67. EMFscientist.org. International EMF scientist appeal. https://emfscientist .org/index.php/emf-scientist-appeal. Published 2019. Accessed November 21, 2019.

68. Ishisaka N. UW Scientist Henry Lai makes waves in the cell phone industry. https://www.seattlemag.com/article/uw-scientist-henry-lai-makes-waves-cell-phone-industry. Published 2011. Accessed February 25, 2019.

69. Oreskes N, Conway EM. *Merchants of Doubt: How a Handful of Scientists Obscured the Truth on Issues from Tobacco Smoke to Climate Change.* New York: Bloomsbury; 2012.

70. deFur PL, Kaszuba M. Implementing the precautionary principle. *The Science of the Total Environment.* 2002;288(1–2):155–165.

71. Szmigielski S. Cancer risks related to low-level RF/MW exposures, including cell phones. *Electromagnetic Biology and Medicine.* 2013;32(3):273–280.

13

Detoxification Methods That Work

Everyone has a doctor in him or her; we just have to help it in its work. The natural healing force within each one of us is the greatest force in getting well.
> —Hippocrates, ancient Greek physician,
> "Father of Medicine" (c. 460–c. 370 BC)

A s you have read throughout the previous chapters, environmental chemicals and radiation are pervasive and have far-reaching known and, of course, still unknown effects on our health. To recap, there are more than 90,000 chemicals in use, and the great majority lack third-party (i.e., independent) or any testing for safety, especially when it comes to safety during pregnancy and in infants, children, and other vulnerable groups, such as those with compromised immune systems. With the cheap cost of plastic and chemical production, no legislative oversight or safety testing, and inefficient waste management causing widespread human and wildlife contamination, it appears that there may be no happy ending to this pollution story any time soon. This is not necessarily so, although it will require work to educate and empower ourselves to make smart choices. These choices include purchasing non-toxic products, making lifestyle changes that help rid the body of toxic chemicals (such as improved sleep, increased exercise, eating and drinking clean food and water), and harnessing the body's innate detoxifying mechanisms that have evolved over millions of years. Despite exposure to thousands of un-regulated chemicals found in everyday stuff that we eat, drink, store food in, lather on, and breathe in, and in the medications we take, there are plenty of reasonable, inexpensive, no-brainer ways to reduce, and even help eliminate, toxins in our bodies.

Problems with Chemical Testing for Environmental Chemicals

Testing your body for harmful environmental chemicals has many challenges, particularly testing for chemicals that are not persistent.

1. These biomonitoring studies are very expensive, and finding information on exposures specific to your body is not easily accomplished, particularly for a non-persistent chemical, results of which for an individual may vary from hour-to-hour and day-to-day, depending on the source of exposure, the length of the exposure, and how long a specific chemical may linger in the body. If methods existed to measure all of the chemicals used in every product, we predict that the number of man-made chemicals that would be detected in our bodies could easily number in the thousands.

2. Some exposures, like eating or drinking from an aluminum can lined with bisphenol A (BPA), are brief compared with persistent organic pollutants (POPs). BPA has a half-life (the time it takes for half of the initial amount to be metabolized) of approximately 6-8 hours when consumed in food. However, when BPA is absorbed through the skin from a thermal receipt coated with it, the BPA lasts in the body for over a week. This shows the complexity of trying to estimate exposures even to a single chemical that is not persistent. Chemicals that remain in the body for years would not be expected to show the day-to-day variability seen when measuring non-persistent chemicals such as BPA.[1]

3. Most clinical lab facilities have the capacity to test only a handful of the several thousand chemicals that can cause harm (via a certified assay). The lack of availability of reagents needed to accurately measure most chemicals has led to the use of *indirect* assay methods that have been shown to lead to inaccurate data.[2]
4. Specialty labs, such as Doctors Data, Genova Diagnostics, and Great Plains Laboratory (see appendix 4) are capable of testing for a broader array of harmful environmental chemicals, but the tests are often not covered by conventional health insurance, and can be quite costly, especially if repeat or serial testing is recommended to monitor blood or urine chemical levels over time. Additionally, the certification requirements and oversight in place for clinical laboratories that measure substances that are part of a routine medical screen (e.g., blood levels of sugar, insulin, white blood cells) do not exist for these "boutique" chemical analysis laboratories—which, in addition to being expensive, may or may not provide patients with accurate information.
5. Interpretation of lab assay results can vary between laboratories and practitioners, particularly if the reviewer has not obtained a thorough environmental health/exposure history from the client. Understanding the biomonitoring data collected requires one to be well versed in the properties of the various chemicals being measured, such as their specific health effects, how long the chemical stays in the body, how a person might have been exposed, and ways to reduce exposure. Environmental medicine is generally not taught in medical schools and requires special postgraduate training (such as that received by author AC). An understanding of the reasons for and the likelihood of a "false positive" result (reporting finding something *not* really there), or reasons for a "false negative" result (reporting not finding something that *is* really there) are also important—all assays have false positive and false negative rates.

Important Takeaway

Routine testing for harmful chemicals is not readily available, and concern over exposures often leads to tremendous worry and sleepless nights. If you are having health problems that may be linked to a specific exposure (for example, new-onset numbness of fingers and toes due to heavy-metal exposure), then discuss this with your primary care doctor to help locate a healthcare provider with the required training and expertise. A request to be tested for reasonable exposures may be warranted if your provider is confident in the ultimate accuracy of the results. Making behavioral changes to reduce the daily body load of known toxic chemicals, as we will discuss in this chapter, should be the primary goal, not costly repetitive screening that may create more questions than answers, and worst of all, may not be accurate.

Avoiding Toxins Is Key: Look to the Precautionary Principle

As discussed in detail in chapter 1, the Precautionary Principle states: "When an activity raises threats of harm to human health or the environment, precautionary measures should be taken even if some cause and effect relationship are not fully established scientifically."[3] In other words, "An ounce of prevention is worth a pound of cure," "Better safe than sorry," and "Look before you leap." Using this principle to guide decisions can be the simplest, most effective way to reduce exposure to harmful environmental toxins. The key point is that we need to act and make reasonable changes, even in the face of uncertainty or without all of the evidence currently required by regulatory agencies. The following recommendations are based on all of the available science, and draw upon the wisdom of the precautionary principle.

Avoid It!

- The smartest and most cost-effective way to reduce exposure to any chemical is not to buy it and/or bring it into your life, right? For example, thousands of potentially toxic chemicals, found in cleaning products, can be avoided altogether by not buying the products in the first place.
- How about pesticides? If you don't buy bug spray, these neurotoxic chemicals are less likely to find their way into the pets and the humans living in your home. Do not spray your yard with herbicides. Insecticide and herbicide use becomes an urgent issue if there is a pregnant woman and/or children in the home (these are also dangerous for pets). Find better ways to get rid of pests, such as putting food away after eating, wiping up spills, and dusting/vacuuming up crumbs. Wipe countertops with white vinegar mixed with real lemon juice, which naturally disinfects and also keeps insects away.

- Laundry detergents are filled with chemicals, and so are fabric softeners (who came up with them anyway?). Purchasing fragrance-free laundry products will keep phthalates and other endocrine disruptors off of skin, and exposures through inhalation will be reduced.
- When it comes to avoiding chemicals in food, stick with whole, unprocessed foods, wash off and soak produce to remove toxic pesticides, cut fat from meat and poultry (fat is where chemicals are stored), remove skin (where the fat is) from fish, and use glass and stainless steel to cook and store food to avoid chemicals leaching into the food from plastics!

Use Less Stuff

- The fewer products one uses on a regular basis, the less likely harmful chemicals will get into your body. For example, using fewer products such as body sprays, lotions, hair gel, after shave, and perfumes correlates with fewer chemicals being found in the urine and blood of those tested (see chapter 8).[4]

Make It Yourself or Buy Cleaner Products

- Make your own personal care and cleaning products (see chapters 8 and 9), or simply look up safer cleaning and personal care products on the websites of vetted groups made up of trained scientists to sort this all out. Some examples:
  Websites: EWG.org, EWG.org/Skindeep
  Apps: Healthy Living, Think Dirty
- More and more studies show that when we use *safer* products, levels of many harmful chemicals drop in the urine and blood of those tested. The Hermosa Study showed a reduction in phthalate, paraben, and phenol exposure in 100 Latina girls who changed out their personal care products to safer options over a 3-day period![5]

Be Proactive about Removing Chemicals

- Whether or not an exposure has occurred for days, weeks, years, or even decades, an adult body has evolved clever ways to reduce and eliminate many of the toxic substances that get into it. Children's bodies, however, are less capable of removing harmful chemicals because their detoxification systems are not fully mature.

- Endocrine disrupting chemicals are a unique category of environmental pollutants that can "trick" the body into thinking that they are hormones produced in your body or they can act like drugs that block hormone production or action. At very low exposures not previously studied by toxicologists in regulatory agencies, numerous EDCs have been shown to interfere with multiple parts of the human endocrine system, such as thyroid, estrogen, and androgen hormone function.

Dietary Removal of Chemicals

Cruciferous Vegetables

- Using the detox properties of many foods is a brilliant way to reduce the amount of chemicals circulating in our bodies. Remember, humans have evolved for millions of years by eating whole foods, such as produce, so why not stick close to foods appropriate for our genetic template? Cruciferous vegetables, for instance (see Box 13.1),

---

Box 13.1

+ Cruciferous Vegetables

- Cabbage
- Chinese cabbage
- Broccoli
- Kohlrabi
- Brussels sprouts
- Turnip greens
- Mustard greens
- Collard greens
- Watercress
- Land cress
- Shepherd's purse
- Cauliflower
- Bok choy
- Kale
- Daikon radish
- Oriental radish
- Horseradish
- Arugula
- Wasabi
- Rutabaga
- Turnip

are a group of vegetables from the Brassicaceae family that have the unique ability to stimulate liver enzymes that are responsible for breaking down harmful chemicals.[6] Along with other nutrients such as folic acid, vitamin C, phytochemicals, carotenoids, calcium, and fiber, brassica vegetables contain large amounts of sulfur-containing compounds called glucosinolates, which may be responsible for their strong detoxification properties. Sulphoraphane is a naturally occurring compound found in cruciferous vegetables; it causes the most efficient part of liver detoxification (phase II conjugation) to "rev up," thereby increasing enzymes that have anti-cancer properties.[7] Indole-3-carbinol (I3C), a natural anti-cancer compound, and DIM (diindolylmethane) are also found in cruciferous veggies. Both of these important compounds have been shown to increase the ratio of the "good" form of estrogen metabolites (2-hydroxyestrogen) to the more harmful form (16α-hydroxyestrogen), reducing the risk of developing estrogen-related cancers, such as breast, prostate, and ovarian cancers.[8,9,10] Try to buy fresh or (cheaper) frozen organic cruciferous vegetables whenever possible, and soak non-organic cruciferous veggies in warm, clean water and baking soda or with a mixture of 1 part white vinegar to 4 parts warm, clean water, to help remove pesticide residue, otherwise you defeat the purpose.

Nutrient "Sufficiency"

Preventing health effects from environmental toxins thus not only involves avoidance of chemicals in various foods, but *also* requires intake of appropriate nutrients that may counteract the harmful effects of chemicals. When humans are nutrient sufficient, they are also better equipped to handle toxin exposures. For example, consider folic acid, a water-soluble B vitamin also known as folate or vitamin B_9. Folic acid is commonly found in most green leafy vegetables and has been shown to offset the damaging effects of BPA in exposed offspring.[11] It is likely that folic acid counteracts other environmental chemical exposures, but this has not been investigated. Omega-3 fatty acids, which are found in fish, eggs, nuts, oils, chia and flax seeds, and leafy greens, offset the toxic effects of BPA, lead, mercury, and dioxin, according to both human and animal studies.[12,13,14,15]

Iodine is also beneficial in reducing risk of toxic chemicals. Appropriate iodine supplementation during pregnancy and while nursing can offset the effects of various environmental pollutants such as nitrate, thiocy-anate, and perchlorate, all of which can disrupt normal thyroid func-tion and thus affect fetal brain development and cognition.[16] Quercetin, an antioxidant flavonoid found in apples and onions, has been shown to be protective against PCBs and methylmercury in animal studies.[17,18] Children with sufficient intake of iron, calcium, and vitamin C absorb less lead, [19,20,21,22] and studies found that children who were iron deficient were more likely to absorb cadmium, which is associated with adverse health effects.[23,24]

To make sure you're nutritionally "sufficient," eat a broad diet filled with good fats (omega-3 fatty acids), green leafy vegetables, a variety of fresh or frozen produce in a variety of colors, and also take a reputable, third-party tested, clean (no coloring, preservatives, fillers, etc.) daily multivitamin that contains adequate iodine (150 micrograms, as potassium iodide) and B vitamins, especially if you are pregnant or breast feeding.[25] In addition to routine laboratory testing, have vitamin and mineral levels (including vitamins D, B12, and folic acid; zinc; selenium; urine iodine; complete blood count for iron deficiency) checked by a healthcare practitioner who can in-terpret the results and make reasonable recommendations.

Filtered Drinking Water

As mentioned in chapter 5, water is also essential for flushing toxins from the body, and as long as it is filtered to reduce harmful contaminants, it remains a critical tool for cleaning the body. How much filtered water (not bottled water, which is likely not filtered and is unregulated) should we be drinking? The National Academies of Sciences, Engineering, and Medicine says that the adequate amount of fluid intake for men is 15.5 cups (3.0 liters) of fluids per day, and 11.5 cups (2.2 liters) for women. About 20% of this daily fluid intake comes from food (as an extreme ex-ample, watermelon and spinach are close to 99% water by weight).[26] If you are pregnant and breast feeding, you will require an even higher daily water intake.[27] Those who live in hot, dry climates; exercise regularly; or are experiencing vomiting and/or diarrhea, are prone to kidney stones or blood clots, should also increase their fluid intake. The take-home mes-sage is that the lack of adequate hydration can cause significant health problems. Remember to carry your filtered water in glass or stainless steel to avoid exposure to plastic chemicals that would leach into your water from reusable plastic water bottles, or you defeat the purpose of filtering your water.

Exercise

Exercise serves many important roles in human physiology: maintaining muscle strength and tone, aiding new bone development, cooling the body through sweating, and increasing the release of serotonin (the "feel-good" neurotransmitter). Sweating and burning fat from fat cells (which store many of the lipophilic or "fat-loving" toxic chemicals) also leads to toxin removal. During aerobic exercise, blood flow increases to the liver, which helps churn up detoxification activity, including an increase in anti-cancer (antioxidant) enzymes and an important detoxification chemical, gluta-thione, in both the liver and lungs. Sweating from physical exercise has been shown to help eliminate lipophilic chemicals such as BPA, PCBs, perfluorinated compounds (used for water-proof and "nonstick" products), and heavy metals.[28–32]

Saunas and Sweating

An enjoyable way to eliminate toxic chemicals from the body is to sweat them out using sauna therapy. In addition to the many health benefits of sauna therapy, such as reducing stress, lowering blood pressure, decreasing pain levels, and increasing feelings of vitality; traditional dry sauna or steam sauna bathing is quite effective in driving toxic chemicals out of the body.[33] For people with severe arthritis of any kind, who have limited ability to move, regular sauna use can be a wonderful way to help detoxify the body.

How does it work? The traditional sauna heats up an enclosed space to a temperatures as high as 160–200 degrees F (70–90 degrees C) with 25% humidity; in comparison, steam rooms are typically heated to 120–130 degrees F at 100% humidity. In response to the heat, blood flow increases to the skin to cool the skin surface down through sweating (evaporative cooling), which also releases excess minerals, water, and toxins onto the skin surface. Studies have shown that people exposed to high levels of heavy metals, industrial chemicals (PCBs, solvents, flame retardants), nonstick and water proof chemicals, airborne chemicals, and even drug overdoses, showed marked health improvements after sauna therapy.[32,34,35] But be sure to replenish loss of trace minerals such as sodium, potassium, and zinc, which are also released into sweat, especially when using a sauna daily or multiple times per week. A great way to do this is by creating a drink (in glass or stainless steel) that has approximately 3 ounces of real juice (for flavor), approximately 17 ounces of clean, filtered water, and a few "turns" of sea salt from a grinder; unprocessed sea salt is filled with important electrolytes and minerals (potassium, chloride, magnesium, and sodium) that are lost during exercise and sweating. You've just made non-toxic Gatorade!

*** It is important to check with your doctor before using sauna therapy or engaging in heavy exercise. Caution should always be undertaken when sauna or steam therapy is considered, particularly if you have a history of heart failure, heart attack, stroke, lung disease (COPD, emphysema), multiple sclerosis or other diseases, or if you are pregnant.[33,36] Never stay in a sauna more than 30 minutes, and hydrate with water (or your own home-made, chemical-free Gatorade, see detox recipes in Appendix 1) both before and after sauna therapy. Hydration is key to avoiding problems.

An alternative for those who cannot tolerate the high temperatures of sauna or steam therapy is the use of infrared sauna (IR), which heats the body while the surrounding temperature remains relatively cool. Infrared saunas, in general, vary by manufacturer, materials, and by wavelength of the radiation emitted. Near-infrared saunas are capable of penetrating deeper below the skin surface, up to 4 cm, without increasing the skin temperature significantly, whereas middle and far-infrared saunas are absorbed mostly in the outermost layers of the skin and increase skin temperature significantly.

Although the type of infrared sauna used (near vs. far) was not specified, studies looking at rheumatoid arthritis, ankylosing spondylitis, and Sjogren's syndrome patients have shown improvement of symptoms with regular use.[37-39] In congestive heart failure (CHF) patients, far-infrared sauna may be beneficial because of the increased release of nitric oxide (NO) into the blood vessels, causing blood vessels to widen and improving blood flow.[39] Another study showed improved quality of life in people with type II diabetes mellitus who used infrared sauna regularly. In Japan and Korea infrared sauna, called Waon therapy, is used extensively, particularly in cardiac care.[40-46]

***Use caution with infrared sauna therapy: the temperature of the skin can increase to more than 104 degrees F (40 degress C) under direct IR irradiation, and regular use may lead to premature skin aging and impaired function, including potentially skin cancer. Pregnant women and those with active infections, a history of skin cancer (or those at high risk for developing skin cancer) should avoid infrared sauna therapy.[47,48]

Sleep

Most of us understand that good quality *and* quantity of sleep are important for our day-to-day ability to function. There are studies showing that the majority of US teenagers are not getting the recommended amount of sleep (see Table 13.1).[49,50] After a bad night's sleep, we might feel groggy, lethargic, and even emotional, especially if we have a bunch of chores or work to do. But, if we experience ongoing sleep deprivation, we can be at increased risk for developing a whole host of medical conditions, including high blood pressure, weight gain, diabetes, elevated cholesterol levels, and even Alzheimer's disease. On the flip side, restful sleep can "reset" our brains and make us feel sharp, energized, and motivated.

Did you know that sleep also plays a vital role in detoxifying our body and especially our brain? Researchers discovered that the human brain has a system similar to the lymphatic system known as the glymphatic system, which helps to clear waste products and toxins from fluid in and around brain cells.[51] At night, we clear harmful chemicals from this fluid, so getting a good

Table 13.1 Recommended Amount of Sleep per Night by Age Group.[52]

Age	Recommended Amount of Sleep
Newborns	16-18 hours a day
Preschool-aged children	11-12 hours a day
School-aged children	At least 10 hours a day
Teens	9-10 hours a day
Adults (including the elderly)	7-8 hours a day

Source: NIH, National Heart, Lung, and Blood Institute

quality and quantity of sleep has even more significance than just a restful night's sleep. Here are some important tips to help improve *your* sleep.

Create a routine: Try to maintain a regular sleep-wake schedule, including on weekends, allowing for 7 to 8 hours of sleep for adults, 9 to 10 hours for teens, and at least 10 hours per night for school-aged children (Table 13.1).

Limit screen time. Turn off your computer, smartphone, and tablet 60 minutes prior to sleep time. Dim your computer light or use blue-blocker apps to restrict exposure to these wavelengths 1 to 2 hours before sleep, to reduce brain stimulation from screen light.

Create a comfortable sleep environment. Keep your bedroom cool, between 65 and 70 degrees, block out all light from windows, under doorways, and from digital clocks, or use an eye mask. Any light can stimulate the pineal gland of the brain, which is how the body recognizes it is time to get up.

Exercise daily. This facilitates the body's natural desire for sleep.

Limit use of sleep medications and stimulants. Many sleeping medications (e.g., Benadryl) and alcohol actually worsen sleep by shortening the most restful sleep period, also called stage 4 or rapid eye movement (REM) sleep. Many sleep medications can also create dependency and require increasing doses. Try to limit alcohol use, particularly after dinner, reduce foods and drinks with caffeine, and stop caffeine intake at least 8-10 hours before sleep time, due to its ability to circulate throughout the body for many hours (the initial half-life—50% cleared from blood—is about 6 hours for caffeine).[53]

Reduce stress. Give daily relaxation routines a try, such as 4-7-8 breathing (4-second inhalation through nose, 7-second hold, 8-second exhalation through the mouth) along with guided meditation (e.g., smartphone apps such as Relax and Rest, Calm, Simply Being, Zen, Insight Timer) and journaling, which is the act of writing down ideas and feelings to "unload" the mind from distraction and allow for stress relief.

Reduce unnecessary chemicals in your sleeping area. Change out your mattress and any bedding made with synthetic materials (polyester, rayon, etc.) with 100% cotton materials and avoid bedding labeled "wrinkle-free" as it is often treated with formaldehyde and other chemicals. Improve bedroom air quality by reducing "off-gassing" of synthetic furnishings, walls, carpeting or vinyl floors. Add a high-efficiency particulate air (HEPA) filtration system, and encourage the addition into the bedroom of ordinary houseplants (e.g., spider plants, peace lilies, areca palm, mother-in-law's tongue, money plant). Consider removing sources of electromagnetic fields from the bedroom (television, stereo, alarm clocks, lamps, etc.) as their emission of electromagnetic radiation suppresses your innate ability to release melatonin.[54,55] Consider replacing your plug-in alarm clock with a battery operated version.

Supplement use for sleep (Preferably, used on a short-term basis):

- **Melatonin.** A dose of 0.3–5 mg orally or sublingually (i.e., under the tongue, for very rapid effect) at bedtime can be used, especially for patients with associated circadian rhythm disorder and for jet lag. A time-release formulation is often most effective due to peak concentration of about 4 hours in short-acting formulations. A low-dose 2 mg SR (slow release) formulation, has been approved in Europe for those over 55 years of age. Take the SR formulation 2 hours *before* bedtime, not at bedtime.

- **Valerian.** For adults: 300 to 900 mg standardized extract of 0.8% valerenic acids or as crude root at a dose of 2 to 3 g steeped for 10 to 15 minutes and taken 30 to 60 minutes before bedtime for 2 to 4 weeks to assess effectiveness. Tea preparations are not very tasty, making adherence an issue. Also, it smells horrible, so look for closed capsules and seal the lid.

- **Magnesium.** Magnesium glycinate, citrate, or magnesium carbonate tablets or powder, 200–400 mg at night, 30–45 minutes prior to bedtime. Other types of magnesium may cause diarrhea or stomach upset (avoid magnesium products in patients with kidney problems and discuss with your doctor).

- **Aromatherapy.** Pure, organic, nonsynthetic oils, such as lavender (Lavandula angustifolia) can be effective for improving sleep quality/hygiene.[56] Rub a small amount on your forearm before bedtime or place onto bedding for a more restful night sleep.

***If you have any of the following conditions, which can contribute to poor sleep quality and quantity, talk to your healthcare provider to test and treat appropriately: chronic pain, abuse of alcohol and drugs, snoring, high blood pressure, restless leg syndrome, severe anxiety/depression, trauma or posttraumatic stress disorder, heavy metal exposure, history of head injury, or seizure disorder.

Air Quality

Clean up the air you breathe with just a few simple changes. Start by not buying air fresheners, "plug-ins," synthetic candles and incense, carpet powders, and products with fragrances (cosmetics, body sprays, aerosol sprays, laundry products).

Do not smoke cigarettes, or if you cannot quit, at least stop smoking indoors or where smoke can affect others (second-hand smoke affects kids, the elderly, and pets). Remember that chemicals from smoke will land on surfaces (third-hand smoke), which can be absorbed through the skin if touched, so smoking while no one else is at home can still cause harm to others and, of course, to you.

Home furnishings, including couches and furniture made with particle board, may contain chemicals that can off-gas into the air, such as formaldehyde, heavy metals, flame-retardant chemicals, and toxins in glue, also known as volatile organic compounds (VOCs). Before buying household furnishings, call the manufacturer to find out if these harmful chemicals are used in production. See resources for buying safer home furnishings in chapter 11.

Use indoor paints that are "VOC-Free," open windows while painting, and use a protective face mask and body covering when handling any paint thinners, paint strippers, or other industrial chemicals.

For those who commute on heavily trafficked roads, engine fumes containing pollutants such as ozone, benzene, mercury, dioxins, and furans can be overwhelming and cause increased risk for headache, COPD, and asthma exacerbation. Avoid automobile exhaust by closing the car's air vents and switch to recirculating interior air using the "recirculate" button (see Figure 13.1), thereby blocking outside air from entering the interior of the car.[57] Plug-in air filters for automobiles are also available commercially. Limit engine idling whenever possible.

Using a quality air purifier in your home or workplace will help reduce indoor fine particulate matter (particles with diameter less than 2.5 μm; $PM_{2.5}$). The purifier should meet high-efficiency particulate air or HEPA filter standards, which state that 99.7% of particles greater than 0.3 μm in size are removed.[58] Check your HVAC system regularly, and change the filter regularly (check them weekly so that you know when they need to be changed). Air filters have a minimum efficiency reporting value (MERV rating) to assess the effectiveness of filters. The MERV rating (from 1 to 16) identifies the size of the particles trapped; the higher the MERV rating, the greater the percentage of particles captured with each pass of air.

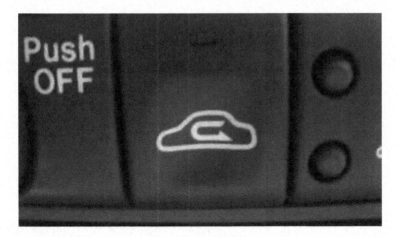

Figure 13.1 Automobile recirculate button.

Check with a certified HVAC professional to see which MERV rated filter is best for your space.

Opening windows daily to circulate fresh air is ideal, particularly in a modern house that allows minimal infiltration of outside air. However, in some environments with high dust levels, such as a house on an unpaved country road or near a freeway with heavy exhaust pollution, this could increase indoor dust or VOC levels and is not advisable. Vacuum weekly for dust removal using a vacuum with a HEPA filter; dust contains an enormous amount of harmful chemicals.[59] The presence in the house of a pet that sheds hair necessitates cleaning more frequently.

Resources

The EPA website https://airnow.gov/ allows you to check air quality index forecast and alerts by zip code.

EPA smartphone app: Air Now

American Lung Association smartphone app: State of Air

Safe Supplements for Detoxification

Many herbal and nutritional supplements have been found to increase elimination of various toxic substances from the human body. Surveys indicate that about 20% of Americans use at least one herbal supplement, and at least 25% of herbal supplement users also take one or more prescription drugs, raising the potential for herb-drug interactions.[60,61] This is important because, unlike prescription drugs, herbal supplements are completely unregulated, so these interactions have likely not been studied. Patients with chronic illnesses use more medications and herbal supplements than the general population, further increasing the risk of medication-supplement interactions.[62,63]

The purity of nutritional and herbal supplements raises particular issues. One recent study presented in *JAMA* revealed the enormous number of unapproved pharmaceutical ingredients making their way into dietary supplements sold across the United States.[64] In addition, herbal supplements from Southeast Asia and China have been found to contain molds, fungi, insects, pesticides, and heavy metals, often due to poor sourcing and manufacturing processes.[65] There is virtually zero oversight in the inspection and testing of supplements and cooking spices produced overseas. These products often contain contaminants such as powdered metals (lead, cadmium, and mercury) to increase the weight of the product, which in turn increases the selling price. Children and adults around the world are unknowingly exposed to these toxic ingredients, believing that they're making *healthy* choices by taking the supplement. The United States can be seen as the "Wild West" when it comes to regulating supplements.

Prebiotics and Probiotics

Humans have been living symbiotically with bacteria for millions of years. Human intestines harbor a very large collection of microscopic "bugs" or microbes—between 10 trillion and 100 trillion organisms. Until recently, medical science had largely ignored this intricate microscopic world, which we now know plays an integral role in maintaining normal human physiology and function.

New research has shown the value of probiotic supplementation for reversal and prevention of a whole host of human illnesses, including type 1 diabetes, ADHD, *Clostridium difficile* infection, bowel diseases (Crohn's disease, irritable bowel syndrome or IBS, ulcerative colitis), and obesity. During and after antibiotic treatment, for instance, the addition of prebiotic ("food" for the bacteria) and probiotic foods (see Box 13.2) may counterbalance the indiscriminate loss of beneficial bacteria. Probiotics are living microorganisms intended to replace or supplement the gut microbiome. Chronic use of both over-the-counter and prescription medications has been discovered to "kill off" good bacteria strains as well (see chapter 6), and it may take up to a full year to restore them in the gut.[66]

Probiotics have been studied as potential detoxification tools for many substances, including heavy metals, BPA, and PCBs.[67] The most commonly studied probiotics include *Lactobacillus rhamnosus* GG, *Lactobacillus reuteri*, *Saccharomyces boulardii*, and various strains of *Bifidobacterium*;

Box 13.2

+ Prebiotic

- Onions
- Jerusalem artichokes
- Garlic leeks
- Leeks
- Bananas
- Jicama
- Chicory root
- Burdock root
- Asparagus
- Dandelion greens
- Peas
- Eggplant
- Chinese chives
- Soybeans
- Sugar maple
- Yogurt, cottage cheese kefir
- Breast milk

Probiotic

- Sauerkraut
- Yogurt
- Kimchi
- Kombucha
- Kefir
- Tempeh
- Breast milk

---

they are commonly used for generalized bowel health and for treatment of irritable bowel syndrome and diarrhea, and they are readily available in most pharmacies.

Glutathione and N-Acetyl-Cysteine

Glutathione (GSH) is an important compound found in all human tissues. Besides maintaining normal functions of the cell, GSH is capable of detoxifying many harmful industrial chemicals that get into the body, as well as monitoring the genes that oversee the growth and death of cancer cells. Glutathione is not available in a supplement form such as a pill that can be absorbed by the body, but it can be taken by intravenous administration.

N-acetyl-cysteine (or NAC), on the other hand, is the "precursor" of glutathione, which means that when NAC is eaten in food or taken as a supplement, it can increase glutathione production. NAC has the ability to repair lung damage in smokers, repair liver damage from Tylenol overdose in animal experiments,[68,69,70] and increase detoxification enzymes in the liver.[71] Food sources of N-acetyl-cysteine include whey protein—as long as the product is not heated or blended, which can change its structure so that it becomes ineffective. In healthy people, use of NAC in supplement form, ranging from 100 to 400 mg daily, can safely be used for counteracting routine chemical exposures and thus for detoxification.

Milk Thistle

Milk thistle (*Silybum marinum*) is an herb that has historically been used to treat liver and gallbladder disorders. It was famously found to counteract the poisonous effects from eating the Amanita mushroom found in many parts of the world.[72] Silymarin, a flavonoid compound in milk thistle, similar to quercetin, genistein, and polyphenols in green tea,[73] is capable of modulating the detoxification system (cytochrome P450, which is a class of enzymes) in the liver to increase the breakdown of many harmful chemicals, especially many known to cause cancer.

Studies have shown milk thistle to have positive effects on acute poisonings, including by organic solvents,[74] to improve liver damage from chronic hepatitis B and C infection, and to protect drinkers from alcoholic liver disease.[75] An increasing number of studies reveal its benefit in protecting the liver from the side effects of cancer treatment.[76] Flavonoids, such as those found in milk thistle, have been shown to have antibacterial, anti-viral, anti-inflammatory, anti-cancer, pain relief, anti-allergy, liver-protective, and both estrogen-promoting and -reducing properties (compounds that can have both effects are not uncommon). The German Commission E, one of the longest-standing authorities on the safe use of herbal therapies, currently recommends the use of milk thistle for abdominal complaints, toxin-induced liver damage, end-stage liver disease, and as a supportive therapy for chronic inflammatory liver conditions.[77] Although it is generally well tolerated, milk thistle can have laxative effects. Additional research is needed before high dose daily use is recommended for prevention of chemical exposure, but safe dosing for liver health is 250 mg once or twice daily (of an extract standardized to provide 80% silymarin).[78]

Diindolylmethane

Diindolylmethane (DIM for short) is a phytonutrient found in cruciferous vegetables including broccoli, brussels sprouts, cabbage, cauliflower, and kale (see "Cruciferous Vegetables" earlier in this chapter). Unlike other plant nutrients, such as soy isoflavones (that have known endocrine-disrupting effects in infants), DIM has unique hormonal benefits. It supports the activity of enzymes that improve breakdown of estrogen and increases the level of "favorable" estrogens (2-hydroxyestrone) while reducing the level of "less-favorable" estrogens (16-α-hydroxyestrone). Given the variability of regular vegetable intake for most busy people, DIM is a useful—yet costly—supplement when a bowl of broccoli isn't handy. DIM can be used safely at doses of 100–200 mg daily.

Resources to Learn More about Herb-Drug Interactions

Herb, Nutrient, and Drug Interactions: Clinical Implications and Therapeutic Strategies, by Mitchell Bebel Stargrove, Jonathan Treasure, and Dwight L. McKee (Mosby, 2007)

Memorial Sloan Kettering Cancer Center: About Herbs, Botanicals & Other Products: https://www.mskcc.org/cancer-care/treatments/symptom-management/integrative-medicine/herbs

---

Mayo Clinic: Drugs and Supplements http://www.mayoclinic.org/drugs-supplements

National Institutes of Health, National Center for Complementary and Integrative Health: Herbs at a Glance: https://nccih.nih.gov/health/herbsataglance.htm

Cleveland Clinic: Herbal Supplements: Helpful or Harmful: http://my.clevelandclinic.org/services/heart/prevention/emotional-health/holistic-therapies/herbal-supplements

Natural Medicines Comprehensive Database: http://naturaldatabase.therapeuticresearch.com/home.aspx?cs=&s=ND

Fasting

Weight loss accomplished via periodic fasting, also known as intermittent fasting, has many benefits for overall health and longevity. Besides its ability to improve cell function, repair or remove molecules damaged by "oxidative stress" and aging, and reduce inflammation at the cellular level, intermittent fasting can also be used for weight loss.[79-84] On the flip side, because fat (adipose) tissue is the storage site for fat-soluble toxic chemicals such as BPA, weight loss can cause increased blood levels of harmful chemicals as they are released from the organs where they are stored, such as fat. In one study, researchers measured levels of chlorinated pesticides in adults undergoing either a calorie-restricted diet or stomach-stapling surgery; they found that the greater the weight loss, the greater the increase of pesticide levels in the blood, at least over the short term.[85] Reasonable intermittent fasting protocols for *healthy individuals* include not eating after dinner for a 10–18 hour period, either daily or a few days out of the week. The window of time between the last and first meal of the day should be increased gradually (over weeks to months), to allow your body to acclimate. Complete fasting, extreme juice fasts, and nutrient-poor fasting regimens may be quite harmful for specific individuals, and are not recommended for those with diabetes or anemia; who are undergoing cancer treatment or are chronically ill; or who are pregnant or nursing, as many chemicals easily cross the placenta into the fetus and also concentrate in breast milk.[86]

***Always consult your healthcare practitioner when considering intermittent fasting or new supplement use, as these can cause more harm than good if not managed properly.

Cleanses

Detoxification programs range from juicing, cleanses, and fasts, to protocols such as chelation therapy, activated charcoal, and bentonite (clay soil) ingestion. Given the potential risks of these variable and often-unsupervised protocols, people should discuss any of these practices in detail with their healthcare providers *before* undertaking them.

Most people believe that various cleanses are safe, however variable practices change the nutrient value of cleanses, which may make them more or less efficacious for overall health. "Juicing cleanses" often include the use of conventional fruits, vegetables, and herbs that may be contaminated with pesticides and heavy metals.[65] Juicing should not remove the fiber portion of the produce, because fiber is necessary for slower transit through the body and helps lower the amount of insulin released from the pancreas; the rate of insulin release is measured as the "glycemic index," which is the blood insulin level divided by the blood glucose level. Thus, the slower food transits, the lower the release of insulin, and therefore the lower the glycemic index, which is good. Many frozen fruits and vegetables have the same or greater levels of nutrients as fresh produce.[25] Frozen produce often costs less, and organic frozen produce, which has fewer pesticides, can now be found in many food stores.

Any juice diet or cleanse that is undertaken for an extended period of time can be harmful and should be discussed with a certified nutritionist or physician who has training in this area. These diets may be devoid of essential micronutrients and vitamins necessary for proper biological activities. For patients who are busy and have limited time to prepare vegetables and fruits, juicing can be a reasonable addition to a complete and balanced diet.

Juicing Tips

Use organic fresh or frozen produce when available, or soak non-organic produce in 1 part vinegar to 4 parts clean filtered water to remove pesticide residues (for detox food and drink recipes see appendix 1).

- Do not remove fiber (the peel or fibrous interior) from produce; this will deplete the overall fiber intake and raise the glycemic index.
- Use vegetables high in water content, such as cucumber and celery, as your base.
- Limiting fruit content will keep juices low in sugar. Use low-fructose fruits such as green apples (fructose when combined with glucose forms sucrose, which is known as sugar) to sweeten your drink. Note that green apples are lower in fructose than red apples. See Table 13.2.
- Avoid added sugar, such as flavored almond milk, which can raise the glycemic index. Some juice blends may have as much sugar as a candy bar!
- Serving size matters. If you have large portions of a fruit-based drink, the sugar content will be increased as well.

Table 13.2 High Fructose (Sugar) Produce versus Low Fructose (Sugar) Produce Options. Eat fewer high sugar fruits that spike blood sugar and eat more low sugar fruits for balanced energy. Adapted from: https://paleodesserts.com/how-much-fruit-t-eat-per-day/

High Sugar Fruits That Spike Blood Sugar	Low Sugar Fruits That Balance Energy
• banana	• grapefruit
• melons	• granny smith apple
• mango	• lemon
• pineapple	• lime
• peach	• kiwi
• watermelon	• tart berries
• plum	• strawberries
• most apples	• blackberries
• grapes	• raspberries
• oranges/orange juice	• blueberries
• raisins, dates, dried fruits	• gooseberries

- Consider adding to your juice healthy fats, such as avocado, extra virgin olive oil, unsweetened coconut milk or oil, and almond or cashew butter.

Chelation for Toxic Metal Exposures

Heavy metals can cause a host of health issues in humans. Lead, arsenic, mercury, and cadmium rank among the top 10 substances on the Agency for Toxic Substances and Disease Registry (ATSDR) Priority List of Hazardous Substances.[87] Exposure to metals comes from many sources. For example, lead is found in residential paint (in homes built before 1978, and still remains in thousands), contaminated herbal medicines, gasoline (disallowed since the mid-1980s except in aviation gas), outdated plumbing, firearms, and cigarette smoke. Arsenic is found in well water, rice (both organic and conventional), and apple juice. Mercury is found in large top-predator fish (tuna, shark). Cadmium can be found in toys, jewelry, rechargeable batteries, and other products from overseas.

In chelation therapy, a compound or "chelator" such as ethylenediaminetetraacetic acid (EDTA) or dimercaptosuccinic acid (DMSA) is used to bind with a metal (e.g., mercury, lead, iron) and eliminate it from the body. Chelation therapy can be given as a pill or intravenously and must be overseen by a trained physician, since this can also reduce levels of elements, such as calcium, needed for normal body functions. Heavy metals, similar to many "fat-loving" environmental chemicals, reside in fat tissue, but are "released" with chelation therapy. Use of this therapy for people exposed to high-dose metal poisoning, such as lead contamination, has proven to be invaluable. Since there is evidence now to show a strong association between metal exposure and increased risk for heart disease, high cholesterol, high blood pressure, and even kidney disease, researchers have studied the potential benefits for routine chelation therapy to prevent heart ailments.

One large study found that patients who were stable after a heart attack and were taking established medical therapy (i.e., statin drugs and aspirin) had a significant reduction in heart complications when treated with a combination of high-dose vitamins and chelation therapy.[88] Even more striking was the finding that patients 50 years of age and older with diabetes who had also suffered a heart attack, had a dramatic reduction in later heart complications with EDTA chelation, including a 43% reduction in deaths over the 5 years they were studied.[89]

Chelation therapy is not without risk. Side effects include dehydration, low calcium levels, kidney damage, elevated liver enzymes, allergic reactions, lowered levels of necessary micronutrients like zinc, and even death.[90]

Certain populations, such as those who have suffered a heart attack and also have diabetes, may benefit from chelation therapy, but more research is needed before this becomes the standard of care. In cases of acute or chronic poisoning, such as those seen with widespread drinking water contamination in Flint, Michigan, chelation therapy determination and management should be performed under the guidance of a trained medical toxicologist or environmental health physician.

Stress Detoxification

Although many people might not consider stress to be an environmental "toxin," it plays a major role in the normal functioning of human cellular processes, hormonal feedback, and mechanisms of detoxification.[91] However, chronic stress can cause harm to our health. Under chronic stress, our body releases the stress hormone cortisol, which has been shown to damage cells in parts of the brain, disrupt normal immune system function, and contribute to the development of dementia.[92,93,94] Increased stress can often interfere with the food choices we make and the quantity of the food we eat, contributing to shifts in weight gain—stress-induced obesity. Stress effects also include reduced feelings of energy, disrupted sleep patterns, and limited social interaction.

Other forms of stress considered harmful to the human body are environmental or situational stressors. Situational stressors can be particularly harmful during pregnancy, which can have health consequences for the mother as well as the baby,[95–99] One extreme example is the Dutch Famine (referred to as the "hunger winter") during WWII when pregnant women were exposed to severe famine, and their offspring were followed by researchers for many years afterward to monitor for health consequences. It was discovered that the children of these underfed women developed higher rates of breast cancer and obesity and were more likely to become smokers; they were also not as physically active as the children born to well-fed mothers during that same time period.[100–104] Newer research has found that childhood stress is linked to increased risk for obesity, high blood pressure, and development of autoimmune disease later in life.[105]

Important Takeaway

A reasonable amount of stress, in short, recoverable time periods is normal and can even be productive; but ongoing, chronic stress can be counterproductive and even debilitating for mental and physical health. There are many ways to help manage and alleviate stress; try these:

- Yoga, Tai Chi, and Reiki
- Mindfulness meditation
- Breathing exercises such as the one shown in this video (https://www.youtube.com/watch?v=sJ04nsiz_M0)
- Physical activity and exercise
- Expressive activities such as dance, arts, and crafts
- Journaling
- Connecting with friends, community, and spiritual support
- Connecting with nature and pets/animals
- Seeking guidance through cognitive therapy
- Acupuncture, energy medicine
- Reducing use of technology, including social media
- Aromatherapy

Noise Detoxification

Most of us don't consider noise a contributor to health issues, but studies show noise can lead to a variety of acute and chronic conditions. Bustling highways and airports are among the most well-studied sources of noise pollution, and research shows that people who live near airports are at increased risk for heart (cardiovascular) disease—and this is separate from the increased risk from air pollution.[106] One study published in the *British Medical Journal* found that people who lived in the noisiest areas had an elevated risk for coronary artery disease, stroke, and cardiovascular disease, even after adjusting for confounding factors such as smoking, road-traffic noise exposure, air pollution, socioeconomic factors, and ethnicity. In addition, the study showed that the risk increased with higher exposure (increased "dose"); the risk was greatest in the 2% of the population who experienced the highest levels of noise.[107] Another study looking at elevated noise levels at 89 US airports sampled found increased admissions to area hospitals for cardiovascular conditions among elderly people on Medicare.[108] Environmental noise is a well-recognized health risk, and the World Health Organization estimates that one million healthy life years are lost annually in Western Europe alone due to noise-related complications!

So what does that tell us? Not only does chronic exposure to loud noise have an effect on restful and restorative sleep, thereby reducing the ability to clear toxins from the brain at night, it can also play a large role in stress and anxiety, potentially leading to increased heart rate, elevated and sustained blood pressure, increased release of stress hormones like cortisol, and increased inflammation.[109] Chronic noise pollution can act as an "obesogen": chronic stress alters the internal clock (circadian rhythms) of the body, disrupting metabolism and leading to weight gain.[110]

How can we reduce noise levels where we live, work, and play? First by being conscious of the health risks, and then being proactive with noise control. Try these simple measures:

- Consider noise-blocking shades and curtains.
- Use noise-reducing earplugs and headsets.
- Purchase a "white noise" machine that plays music or sounds of nature to override uncomfortable noise.
- Reduce time spent outdoors when traffic or other noise levels are at their highest.
- Add sound-reducing materials to your home such as specialized insulation, thickened sheet rock, stone or ceramic wall covering, hanging wool, and harder woods.

Bottom Line

Humans have evolved many remarkable ways to reduce harm from many toxic environmental exposures through physiologic means. But when it comes to the environmental harm from modern-day living (poor diet, food and drinking water contaminants, poor sleep, increased stress, synthetic light, noise pollution, lack of nature, socialization, community, and spiritual connection), we require awareness and proactive methods to truly thrive.

For reliable environmental health and wellness information, practical tips, and recommendations, follow Dr. Cohen's platform, *The Smart Human* on Facebook, Twitter, and Instagram, and sign up for The Smart Human newsletter at TheSmartHuman.com and listen to The Smart Human podcast.

References

1. Ye X, Wong LY, Bishop AM, Calafat AM. Variability of urinary concentrations of bisphenol A in spot samples, first morning voids, and 24-hour collections. *Environ Health Perspect.* 2011;119(7):983–988.

2. Gerona R, vom Saal FS, Hunt PA. BPA: have flawed analytical techniques compromised risk assessments? *The Lancet Diabetes & Endocrinology.* 2020;8(1):11–13.

3. deFur PL, Kaszuba M. Implementing the precautionary principle. *The Science of the Total Environment.* 2002;288(1–2):155–165.

4. Duty SM, Ackerman RM, Calafat AM, Hauser R. Personal care product use predicts urinary concentrations of some phthalate monoesters. *Environ Health Perspect.* 2005;113(11):1530–1535.

5. Harley KG, Kogut K, Madrigal DS, et al. Reducing Phthalate, Paraben, and Phenol Exposure from Personal Care Products in Adolescent Girls: Findings from the HERMOSA Intervention Study. *Environ Health Perspect.* 2016.

6. Nho CW, Jeffery E. The synergistic upregulation of phase II detoxification enzymes by glucosinolate breakdown products in cruciferous vegetables. *Toxicol Appl Pharmacol.* 2001;174(2):146–152.

7. Atwell LL, Beaver LM, Shannon J, Williams DE, Dashwood RH, Ho E. Epigenetic regulation by sulforaphane: opportunities for breast and prostate cancer chemoprevention. *Current Pharmacology Reports.* 2015;1(2):102–111.

8. Acharya A, Das I, Singh S, Saha T. Chemopreventive properties of indole-3-carbinol, diindolylmethane and other constituents of cardamom against carcinogenesis. *Recent Patents on Food, Nutrition & Agriculture.* 2010;2(2):166–177.

9. Caruso JA, Campana R, Wei C, et al. Indole-3-carbinol and its N-alkoxy derivatives preferentially target ERalpha-positive breast cancer cells. *Cell Cycle (Georgetown, Tex).* 2014;13(16):2587–2599.

10. Kapusta-Duch J, Kopec A, Piatkowska E, Borczak B, Leszczynska T. The beneficial effects of Brassica vegetables on human health. *Rocz Panstw Zakl Hig.* 2012;63(4):389–395.

11. Dolinoy DC, Huang D, Jirtle RL. Maternal nutrient supplementation counteracts bisphenol A-induced DNA hypomethylation in early development. *Proceedings of the National Academy of Sciences of the United States of America.* 2007;104(32):13056–13061.

12. Hebatalla I, Ahmed EE, Amany AA. The possible protective effects of some antioxidants against growth retardation and malformation induced by bisphenyl-A in rats,. *Life Science Journal.* 2013;10(4):1575–1586.

13. McConaha ME, Ding T, Lucas JA, Arosh JA, Osteen KG, Bruner-Tran KL. Preconception omega-3 fatty acid supplementation of adult male mice with a history of developmental 2,3,7,8-tetrachlorodibenzo-p-dioxin exposure prevents preterm birth in unexposed female partners. *Reproduction*. 2011;142(2):235–241.

14. Myers GJ, Davidson PW, Strain JJ. Nutrient and methyl mercury exposure from consuming fish. *J Nutr*. 2007;137(12):2805–2808.

15. Rice DC. Overview of modifiers of methylmercury neurotoxicity: chemicals, nutrients, and the social environment. *Neurotoxicology*. 2008;29(5):761–766.

16. Rogan WJ, Paulson JA, Baum C, et al. Iodine deficiency, pollutant chemicals, and the thyroid: new information on an old problem. *Pediatrics*. 2014;133(6):1163–1166.

17. Barcelos GR, Grotto D, Serpeloni JM, et al. Protective properties of quercetin against DNA damage and oxidative stress induced by methylmercury in rats. *Arch Toxicol*. 2011;85(9):1151–1157.

18. Rocha de Oliveira C, Ceolin J, Rocha de Oliveira R, et al. Effects of quercetin on polychlorinated biphenyls-induced liver injury in rats. *Nutr Hosp*. 2014;29(5):1141–1148.

19. Jiao J, Lu G, Liu X, Zhu H, Zhang Y. Reduction of blood lead levels in lead-exposed mice by dietary supplements and natural antioxidants. *J Sci Food Agric*. 2011;91(3):485–491.

20. Sandstrom B. Micronutrient interactions: effects on absorption and bioavailability. *Br J Nutr*. 2001;85 Suppl 2:S181–185.

21. Suarez-Ortegon MF, Mosquera M, Caicedo DM, De Plata CA, Mendez F. Nutrients intake as determinants of blood lead and cadmium levels in Colombian pregnant women. *American Journal of Human Biology: The Official Journal of the Human Biology Council*. 2013;25(3):344–350.

22. Zentner LE, Rondo PH, Duran MC, Oliveira JM. Relationships of blood lead to calcium, iron, and vitamin C intakes in Brazilian pregnant women. *Clinical Nutrition (Edinburgh, Scotland)*. 2008;27(1):100–104.

23. Silver MK, Lozoff B, Meeker JD. Blood cadmium is elevated in iron deficient U.S. children: a cross-sectional study. *Environmental Health: A Global Access Science Source*. 2013;12:117.

24. Suh YJ, Lee JE, Lee DH, et al. Prevalence and relationships of iron deficiency anemia with blood cadmium and vitamin D levels in Korean Women. *Journal of Korean Medical Science*. 2016;31(1):25–32.

25. Rabin R. Are frozen fruits and vegetables as nutritious as fresh? https://well.blogs.nytimes.com/2016/11/18/are-frozen-fruits-and-vegetables-as-nutritious-as-fresh/?mcubz=1. Published 2016. Accessed February 10, 2019.

26. Manore MM. Exercise and the Institute of Medicine recommendations for nutrition. *Current Sports Medicine Reports.* 2005;4(4):193–198.

27. Kenefick RW, Cheuvront SN. Hydration for recreational sport and physical activity. *Nutr Rev.* 2012;70 Suppl 2:S137–142.

28. Bulow J. Adipose tissue blood flow during exercise. *Danish Medical Bulletin.* 1983;30(2):85–100.

29. Duncan K, Harris S, Ardies CM. Running exercise may reduce risk for lung and liver cancer by inducing activity of antioxidant and phase II enzymes. *Cancer Letters.* 1997;116(2):151–158.

30. Leeuwenburgh C, Hollander J, Leichtweis S, Griffiths M, Gore M, Ji LL. Adaptations of glutathione antioxidant system to endurance training are tissue and muscle fiber specific. *The American Journal of Physiology.* 1997;272(1 Pt 2):R363–369.

31. Yiamouyiannis CA, Sanders RA, Watkins JB, 3rd, Martin BJ. Chronic physical activity: hepatic hypertrophy and increased total biotransformation enzyme activity. *Biochem Pharmacol.* 1992;44(1):121–127.

32. Genuis SJ, Birkholz D, Ralitsch M, Thibault N. Human detoxification of perfluorinated compounds. *Public health.* 2010;124(7):367–375.

33. Hannuksela ML, Ellahham S. Benefits and risks of sauna bathing. *Am J Med.* 2001;110(2):118–126.

34. Ross GH, Sternquist MC. Methamphetamine exposure and chronic illness in police officers: significant improvement with sauna-based detoxification therapy. *Toxicology and Industrial Health.* 2012;28(8):758–768.

35. Genuis SJ, Sears ME, Schwalfenberg G, Hope J, Bernhoft R. Clinical detoxification: elimination of persistent toxicants from the human body. *The Scientific World Journal.* 2013;2013:238347.

36. Crinnion WJ. Toxic effects of the easily avoidable phthalates and parabens. *Alternative Medicine Review: A Journal of Clinical Therapeutic.* 2010;15(3):190–196.

37. Oosterveld FG, Rasker JJ, Floors M, et al. Infrared sauna in patients with rheumatoid arthritis and ankylosing spondylitis. A pilot study showing good tolerance, short-term improvement of pain and stiffness, and a trend towards long-term beneficial effects. *Clinical Rheumatology.* 2009;28(1):29–34.

38. Tei C, Orihara FK, Fukudome T. Remarkable efficacy of thermal therapy for Sjogren syndrome. *Journal of Cardiology.* 2007;49(5):217–219.

39. Vatansever F, Hamblin MR. Far infrared radiation (FIR): its biological effects and medical applications. *Photonics & Lasers in Medicine.* 2012;4:255–266.

40. Taylor J. Recent pioneering cardiology developments in Japan: Japanese cardiologists have discovered waon therapy for severe or refractory heart failure and extracorporeal cardiac shock wave therapy for severe angina pectoris. *European Heart Journal.* 2011;32(14):1690–1691.

41. Miyata M, Tei C. Waon therapy for cardiovascular disease: innovative therapy for the 21st century. *Circulation Journal: Official Journal of the Japanese Circulation Society.* 2010;74(4):617–621.

42. Miyata M, Kihara T, Kubozono T, et al. Beneficial effects of waon therapy on patients with chronic heart failure: results of a prospective multicenter study. *Journal of Cardiology.* 2008;52(2):79–85.

43. Kihara T, Miyata M, Fukudome T, et al. Waon therapy improves the prognosis of patients with chronic heart failure. *Journal of Cardiology.* 2009;53(2):214–218.

44. Kuwahata S, Miyata M, Fujita S, et al. Improvement of autonomic nervous activity by waon therapy in patients with chronic heart failure. *Journal of Cardiology.* 2011;57(1):100–106.

45. Kubozono T, Miyata M, Tei C. [The cutting-edge of medicine; waon therapy for cardiovascular disease]. *Nihon Naika Gakkai Zasshi The Journal of the Japanese Society of Internal Medicine.* 2011;100(4):1067–1075.

46. Fujita S, Ikeda Y, Miyata M, et al. Effect of waon therapy on oxidative stress in chronic heart failure. *Circulation Journal: Official Journal of the Japanese Circulation Society.* 2011;75(2):348–356.

47. Schieke SM, Schroeder P, Krutmann J. Cutaneous effects of infrared radiation: from clinical observations to molecular response mechanisms. *Photodermatology, Potoimmunology & Photomedicine.* 2003;19(5):228–234.

48. Robert C, Bonnet M, Marques S, Numa M, Doucet O. Low to moderate doses of infrared A irradiation impair extracellular matrix homeostasis of the skin and contribute to skin photodamage. *Skin Pharmacology and Physiology.* 2015;28(4):196–204.

49. Centers for Disease Control and Prevention (CDC). Sleep in middle and high school students. https://www.cdc.gov/features/students-sleep/index.html. Published 2018. Accessed January 16, 2020.

50. CDC. Geographic variation in short sleep duration data and statistics. https://www.cdc.gov/sleep/data_statistics.html. Published 2017. Accessed January 16, 2020.

51. Xie L, Kang H, Xu Q, et al. Sleep drives metabolite clearance from the adult brain. *Science (New York, NY).* 2013;342(6156):373–377.

52. Paruthi S, Brooks LJ, D'Ambrosio C, et al. Consensus statement of the American Academy of Sleep Medicine on the recommended amount of sleep for healthy children: methodology and discussion. *J Clin Sleep Med.* 2016;12(11):1549–1561.

53. Nehlig A. Effects of coffee/caffeine on brain health and disease: what should I tell my patients? *Practical Neurology.* 2015.

54. Lewczuk B, Redlarski G, Zak A, Ziolkowska N, Przybylska-Gornowicz B, Krawczuk M. Influence of electric, magnetic, and electromagnetic fields

on the circadian system: current stage of knowledge. *BioMed Research International.* 2014;2014:169459.

55. Singh S, Mani KV, Kapoor N. Effect of occupational EMF exposure from radar at two different frequency bands on plasma melatonin and serotonin levels. *International Journal of Radiation Biology.* 2015;91(5):426–434.

56. Lillehei AS, Halcon LL, Savik K, Reis R. Effect of inhaled lavender and sleep hygiene on self-reported sleep issues: a randomized controlled trial. *J Altern Complement Med.* 2015;21(7):430–438.

57. Hudda N, Fruin SA. Models for predicting the ratio of particulate pollutant concentrations inside vehicles to roadways. *Environmental Science & Technology.* 2013;47(19):11048–11055.

58. Park HK, Cheng KC, Tetteh AO, Hildemann LM, Nadeau KC. Effectiveness of air purifier on health outcomes and indoor particles in homes of children with allergic diseases in Fresno, California: a pilot study. *The Journal of Asthma: Official Journal of the Association for the Care of Asthma.* 2016:1–6.

59. Rudel RA, Camann DE, Spengler JD, Korn LR, Brody JG. Phthalates, alkylphenols, pesticides, polybrominated diphenyl ethers, and other endocrine-disrupting compounds in indoor air and dust. *Environmental Science & technology.* 2003;37(20):4543–4553.

60. Bardia A, Nisly NL, Zimmerman MB, Gryzlak BM, Wallace RB. Use of herbs among adults based on evidence-based indications: findings from the National Health Interview Survey. *Mayo Clinic Proceedings.* 2007;82(5):561–566.

61. Eisenberg DM, Davis RB, Ettner SL, et al. Trends in alternative medicine use in the United States, 1990-1997: results of a follow-up national survey. *JAMA.* 1998;280(18):1569–1575.

62. Miller MF, Bellizzi KM, Sufian M, Ambs AH, Goldstein MS, Ballard-Barbash R. Dietary supplement use in individuals living with cancer and other chronic conditions: a population-based study. *Journal of the American Dietetic Association.* 2008;108(3):483–494.

63. White CP, Hirsch G, Patel S, Adams F, Peltekian KM. Complementary and alternative medicine use by patients chronically infected with hepatitis C virus. *Canadian Journal of Gastroenterology.* 2007;21(9):589–595.

64. Tucker J, Fischer T, Upjohn L, Mazzera D, Kumar M. Unapproved pharmaceutical ingredients included in dietary supplements associated with US Food and Drug Administration warnings. *JAMA Network Open.* 2018;1(6):e183337.

65. Posadzki P, Watson L, Ernst E. Contamination and adulteration of herbal medicinal products (HMPs): an overview of systematic reviews. *European Journal of Clinical Pharmacology.* 2013;69(3):295–307.

66. Maier L. Pruteanu M, Kuhn M, et al. Extensive impact of non-antibiotic drugs on human gut bacteria. *Nature*. 2018;555(7698):623–628.

67. Ibrahim F, Halttunen T, Tahvonen R, Salminen S. Probiotic bacteria as potential detoxification tools: assessing their heavy metal binding isotherms. *Canadian Journal of Microbiology*. 2006;52(9):877–885.

68. De Flora S, Izzotti A, D'Agostini F, Balansky RM. Mechanisms of N-acetylcysteine in the prevention of DNA damage and cancer, with special reference to smoking-related end-points. *Carcinogenesis*. 2001;22(7):999–1013.

69. Murray TV, Dong X, Sawyer GJ, et al. NADPH oxidase 4 regulates homocysteine metabolism and protects against acetaminophen-induced liver damage in mice. *Free Radical Biology & Medicine*. 2015;89:918–930.

70. Rahman Q, Abidi P, Afaq F, et al. Glutathione redox system in oxidative lung injury. *Critical reviews in toxicology*. 1999;29(6):543–568.

71. Jan AT, Azam M, Siddiqui K, Ali A, Choi I, Haq QM. Heavy metals and human health: mechanistic insight into toxicity and counter defense system of antioxidants. *International Journal of Molecular Sciences*. 2015;16(12):29592–29630.

72. Ward J, Kapadia K, Brush E, Salhanick SD. Amatoxin poisoning: case reports and review of current therapies. *The Journal of Emergency Medicine*. 2013;44(1):116–121.

73. Srinivasan P, Suchalatha S, Babu PV, et al. Chemopreventive and therapeutic modulation of green tea polyphenols on drug metabolizing enzymes in 4-Nitroquinoline 1-oxide induced oral cancer. *Chem Biol Interact*. 2008;172(3):224–234.

74. Szilard S, Szentgyorgyi D, Demeter I. Protective effect of Legalon in workers exposed to organic solvents. *Acta medica Hungarica*. 1988;45(2):249–256.

75. Rambaldi A, Jacobs BP, Gluud C. Milk thistle for alcoholic and/or hepatitis B or C virus liver diseases. *The Cochrane database of systematic reviews*. 2007(4):Cd003620.

76. Greenlee H, Abascal K, Yarnell E, Ladas E. Clinical applications of Silybum marianum in oncology. *Integrative Cancer Therapies*. 2007;6(2):158–165.

77. Blumenthal M, Busse WR, Goldberg A, et al. *The Complete German Commisssion E Monographs: Therapeutic Guide to Herbal Medicines*. Baltimore, Md: Lippincott Williams & Wilkins; 1999.

78. Hodek P, Trefil P, Stiborova M. Flavonoids—potent and versatile biologically active compounds interacting with cytochromes P450. *Chem Biol Interact*. 2002;139(1):1–21.

79. Longo VD, Mattson MP. Fasting: molecular mechanisms and clinical applications. *Cell Metab*. 2014;19(2):181–192.

80. Mattson MP. Challenging oneself intermittently to improve health. *Dose-Response: A Publication of International Hormesis Society.* 2014;12(4):600–618.

81. Mattson MP. Lifelong brain health is a lifelong challenge: from evolutionary principles to empirical evidence. *Ageing Research Reviews.* 2015;20:37–45.

82. van Praag H, Fleshner M, Schwartz MW, Mattson MP. Exercise, energy intake, glucose homeostasis, and the brain. *J Neurosci.* 2014;34(46):15139–15149.

83. Johnstone A. Fasting for weight loss: an effective strategy or latest dieting trend? *International Journal of Obesity (2005).* 2015;39(5):727–733.

84. Effects of intermittent fasting on health, aging, and disease. *The New England Journal of Medicine.* 2020;382(3):298.

85. Hue O, Marcotte J, Berrigan F, et al. Increased plasma levels of toxic pollutants accompanying weight loss induced by hypocaloric diet or by bariatric surgery. *Obesity Surgery.* 2006;16(9):1145–1154.

86. Pizzorno JE, Murray MT. *Textbook of Natural Medicine.* Elsevier, 2013;4th Edition:pg 480.

87. United States Agency for Toxic Substances and Disease Registry (ATSDR). Priority list of hazardous substances 2015. http://www.atsdr.cdc.gov/SPL/index.html. Published 2015. Accessed April 4, 2016.

88. Lamas GA, Boineau R, Goertz C, et al. EDTA chelation therapy alone and in combination with oral high-dose multivitamins and minerals for coronary disease: The factorial group results of the Trial to Assess Chelation Therapy. *American Heart Journal.* 2014;168(1):37–44.e35.

89. Escolar E, Lamas GA, Mark DB, et al. The effect of an EDTA-based chelation regimen on patients with diabetes mellitus and prior myocardial infarction in the Trial to Assess Chelation Therapy (TACT). *Circulation Cardiovascular Quality and Outcomes.* 2014;7(1):15–24.

90. American College of Medical Toxicology. Use and misuse of metal chelation therapy. http://www.acmt.net/cgi/page.cgi/Use_Misuse_of_Metal_Chelation_Therapy_Webinar.html. Published 2012. Accessed April 4, 2016.

91. Sawa T, Naito Y, Katoh H, Amaya F. Cellular stress responses and monitored cellular activities. *Shock (Augusta, Ga).* 2016.

92. Stein-Behrens BA, Sapolsky RM. Stress, glucocorticoids, and aging. *Aging (Milan, Italy).* 1992;4(3):197–210.

93. Andel R, Crowe M, Hahn EA, et al. Work-related stress may increase the risk of vascular dementia. *Journal of the American Geriatrics Society.* 2012;60(1):60–67.

94. Crowe M, Andel R, Pedersen NL, Gatz M. Do work-related stress and reactivity to stress predict dementia more than 30 years later? *Alzheimer Disease and Associated Disorders.* 2007;21(3):205–209.

95. Ostlund BD, Conradt E, Crowell SE, Tyrka AR, Marsit CJ, Lester BM. Prenatal stress, fearfulness, and the epigenome: exploratory analysis of sex differences in DNA methylation of the glucocorticoid receptor gene. *Frontiers in Behavioral Neuroscience.* 2016;10:147.

96. Kitsiou-Tzeli S, Tzetis M. Maternal epigenetics and fetal and neonatal growth. *Current Opinion in Endocrinology, Diabetes, and Obesity.* 2016.

97. McCreary JK, Erickson ZT, Hao Y, Ilnytskyy Y, Kovalchuk I, Metz GA. Environmental intervention as a therapy for adverse programming by ancestral stress. *Scientific Reports.* 2016;6:37814.

98. Lobel M, Cannella DL, Graham JE, DeVincent C, Schneider J, Meyer BA. Pregnancy-specific stress, prenatal health behaviors, and birth outcomes. *Health Psychology: Official Journal of the Division of Health Psychology, American Psychological Association.* 2008;27(5):604–615.

99. O'Donnell KJ, Glover V, Jenkins J, et al. Prenatal maternal mood is associated with altered diurnal cortisol in adolescence. *Psychoneuroendocrinology.* 2013;38(9):1630–1638.

100. Entringer S, Buss C, Wadhwa PD. Prenatal stress, development, health and disease risk: a psychobiological perspective-2015 Curt Richter Award Paper. *Psychoneuroendocrinology.* 2015;62:366–375.

101. Harris A, Seckl J. Glucocorticoids, prenatal stress and the programming of disease. *Hormones and Behavior.* 2011;59(3):279–289.

102. Fransen HP, Peeters PH, Beulens JW, et al. Exposure to famine at a young age and unhealthy lifestyle behavior later in life. *PLoS One.* 2016;11(5):e0156609.

103. Elias SG, Peeters PH, Grobbee DE, van Noord PA. Breast cancer risk after caloric restriction during the 1944–1945 Dutch famine. *Journal of the National Cancer Institute.* 2004;96(7):539–546.

104. van Noord PA. Breast cancer and the brain: a neurodevelopmental hypothesis to explain the opposing effects of caloric deprivation during the Dutch famine of 1944–1945 on breast cancer and its risk factors. *J Nutr.* 2004;134(12 Suppl):3399s–3406s.

105. Song H, Fang F, Tomasson, G, et al. Association of stress-related disorders with subsequent autoimmune disease. *Journal of the American Medical Association.* 2018;319:2388–2400.

106. Munzel T, Schmidt FP, Steven S, Herzog J, Daiber A, Sorensen M. Environmental noise and the cardiovascular system. *J Am Coll Cardiol.* 2018;71(6):688–697.

107. Hansell AL, Blangiardo M, Fortunato L, et al. Aircraft noise and cardiovascular disease near Heathrow airport in London: small area study. *BMJ (Clinical research ed).* 2013;347:f5432.

108. Correia AW, Peters JL, Levy JI, Melly S, Dominici F. Residential exposure to aircraft noise and hospital admissions for cardiovascular diseases: multi-airport retrospective study. *BMJ (Clinical research ed)*. 2013;347:f5561.

109. Daiber A, Kroller-Schon S, Frenis K, et al. Environmental noise induces the release of stress hormones and inflammatory signaling molecules leading to oxidative stress and vascular dysfunction–Signatures of the internal exposome. *Biofactors*. 2019;45(4):495–506.

110. Coborn JE, Lessie RE, Sinton CM, Rance NE, Perez-Leighton CE, Teske JA. Noise-induced sleep disruption increases weight gain and decreases energy metabolism in female rats. *International Journal of Obesity (2005)*. 2019;43(9):1759–1768.

Appendix 1

Detox Recipes

Whenever possible, use USDA organic ingredients, filtered water, and cookware, bakeware, and utensils that are glass, high-quality ceramics, copper, and/or stainless steel. Many of the following recipes use cruciferous vegetables and produce high in antioxidants for greater detoxification properties.

ALY'S NON-TOXIC GATORADE

All of the electrolytes, without the fake food additives and packaging chemicals!

Ingredients

- 3 ounces juice (without added synthetic sweeteners, preferably bought in a glass bottle)
- 17 ounces filtered water
- 2 pinches or 3 turns of a grinder of Himalayan or Kosher unprocessed sea salt

Yields 1 serving

Instructions

Add all ingredients to a 20 oz glass or stainless steel water bottle and stir. Should stay fresh for about seven days when kept refridgerated.

The following recipes are adapted and modified from:
TheSuppersPrograms.org

SOUPS

Creamy Cauliflower Soup

https://www.thesuppersprograms.org/content/creamy-cauliflower-soup

Ingredients

- 3 tablespoons coconut oil
- 1 teaspoon salt (or to taste)
- 3 leeks (trimmed, washed, and thinly sliced)
- 2 cloves garlic (peeled and roughly chopped)
- 1 2-inch piece of ginger (peeled and grated)
- 1 medium head cauliflower (roughly cut into chunks)
- 1/2 cup raw cashews (soaked for 2 hours or overnight, drained and rinsed)
- 4 cups broth (vegetable or chicken)
- 1 tablespoon apple cider vinegar (or fresh lemon juice)

Yields 8 servings

Instructions

Melt coconut oil in a large soup pot over medium heat. Add salt and leeks and sauté for 5 minutes. Add garlic, ginger, and cauliflower and sauté for another 5 minutes. Add cashews and broth. Bring to a boil, reduce heat, cover, and simmer for 30 minutes. Remove from heat and let cool for an hour or longer.

Purée in a high-speed blender until creamy. Season with vinegar or lemon juice, and salt to taste. Serve with hot sauce if desired.

Butternut Squash Puréed Soup

https://www.theuppersprograms.org/content/butternut-squash-puréed-soup

Ingredients

2 tablespoons coconut oil (enough to coat the bottom of a large soup pot)
1 onion (chopped)
1 tablespoon ground cumin
1 teaspoon ground cardamom
1/8 teaspoon cayenne pepper
1 butternut squash (peeled, seeded, and cubed)
2 yellow summer squash (diced; or use 2 parsnips for a sweeter soup)
3 carrots (roughly chopped)
1 1/2 quart vegetable stock

Yields 10 servings

Instructions

Melt the coconut oil over medium heat. Add onion and sauté for 5 minutes until translucent. Add the spices, stir, and sauté for 1 minute. Stir in the chopped vegetables and sauté for another minute. Add the broth, bring to a boil, reduce heat to low, and simmer for about 15 minutes until butternut squash is soft. Remove from heat and carefully process in with an immersion blender, food processor, or traditional blender until smooth.

IMPORTANT: Always use great caution when puréeing hot liquids. If you have time, allow the soup to cool before blending. Never fill the container more than half full and cover the lid with a folded kitchen towel and hold it in place before you turn on the blender.

Barley Miso Soup

https://www.theuppersprograms.org/content/barley-miso-soup

Barley is a gluten grain and should not be eaten by anyone who is completely avoiding gluten.

Ingredients

12 cups water
2 tablespoons tamari (soy sauce)

1 strip of kombu

1/3 cup dried shiitake mushrooms (soaked according to package directions)

1/4 cup dried seaweed (wakame or arame)

1/4 block of tofu (chopped into small cubes)

1/2 cup barley miso (or more to taste)

Yields 4 servings

Instructions

Bring the water to a simmer with the kombu and tamari. Add mushrooms and seaweed, and simmer about 10 minutes. Add tofu and turn off the heat. Mix a little broth into the miso to dissolve. Break up clumps and return it to the pot. Do not heat after the miso goes in. Different miso pastes have different flavors and saltiness. Taste the broth and if it tastes too watery, add more dissolved miso.

Additional Notes

Kombu is a type of kelp or seaweed that can improve the digestibility of beans and legumes. It can be found in some grocery and most "health food" stores.

Carrot Ginger Soup

https://www.thesuppersprograms.org/content/carrot-ginger-soup

Ingredients

2 tablespoons coconut oil (or olive oil)

2 onions (peeled and chopped)

1 1/2 pound carrots (peeled and sliced)

1 tablespoon grated fresh ginger

1 quart vegetable stock or water

salt and pepper (to taste)

Yields 4 servings

Instructions

In a large soup pot, melt coconut oil over medium heat. Sauté the onion for 5 minutes, without browning. Add the carrots, ginger, and a sprinkling of salt. Cover and cook for another 10 minutes. Stir occasionally and do not allow vegetables to brown. Add the stock or water and bring to a boil, reduce heat, and simmer gently for about 15 minutes, until the carrots are tender.

Using an immersion blender, food processor, or traditional blender, purée the soup. Return the soup to the pan, reheat gently, and season to taste with salt and pepper.

Quick Gazpacho

https://www.thesuppersprograms.org/content/quick-gazpacho

Ingredients

- 1 clove garlic (peeled and mashed)
- 1 tablespoon olive oil
- 2 tablespoons lemon or lime juice (or 1–2 tablespoons vinegar)
- 1 red bell pepper (cored, seeded, and cut into 1/2-inch pieces)
- 1 medium cucumber (peeled, seeded, and cut into 1/2-inch pieces)
- 2 tomatoes (cored and cut into 1/2-inch pieces)
- 8 ounces vegetable juice (Kundsen Very Veggie [low carb and low sodium], V-8, or any tomato juice)
- 1 pinch sea salt
- 1 red onion (finely chopped, optional)
- 1 celery stalk (cut into 1/4-inch dice, optional)
- 1 parsley, basil, or cilantro (stemmed and roughly chopped, optional)
- hot sauce (optional)

Yields 4 servings

Instructions

Place the garlic, oil, and citrus juice or vinegar in a food processor and pulse to mince the garlic. Add the pepper and cucumber. Pulse to chop. Add the tomatoes and vegetable juice and process just to blend. It should still be a bit chunky. Taste and add salt if needed.

Serve in individual bowls. Garnish with red onion, celery, and chopped herbs. Serve with hot sauce on the side.

SALADS

Broccoli Slaw

https://www.thesuppersprograms.org/content/broccoli-slaw
Source: Based on a recipe from thekitchn.com

Ingredients

Slaw

> 2 pounds broccoli (about 1 large head)
> 1 red cabbage (small)
> 1 jicama
> 1/2 red onion (finely chopped)

Dressing

> 1/2 cup paleo mayonnaise (made with olive or avocado oil)
> 2 tablespoons lemon juice
> 2 tablespoons apple cider vinegar
> 1 teaspoon salt
> freshly ground black pepper

Yields 12 servings

Instructions

Shred broccoli, cabbage, and jicama in food processor using the grater disc. In a large bowl, combine the shredded broccoli, cabbage, jicama, and the chopped red onion.

Whisk together the mayonnaise, lemon juice, vinegar, salt, and a generous quantity of fresh pepper. Pour the dressing over the broccoli mixture and stir to combine. Taste and add more salt or pepper, if needed.

Allow to sit for at least 30 minutes (or an hour in the fridge) so the flavors can mingle. (Up to 24 hours would be okay.) Serve with sliced avocado.

Apple Bok Choy Salad

https://www.thesuppersprograms.org/content/apple-bok-choy-salad

Ingredients

Salad

6 cups finely chopped bok choy (1 large head)
1 large apple (cored and shredded or chopped)
1 large carrot (shredded or chopped)
1/2 cup unsweetened almond, hemp, or soy milk

Dressing

1/2 cup raw cashews (or 1/4 cup raw cashew butter)
1/4 cup apple cider vinegar
1/4 cup raisins
1 teaspoon Dijon mustard

Yields 6 servings

Instructions

Combine bok choy, apple, and carrot in a large bowl. Blend almond milk, cashews, vinegar, raisins, and mustard in a food processor or high-powered blender. Pour dressing over salad and toss to combine.

Dandelion, Jicama, and Orange Prebiotic Salad

https://www.thesuppersprograms.org/content/dandelion-jicama-and-orange-prebiotic-salad

Ingredients

1 jicama (diced)
1/2 bunch dandelion greens (chopped)
3 oranges (peeled and chopped)
2 tablespoons extra virgin olive oil
2 tablespoons balsamic vinegar (more to taste)
salt and freshly ground black pepper (to taste)

Yields 4 servings

Instructions

Combine jicama, greens, and oranges. Drizzle with oil and vinegar. Salt and pepper to taste. Toss gently and serve.

Lemony Brussels Sprouts Slaw

https://www.thesuppersprograms.org/content/annas-lemony-brussels-sprouts-slaw

Ingredients

Slaw

1 1/2 pounds Brussels sprouts
1 granny smith apple
1 daikon radish
1 watermelon radish
4 carrots
1/2 red onion (or shallot)

Dressing

2 tablespoons mayonnaise
1 teaspoon Dijon mustard
2 tablespoons fresh lemon juice
1 tablespoon lemon zest
1/4 cup extra virgin olive oil
salt and pepper (to taste)

Yields 8 servings

Instructions

Use a food processor to shred the raw vegetables. Toss the shredded vegetables in a large bowl to combine well.

Make the dressing by measuring all the ingredients into a jar with a fitted lid. Cover and shake vigorously.

Dress the veggie slaw, taste, and adjust seasoning by adding more salt or pepper. Let the slaw sit in the fridge for about an hour, then stir and taste again. When it's time to serve, garnish with fresh mint.

Paleo Bok Choy Salad

https://www.thesuppersprograms.org/content/paleo-bok-choy-salad

Ingredients

Salad

8 baby bok choy (cleaned and sliced thin on diagonal)
8 celery stalks (cleaned and sliced thin on diagonal)

1/2 cup olive oil
1/4 cup fresh lime juice

Dressing

1 teaspoon mustard
1 teaspoon fresh grated ginger (more to taste)
1 teaspoon honey
salt (to taste)
1/2 cup toasted almonds, walnuts, or pumpkin seeds (for garnish)

Yields 8 servings

Instructions

Mix the bok choy and celery in a bowl. Whisk together dressing ingredients and combine with vegetables. Garnish with nuts or seeds.

VEGETABLES

Cauliflower Risotto

https://www.thesuppersprograms.org/content/cauliflower-risotto

Ingredients

1 head cauliflower (trimmed into florets, stem discarded)
1 tablespoon coconut oil
1 leek (well cleaned and thinly sliced)
salt (to taste)
2 cloves garlic (minced)
2 cups seasonal vegetables (optional; such as asparagus, peas, snap peas, bell peppers, mushrooms, sundried tomatoes; cut into small dice)
1 1/2 tablespoon tahini
1 tablespoon nutritional yeast
1 tablespoon miso paste
1 1/2 cup vegetable broth
1 1/2 cup quinoa (cooked according to package directions)
1/2 tablespoon lemon juice
pepper (to taste)
parsley (roughly chopped, for garnish)

Yields 8 servings

Instructions

Pulse the cauliflower florets in small batches in the bowl of a food processor until the size of grains of rice.

Heat the oil in a large skillet. Add the leeks and a sprinkle of salt and sauté until softened. Add the garlic and sauté a few minutes more, until fragrant. If using the optional vegetables, add them now, first adding those that will take longer to cook, then any others. When the leeks are tender and the other vegetables almost done, add the cauliflower.

Meanwhile, whisk together the tahini, nutritional yeast, miso paste, and broth.

Cook for a few minutes more, then add the broth mixture and the cooked quinoa. Simmer for a few minutes more to thicken but do not overcook.

Remove from heat and stir in the lemon juice. Adjust the seasonings and serve garnished with parsley.

Curried Cauliflower

https://www.thesuppersprograms.org/content/curried-cauliflower

Ingredients

2 tablespoons olive oil (enough to coat large sauté pan)
1 large red onion (finely chopped)
1 2-inch piece fresh ginger (peeled and minced)
2 cloves garlic (peeled and minced)
1 head of cauliflower (roughly chopped)
1 14-oz can full-fat coconut milk
1 tablespoon curry paste
1/4 teaspoon salt

Yields 4 servings

Instructions

Heat olive oil in a large sauté pan over medium heat. Sauté onion and ginger until softened, then add garlic and continue cooking until fragrant. Add cauliflower and sauté another 5 minutes. Stir in coconut milk, curry paste, and salt. Cover and simmer 15 minutes to allow flavors to infuse and the cauliflower to soften.

Note:
Curry paste can be found in the Asian foods aisle of most supermarkets.

Mexican "Rice"

https://www.thesuppersprograms.org/content/mexican-%E2%80%9Crice%E2%80%9D

Ingredients

- 1 head cauliflower (proccesed in small batches to the size of rice grains)
- 1 cup grape tomatoes (quartered)
- 4 radishes (diced fine)
- 1 red bell pepper (diced fine)
- 1 bunch cilantro (stemmed and chopped)
- 1 lime (juiced)
- 1 tablespoon onion or scallion (minced)
- 1 tablespoon olive oil
- 1/2 teaspoon cumin
- 1 avocado (diced, optional garnish)
- 1 jalapeno (minced, optional garnish)
- hot sauce (optional garnish)

Yields 6 servings

Instructions

Combine the first nine ingredients and toss with lime juice and olive oil. Taste for salt. If desired, top with diced avocado and garnish with jalapeno and hot sauce.

Roasted Brussels Sprouts

https://www.thesuppersprograms.org/content/roasted-brussels-sprouts

Ingredients

- 1 pound Brussels sprouts (washed, trimmed, and halved)
- 1 tablespoon coconut oil or olive oil
- 1/2 teaspoon salt
- 1 tablespoon apple cider vinegar
- 1/2 teaspoon honey (or 5 drops monkfruit extract)

Yields 4 servings

Instructions

Preheat oven to 425 degrees. Toss Brussels sprouts with salt and oil. Roast on a parchment-lined baking sheet for 30 minutes, tossing every 10 minutes or so. Season with vinegar, honey or monkfruit extract, and salt to taste.

Asparagus in Balsamic Butter

https://www.thesuppersprograms.org/content/asparagus-balsamic-butter

Ingredients

- 3 bunches asparagus
- 1 tablespoon extra virgin olive oil
- salt and pepper
- 4 tablespoons butter (use olive oil if avoiding dairy)
- 1 tablespoon tamari
- 1 tablespoon golden balsamic vinegar
- 2 hard-boiled eggs (grated or crumbled)

Instructions

Preheat oven to 400 degrees. Snap off the tough end of the asparagus. Spread the asparagus in a single layer in 1 or 2 baking dishes. Drizzle with olive oil, and sprinkle with salt and pepper. Bake for 10-12 minutes. In a small saucepan melt the butter (or heat the olive oil) and stir in the tamari and vinegar. Arrange the asparagus on the serving plate, drizzle with the dressing, and sprinkle with the egg.

MAIN DISHES

Moroccan Style Chicken Stew

https://www.thesuppersprograms.org/content/moroccan-style-chicken-stew

Ingredients

- 4 cups chicken broth
- 1 can tomato paste
- 2 teaspoons ground cumin
- 1/4 teaspoon cayenne pepper
- 1 teaspoon salt (or to taste)
- 1/8 teaspoon ground cinnamon
- 1/2 cup raisins
- 1 large onion (finely chopped)
- 2 tablespoons chopped fresh garlic
- 2 pounds yams or sweet potatoes (peeled and cut into small chunks)
- 2 cans chickpeas (rinsed and drained)
- 3 pounds skinless boneless chicken (cut into small chunks)
- 2 cups green vegetables of your choice (broccoli, zucchini, green beans, etc.)
- 3 cups cooked rice or millet

Yields 8 servings

Instructions

In a large soup pot, combine broth, tomato paste, salt, and spices. Whisk until blended. Add raisins, onion, garlic, yams, chickpeas, and chicken. Bring to a gentle boil. Reduce heat to low, then cover and simmer for 20 minutes. Add green vegetables and cook another 10 minutes or until chicken is no longer pink and yams are soft. Serve stew over rice or millet.

Breakfast Challenge Turkey Chili

https://www.thesuppersprograms.org/content/breakfast-challenge-chili

Ingredients

- 2 tablespoons olive oil (enough to coat pan)
- 1 1/2 pounds ground turkey
- 1 tablespoon chili powder
- salt (to taste)
- 8 cups chopped high-fiber vegetables (e.g., celery, cauliflower, mushrooms, kale, zucchini, cabbage, turnips)
- 2 cans preferred beans, rinsed and drained (omit for low-carb option)

1 jar of tomato sauce (check for no added sugar)
1 jar of salsa (check for no added sugar)
broth or water (as needed for consistency)
2 tablespoons apple cider vinegar (to taste)
1 teaspoon honey or 6 drops monkfruit extract

Yields 6 servings

Instructions

Coat bottom of soup pot with oil. Over medium heat, brown the ground turkey. Add chili powder and 1 teaspoon salt and sauté for another minute. Add the vegetables, beans (if using), salsa and tomato sauce. Stir and bring to a simmer. Depending on the amount of liquid in the salsa, you may need to add some water or broth. Bring to a boil, reduce heat to low and simmer until the water steams off and it is the consistency you like, about 20 minutes. Balance the flavor with 1 to 2 tablespoons of vinegar, honey or monkfruit, and salt to taste.

Paleo Grass-fed Beef or Lamb Hash

https://www.thesuppersprograms.org/content/paleo-grass-fed-beef-or-lamb-hash

Ingredients

2 tablespoons coconut oil (to coat the pan)
1 teaspoon salt
1 tablespoon ras el hanout (Moroccan spice blend) or curry powder (optional)
1 onion (diced)
3 cloves garlic (minced)
1 red pepper (diced)
1 pound grass-fed ground beef or lamb
4 cups low-starch veggies (e.g., shredded greens, cabbage, diced summer squash, baby spinach)
water or coconut milk (as needed to steam)
lemon juice, salt, pepper (to taste)

Yields 4 servings

Instructions

Heat the oil and add salt and spice, if using. Stir constantly for half a minute—don't let spices get smoky. Place onion in the spice; turn down the heat and cook at least 10 minutes, stirring occasionally. Add garlic and pepper and continue to cook. Add beef or lamb and brown the meat. Add the vegetables and a few tablespoons of water or coconut milk, just enough to steam. Cover and cook 10-15 minutes until vegetables are soft, adding water or coconut milk if needed to steam. Balance flavor with a little lemon juice, salt, and black pepper.

Pulled Chicken, Squash, and Greens

https://www.thesuppersprograms.org/content/pulled-chicken-squash-greens

This is a good recipe for a crowd if doubled or tripled.

Ingredients

- 1 whole roasted or rotisserie chickens (boned and shredded by hand)
- 2 teaspoons coconut oil
- 1 teaspoon salt
- 2 large leeks
- 1/4 cup minced ginger
- 1 large butternut squash, peeled, seeded, and diced
- 2 bunches greens (kale, collards, chard; stems removed, leaves and stems chopped separately)
- 1 quart chicken broth
- salt and pepper to taste
- 1 tablespoon cider vinegar

Yields 6 servings

Instructions

In a large soup pot over medium heat, add coconut oil and salt. Sauté leeks and ginger until they start to color. Add diced squash and sauté for a couple of minutes. Add the broth and chopped stems. Bring to a boil, reduce heat, and simmer for 15 minutes. Add the chopped leaves and shredded chicken and simmer for an additional 5 minutes. Season with salt, pepper, and a splash of cider vinegar to taste.

Miso Crusted Salmon

https://www.thesuppersprograms.org/content/miso-crusted-salmon

Ingredients

- 1 large bunch cilantro (minced)
- 1 bunch scallions (green and white parts, minced)
- 3/4 cups brown or red miso (unpasteurized, more if needed)
- 3 tablespoons freshly grated ginger
- 4 lemons, zested and juiced (zest and juice separated)
- 2 pounds wild salmon filet (skinned and cleaned)

Yields 6 servings

Instructions

Preheat oven to 375 degrees and line a baking sheet with parchment paper. In a large bowl, combine minced cilantro, scallions, miso paste, ginger, lemon zest, and 2 tablespoons of lemon juice. Mixture should be a thick paste. Place prepared salmon filet on lined baking sheet and cover salmon with a thick layer of paste. Bake for 20–25 minutes and check salmon for doneness. Enjoy warm.

DESSERTS / TREATS

Blueberry Chia Seed Pudding

https://www.thesuppersprograms.org/content/blueberry-chia-seed-pudding

Ingredients

- 2 cups vanilla almond milk
- 3/4 cups blueberries (fresh or frozen)
- 1/2 cup chia seeds
- 1 teaspoon ground cinnamon
- 1/2 teaspoon almond extract
- 2 tablespoons honey (or 8 drops of monkfruit extract)
- 1 cup fresh blueberries (garnish)
- 1/4 cup slivered almonds (garnish)

Yields 10 servings

Instructions

Process the almond milk and 3/4 cup of blueberries until smooth. Pour into a large bowl and add chia seeds, cinnamon, almond extract, and honey or monkfruit. Cover and refrigerate (stirring occasionally) for at least 2 and up to 24 hours before serving. Garnish with fresh blueberries and slivered almonds.

Gluten Free Banana Bread

https://www.thesuppersprograms.org/content/gluten-free-banana-bread

Ingredients

1 cup almond butter
1/4 cup honey (optional)
3 bananas (very ripe)
2 eggs
1 cup almond meal
1 teaspoon baking soda
1 teaspoon baking powder
1/4 teaspoon salt
1/4 cup chocolate chips (optional)

Yields 1 loaf

Instructions

Preheat oven to 350 degrees. Line a loaf pan with parchment paper. In a large bowl, mash bananas. Add in the almond butter, eggs, and honey if using. Mix well and add the almond flour, baking soda, baking powder, and salt. Stir until just blended and then fold in the chocolate chips. Pour batter into the prepared loaf pan and bake at 350 for 60 minutes.

Ginger Lemon Truffles

https://www.thesuppersprograms.org/content/ginger-lemon-truffles

Ingredients

6 inches fresh ginger (grated with microplane)
1 pound dried coconut
5 lemons (zested and juiced)
1/4 cup maple syrup (or sweetener of choice: honey, stevia, monkfruit extract, etc.)
1 teaspoon alcohol-free vanilla
1 jar organic cashew butter
1/4 teaspoon pink Himalayan sea salt
1 1/2 cup pulled hemp seeds

Yields 60 truffles

Instructions

With a kitchen mixer or by hand, combine all ingredients except hemp seeds and spin on low until ingredients are well mixed. Taste to balance. Using a 1 oz cookie scoop, scoop out truffles and roll into little balls with gloved hands. Then, drop into a bowl of pulled hemp seeds and toss until coated well. Keep chilled until serving. Keeps up to one week.

Avocado & Berry Ice Cream

https://www.thesuppersprograms.org/content/avocado-berry-ice-cream

Ingredients

1 Haas (if available) avocado (ripe)
2 bananas
1 cup frozen blackberries or other berries (12 oz bag)
pinch of salt
1 teaspoon lemon juice (to taste)
1/2 can full fat coconut milk (15 oz can)

Yields 4 servings

Instructions

Cut avocados and bananas into 1-inch pieces and freeze both for 2–3 hours. Once frozen, combine with remaining ingredients in a blender or food processor and process until smooth, adding water as needed for desired consistency. Serve immediately.

Fudgy Maple Black Bean Brownies

https://www.thesuppersprograms.org/content/fudgy-maple-black-bean-brownies

Sometimes you simply need a treat! These devilishly delicious brownies have no additives, preservatives, gluten, dairy, or refined sugar. But the best part is, you'd never know it! Plus they pack a protein punch with the black beans!

Ingredients

1 15 ounce can of black beans, drained and rinsed
3 eggs
1/3 cup coconut oil or butter (melted)
1/4 cup raw cacao powder
1/8 teaspoon sea salt
1 teaspoon pure vanilla extract (alcohol-free)
1/4 cup pure maple syrup
1/3 cup gluten-free chocolate (chips or chunks)
1/3 cup chopped raw walnuts

Yields 16 brownies

Instructions

Preheat the oven to 350 degrees. Grease an 8 × 8-inch baking pan with coconut oil or butter. Place beans, eggs, coconut oil, cacao powder, salt, vanilla, and maple syrup in food processor and blend until smooth. Remove the blade and gently stir in chocolate chips and walnuts. Transfer mixture to prepared pan. Bake for 35 minutes, or until brownies are set in the center and a toothpick comes out clean. When cool, cut into 9 squares. Best served warm.

BEVERAGES

Super Simple Smoothie

https://www.thesuppersprograms.org/content/super-simple-smoothie

Ingredients

1/2 ripe avocado
1 cup organic strawberries (hulled)
1 ripe banana
2 cups almond or coconut milk

Yields 2 servings

Instructions

Blend all ingredients together.

Green Detox Smoothie

https://www.thesuppersprograms.org/content/green-detox-smoothie

Ingredients

1 cup frozen berries
2 cups spinach leaves
1/2 teaspoon cinnamon
1/4 teaspoon turmeric
1 tablespoon cocoa powder
1/4 teaspoon cayenne pepper (optional)
1/4 cup full-fat coconut milk
1 cup unsweetened green tea (iced or room temperature; use more if needed)

Yields 1 large serving

Instructions

Blend all ingredients in a high-speed blender until puréed.

Cinnamon Warming Tea

https://www.thesuppersprograms.org/content/cinnamon-warming-tea

Ingredients

8 cinnamon sticks
2 quarts water
2 green tea bags
honey (to taste)

Yields 8 servings

Instructions

Bring the water and cinnamon sticks to a boil. Reduce the heat and simmer for 20–30 minutes. Pour into a tea pot with the green tea bags. Steep for 10 minutes. Serve with local raw honey for added antimicrobial benefits and sweetness.

Golden Milk

https://www.thesuppersprograms.org/content/golden-milk

Ingredients

- 1 13 ounce can full-fat coconut milk
- 1 cup water
- 2 tablespoons turmeric powder (or 4-inch piece of fresh turmeric, grated)
- 2 tablespoons honey (or 16 drops monkfruit extract)
- 1 2-inch piece of ginger (grated)
- 2 cinnamon sticks
- 5 peppercorns

Yields 4 servings

Instructions

Combine all ingredients in a saucepan over medium heat. Simmer for 20 minutes. Strain through a fine mesh or cheesecloth into mugs. Serve hot.

Appendix 2
Travel Tips

Airplanes and Drinking Water

On commercial flights . . . don't drink the water! Studies have consistently shown that water from airplane water tanks, used to serve water for coffee and tea, ice cubes, as well for handwashing in the bathroom sink, is grossly contaminated. Studies show tanks are not cleaned regularly or effectively, testing for contaminants is limited to only a handful of bacteria and industrial chemicals, and often the only remedy is a chlorine tablet dropped in to the water tank.

Implemented in 2011, the federal government's Aircraft Drinking Water Rule (ADWR) requires airlines to provide passengers and flight crew with safe drinking water. The ADWR requires airlines to take samples from their water tanks to test for possible coliform bacteria and *E. coli*. Airlines are also required to disinfect and flush each aircraft's water tank *four times per year*. Alternatively, *an airline may choose to disinfect and flush once a year*, but then it must test monthly.

- In recent study looking at contaminants in many commercial airlines. The 2019 Airline Water Study ranks 10 major and 13 regional airlines mainly by the quality of water they provided onboard its flights.[1] The major airlines receiving the highest Airline Water Health Score are

Allegiant and Alaska. Spirit and JetBlue tied for the lowest score. Nearly all regional airlines, except Piedmont, have poor Water Health Scores and a large number of ADWR violations. Republic Airways (which flies for United Express, Delta Connection, and American Eagle) had the lowest score and ExpressJet the second-lowest. ExpressJet averaged 3.36 ADWR violations per aircraft.

- The 2019 Airline Water Study also found that the Environmental Protection Agency—one of the federal agencies responsible for ensuring safe aircraft drinking water—rarely levies civil penalties on airlines in violation of the ADWR.

The researchers for this study recommend that you:

- NEVER drink any water onboard that isn't in a sealed bottle.
- Do not drink coffee or tea onboard (which uses tank water).
- Do not wash your hands in the bathroom (which uses tank water); bring hand sanitizer with you instead.

Additional Travel Tips

- Travel with a glass or stainless steel drinking water bottle without plastic sipping lid or plastic flip straw. There are now many water refilling stations in airports and rail stations nationally and internationally as part of a global effort to reduce the purchase and use of plastic water bottles. Consider purchasing a water bottle with a built-in carbon filter.
- When traveling bring your own filtered drinking water from home whenever possible.
- Avoid using sample shampoos, conditioners, soaps, body washes, and lotions from hotels. These samples contain a variety of harmful chemicals, and many bottles do not list their ingredients. These small plastic bottles also contribute to the worldwide plastic burden and are not recycled.
- Bring your own safe, vetted shampoo, conditioner, soap, and lotions (see chapter 8). Many stores sell TSA-approved, 3 oz bottles for travel, which can be refilled over and over again and stored in a resealable bag to avoid spilling contents onto clothing.

- Fill a 3 oz travel bottle with rubbing alcohol (ethyl alcohol) to wipe down the remote control in your hotel room, which is often the dirtiest item in hotel rooms.
- Call ahead to your hotel and ask housekeeping NOT to use any unnecessary chemicals, such as air fresheners or carpet powder in your hotel room before and during your stay, due to allergies and/or chemical sensitivity.
- Bring or buy a set of stainless steel cutlery and straws to reduce the use of plastic food contamination and to reduce global plastic waste.
- Bring sandals or flip flops to avoid walking on pesticide-laden grass, or newly washed floors with chemical cleaners.
- Choose bottled water, food, and drinks in glass containers.
- Bring your favorite non-toxic, organic tea or coffee in a resealable bag along with stainless steel tea infuser.
- Bring safe sweeteners (i.e., stevia vs. harmful saccharin or aspartame), condiments, and snacks, to reduce the odds of making poor choices where safe or healthy options are limited.
- Reduce unnecessary EMF radiation; some large hotel chains are now offering rooms *without* WiFi due to customer complaints of WiFi sensitivity, such as headache, cognitive changes, and tinnitus.
- Turn off WiFi servers while sleeping at Airbnbs, condos, and rental apartments.
- Put phones on airplane mode at night while sleeping. Alarms are able to sound while in airplane mode on most phones.

Reference

1. Ph.D CP. Airline Water Study 2019. Hunter College NYC Food Policy Center. https://www.dietdetective.com/airline-water-study-2019/. Published 2019. Accessed October 4, 2019.

Appendix 3

Gym Tips

- When going to the gym, avoid using sample shampoos, conditioners, soaps, and body washes found in showers as well as body lotions from large dispensers. These products contain a variety of harmful chemicals, and many bottles do not list their ingredients. It defeats the purpose to exercise, sweat, and use a sauna to detox from toxic chemicals . . . and then put them right back onto your body after a great workout! (see chapter 8).
- Bring your own filtered drinking water from home.
- Use glass or stainless steel water bottle, without plastic sipping lid or plastic flip straw, especially in a sauna or steam room where plastic chemicals can leach into the water under high temperatures.
- Wear flip flops at the gym; many harmful chemicals, especially chlorinated cleaning chemicals, are used to clean gym floors and equipment, saunas, steam rooms, pools, and hot tubs.
- Do pushups on towels as opposed to vinyl flooring to avoid skin contact with plastic and cleaning chemicals.

Appendix 4
Reputable Labs

Toxin Testing

(not typically covered by commercial health insurance and often requires a physician to order)

Genova Diagnostics

www.gdx.net/product/toxic-effects-core-test-urine-blood
    Toxic Effects CORE: This test requires both urine and blood samples to assess pesticide, plasticizers (phthalates and parabens), PCBs, and volatile solvents.

Quicksilver Scientific

www.quicksilverscientific.com
    Blood Metals Panel: Used to measure heavy metals (arsenic, cadmium, cobalt, lead and mercury)
    Tri-Test: Measures both inorganic mercury and methyl mercury (a more toxic form)

Great Plains Lab

www.greatplainslaboratory.com/gpl-tox

Toxic Non-Metal Chemical Profile (GPL-Tox): This test screens for 172 different chemicals.

Water Testing Labs

Well water and municipal tap: Doctors Data (www.doctorsdata.com) can test for toxic metals.

Great Plains Laboratory (www.greatplainslaboratory.com) can test for many other chemicals.

Appendix 5

Abbreviations

BPA	Bisphenol A
CDC	Centers for Disease Control and Prevention
DDT	Dichloro-diphenyl-trichloroethane
DES	Diethylstilbestrol
EDCs	endocrine-disrupting chemicals or compounds
EMF	Electromagnetic fields
EWG	Environmental Working Group
FDA	Food and Drug Administration
GMOs	genetically modified organisms
GRAS	generally regarded as safe
NHANES	National Health and Nutrition Examination Survey
PBDEs	polybrominated diphenyl ethers
PCBs	polychlorinated biphenyls
PFAS	polyfluoroalkyl substances
PFCs	perfluorinated compounds
POPs	persistent organic pollutants
PVC	polyvinyl chloride
SDWA	Safe Drinking Water Act
TSCA	Toxic Substances Control Act
VOCs	volatile organic compounds
WHO	World Health Organization

Appendix 6

Glossary

Absorption: the process by which an agent is taken into an organism's cells or blood supply

Acute exposure: a single exposure to a chemical, drug or radiation

Acute toxicity: the undesirable effects of an acute exposure

Bioaccumulation: the accumulation of a substance, such as a toxic chemical, in various tissues of a living organism (e.g., methylmercury in fish in muscle, PCBs in human fat cells)

Biomagnification: the increasing concentration of a substance, such as a toxic chemical, in the tissues of organisms at successively higher levels of a food chain. As a result of biomagnification, organisms at the top of the food chain generally suffer greater harm from a persistent toxin or pollutant than those at lower levels.

Biomonitoring: the scientific technique that assesses a person's exposure to natural and synthetic chemicals through the evaluation body fluids and tissues, most commonly blood, urine, breast milk, and expelled air.

Biotransformation: the ability of an organism to transform one substance into another, often (but not always) to reduce toxicity or increase excretion (e.g., bacteria can transform mercury into methylmercury)

Carcinogen: any substance that causes cancer (e.g., asbestos, benzene)

Chromosome: DNA and associated proteins located in the nucleus of a cell

Chronic toxicity: health effects from long-term exposure

Corrosive: to eat away or deteriorate, such as with skin

DEHP (di-2-ethyl-hexyl phthalate): one of the many chemicals classified as phthalates; a plasticizer added to materials to make them more flexible; one of the most common phthalates to be studied for health effects among independent researchers; a known endocrine-disrupting chemical

Detoxification: the biochemical process of neutralizing, metabolizing, or excreting a toxic substance (e.g., alcohol breakdown in the liver)

Distribution: how a chemical agent disseminates throughout the body

Dose: a measured amount of exposure, usually relative to body weight or surface area

Dose-response: the effect or response of an agent is related to the dose or amount of exposure

Endocrine-Disrupting Chemical (EDC): substance in the environment (air, soil, water supply), food sources, personal care products, or industrial chemicals that interfere with the normal function of the endocrine system, causing disruption of hormone synthesis, release, and/or function

Epigenetics: The inheritance of patterns of DNA and RNA activity that do not depend on the DNA sequence. By "inheritance," we mean a memory of such activity transmitted from one generation to the next.

Excretion: the process of removing waste or breakdown products from the body

Exposure: duration and type of contact with an agent, which depends on the route [dermal (skin), stomach (ingestion), or inhalation (lung)]; frequency (how often the exposure occurs and time between exposures); and duration (how long the exposure occurs)

Formaldehyde: a breakdown product of many chemicals, such as the artificial sweetener aspartame and quaternium-15; used as a preservative in many cosmetics, shampoos, and hair-straightening processes; declared a known human carcinogen by the US federal government in 2011

Half-life: the time required to reduce the amount of an agent by one half of its original amount

Hazard: an agent or situation capable of causing an adverse effect or harm

Insulin resistance: condition in which insulin, made by the pancreas, is not able to keep blood glucose levels normal, which may eventually lead to diabetes

Leukemia: cancer of the white blood cells that are formed from bone marrow

Maximum contaminant level (MCL): the highest amount of a specific contaminant allowed in public drinking water

Metabolism: when one substance is changed into another, usually to reduce toxicity or to increase excretion from the body

Milligram (mg): one thousandth of a gram (1×10^{-3})

Microgram (µg): one millionth of a gram (1×10^{-6})

Minimal risk levels (MRLs): an estimate of the daily human exposure to a hazardous substance that is not likely to cause appreciable risk of adverse non-cancer health effects, over a specific duration of exposure

Multigenerational exposure: an exposure that occurs with multiple generations simultaneously; when a pregnant woman has an exposure, three generations are exposed: mother, fetus, and the fetal germ cells (eggs in female fetus and cells that give rise to sperm cells in a male fetus)

Mutagen: a substance that causes alterations in cellular DNA (e.g., radiation)

Nanogram: one billionth of a gram $(1 \times 10\text{-}9)$ as used in nanotechnology

Neurotoxicity: adverse changes in the structure or function of the nervous system (e.g., brain, spinal cord, nerves) following exposure to a chemical (e.g., mercury, lead, heroin, pesticides) or physical agent (e.g., radiation)

Neurotransmitter: chemical used to communicate information between cells of the nervous system

Osmosis: a process by which molecules move from an area of less concentrated solution into a more concentrated one across a membrane, thus equalizing the concentrations on each side of the membrane

PBDEs (polybrominated diphenyl ethers): group of chemicals used as flame retardants; classified according to the average number of bromine atoms in the molecule, differentiating their individual structural name (e.g., deca-PBDE has 8-10 bromine atoms)

PCBs (polychlorinated biphenyls): group of chemicals used as cooling agents in electrical transformers (e.g., on top of electricity poles along roads) because they have low flammability

Pesticide: any substance or mixture of substances intended for preventing, destroying, repelling or mitigating any insects, rodents, nematodes, fungi, or weeds or any other form of life declared to be pests

Pharmacology: the study of beneficial and adverse effects of drugs (e.g., aspirin, acetaminophen, caffeine)

Pollutant: an agent, often released by human activity, which adversely affects the environment (e.g., mercury, lead, DDT, PCBs)

Persistence: continued measurable amount of a chemical, from a previous or finite exposure

Precautionary principle: when an activity raises threats of harm to human health or the environment, precautionary measures should be taken even if some cause and effect relationships are not fully established scientifically

"Prop 65": Proposition 65, also known as The Safe Drinking Water and Toxic Enforcement Act of 1986, is a California law passed in 1986. Its goals are to protect drinking water sources from toxic substances that cause cancer and birth defects and to reduce or eliminate toxic chemicals from consumer products, by requiring warnings on products. Prop 65 also requires signs to be posted on businesses, stating whether any products or materials found in that building are listed on the Prop 65 list of toxic chemicals. An official list of substances covered by Proposition 65 is publicly available, and chemicals are added to or removed from the official list based on California's analysis of current scientific data

Pseudo-persistence: continued levels of measurable chemical in the body, despite a short half-life, due to chronic presence and exposure in one's surroundings

Prevalence: the number of people in a population that have a condition relative to all of the people in the population; prevalence is typically shown either as a percentage (e.g., 1%) or a proportion (e.g., 1 in 100)

Reference Dose (RfD): a daily exposure level (dose) that is not expected to cause any adverse health effects in humans throughout the lifetime

Response: the reaction to an exposure

Therapeutic Index: the measure of a drug's benefit and safety; a narrow index indicates that a drug has many toxic effects at high dose levels, a wide index indicates few toxic effects at high dose levels

Toxic: (noun) a poisonous substance that is created through an artificial process, and not from a living cells or organisms

Toxic effect: the adverse reaction (e.g., cancer, learning disability, rash) to an agent

Toxic substance: any substance that can cause acute or chronic injury to the human body or is suspected to do so

Toxicant: an agent capable of causing toxicity; a poison (e.g., DDT, lead, solvents, noise, food additives, ozone)

Toxin: a poisonous substance produced within living cells or organisms (arising from, e.g., plants, animals, bacteria, or fungi)

Transgenerational exposure: an exposure that creates a genetic or epigenetic mutation found in offspring, two or more successive generations from the exposed generation

Xenobiotic: a foreign substance that is not naturally produced by an organism (e.g., xenoestrogen is an estrpgem produced outside the body)

Appendix 7

Tear-Off Refrigerator Sheet

☐ Reduce consumption of foods and drinks with pesticides, coloring, preservatives, or GMO ingredients.

☐ Reduce consumption of canned foods and drinks (buy fresh and/or frozen organics).

☐ Create a healthy water system by choosing a safe water filter from EWG .org/guide to water filters, filling up at home, and using stainless steel or glass water bottles to carry your water.

☐ Avoid cookware and food-storage containers that are nonstick or plastic (use stainless steel and glass).

☐ If you must use plastics, avoid storing food in and eating from plastic containers with recycling codes #3, #6, and #7 (remember: "5,4,1,2 all the rest are bad for you!").

   ***But *all* plastics are mixtures of chemicals with potential for harm

☐ Never heat or microwave food or drinks in plastic; switch to heat-resistant glass.

- ☐ Use fewer personal care products overall and check product safety at EWG.org/skindeep.
- ☐ Open windows daily to ventilate and avoid products that are either aerosolized sprays or loose powders.
- ☐ Avoid air fresheners: plug-ins, aerosols, and incense with synthetic fragrances.
- ☐ Avoid pesticides, such as bug sprays, lawn treatment and fumigation services; there are safer alternatives.
- ☐ Buy couches, mattresses, and other home furnishings without flame retardant chemicals.
- ☐ Ask your healthcare practitioner if your medications are safe, effective and necessary.
- ☐ Wet mop with water, dust, and vacuum 1-2x/week to reduce dust, which harmful chemicals stick to.
- ☐ Choose safe cleaning products from EWG's Guide to Healthy Cleaning (www.EWG.org), or make your own with baking soda, white vinegar, and lemon juice.
- ☐ Take shoes off and put on slippers at the door to reduce the amount of chemicals tracked into your home.
- ☐ Limit radiation exposure by keeping laptop computers, tablets, and cell phones far from the body (especially the chest and groin areas).
- ☐ Turn cellphones on "airplane mode" and turn off WiFi servers when not in use or while sleeping

For regular environmental health and wellness information, practical tips, and recommendations, follow Dr. Cohen's platform, *The Smart Human* on Facebook, Twitter, and Instagram and sign up for her newsletter at TheSmartHuman.com, and listen to her podcast "The Smart Human.

About the Authors

Dr. Aly Cohen is a board certified rheumatologist and integrative medicine specialist, as well as an environmental health expert in Princeton, New Jersey. She has collaborated with the Environmental

Working Group, Cancer Schmancer, and other disease-prevention organizations, and is coeditor of the textbook, *Integrative Environmental Medicine*, part of the Oxford University Press *Weil Integrative Medicine Library*. In 2015, she created TheSmartHuman.com to share environmental health, disease prevention, and wellness information with the public. She lectures nationally on environmental health topics for elementary/high schools, colleges/universities, medical schools, and physician-training programs, and she is a regular expert guest for television, print, and podcasts. In 2015 she received the NJ Healthcare Heroes Award in Education for The Smart Human educational platform and she was awarded the 2016 Burton L. Eichler Award for humanitarianism.

Dr. Cohen is working to educate and empower the next generation to make safer, smarter lifestyle choices through the creation of environmental health and prevention curricula for schools nationally. Her TEDx talk, "How to Protect Your Kids from Toxic Chemicals" can be found on YouTube, and you can follow her health and wellness tips and recommendations on Facebook at The Smart Human, Twitter, and Instagram: @thesmarthuman. Sign up for The Smart Human newsletter, read her latest posts at TheSmartHuman.com, and listen to her podcast The Smart Human.

Dr. Cohen lives on a farm in New Jersey with her husband, two sons and lots of furry friends.

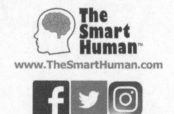

www.TheSmartHuman.com

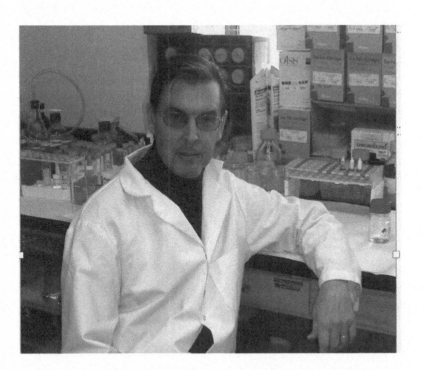

Dr. Fred vom Saal is a Curators' Distinguished Professor of Biology at the University of Missouri-Columbia (MU). After college he taught biology as a Peace Corps Volunteer in Somalia and after the revolution there, he also taught biology in Kenya and then Paris before entering graduate school. Dr. vom Saal has mentored numerous undergraduate and graduate students since joining the MU faculty in 1979 and has published over 250 articles and reviews on his research, which have been funded by grants from NIH, NSF, USDA, EPA, FDA, and NATO, as well as a number of foundations. He served on the National Academy of Sciences Committee on Hormonally Active Agents in the Environment, is an elected fellow of the American Association for the Advancement of Science, and is a recipient of the Heinz Foundation Award in Environmental Science, the Upstream Award from the Jenifer Altman Foundation, the Environmental Health Hero Award from the CleanMed Association, and the University of Missouri Alumni Association Faculty Award.

Dr. vom Saal has served on the editorial boards of numerous scientific journals and federal research review panels both in the United States and abroad. In the mid-1990s, Dr. vom Saal and his colleagues at MU discovered that the endocrine-disrupting chemical bisphenol A (BPA) disrupted fetal development at doses thousands of times lower than had been previously estimated by the FDA and EPA to cause no effect. Because his research has challenged the approaches used by regulatory agencies to assess chemical safety, he has testified about the hazards posed by environmental endocrine-disrupting chemicals in numerous state legislatures, the US House of Representatives, and the US Senate, as well as the EU Parliament. Dr. vom Saal, together with his wife Kathi, enjoys flying around the United States and Canada in their airplane, particularly visiting their families and grandson Charlie.

Acknowledgments

Aly Cohen, MD

I would like to acknowledge many people and pets who have helped me along on this journey:

Truxtun, my dog, whose illness set me on this journey to understand environmental health; Johanna Congleton PhD, former Senior Scientist at the Environmental Working Group for seeing my potential to help educate other physicians on environmental health topics; Dr. Victoria Maizes, Dr. Tieraona Low Dog, and Dr. Andrew Weil for teaching me the logic and beauty of integrative medicine; Fran Drescher and Susan Holland and the team at Cancer Schmancer for their continued support and promotion of my work; Cherry Sprague, former head of Science at Princeton High School who literally and figuratively opened the doors of her high school to let me in; Dorothy Mullen (*thesuppersprograms.org*), my North Star, for your tenacity and fearlessness to pursue TRUTH; Norris Clark for totally getting my "big idea" for my TEDx talk, *How to Protect Your Kids from Toxic Chemicals*; Dr. Fred vom Saal, my coauthor and mentor, for inviting me into the endocrine-disrupting chemical world and enthusiastically supporting all of my environmental health education projects; Dr. Andrew Weil for trusting me to share this critical information with the world through both his academic and consumer book series; my patients who patiently allow me to share with them new information as I grow and evolve as a physician; and The Smart Human community on social media who support and challenge me every day.

Finally, I would like to thank my entire family, especially my amazing parents and big brother; my true and steadfast "partner in crime" husband, Stephen; my beautiful, crazy boys Asher and Landon; and my furry buddies, Truxtun, Kitty, Oliver, and Charlie, for being the greatest cheerleaders of them all.

Fred vom Saal, PhD

My first experience teaching biology was as a Peace Corps volunteer in a high school in northwest Somalia. After there was a revolution, and diplomatic relations with the United States were severed, I transferred to western Kenya, again teaching biology, but in a region where the children were severely nutritionally stressed due to very limited protein in their diet (consisting primarily of cassava root). The adverse effect this had on their health and ability to learn set me on a path of discovery over the last 50 years, focusing on how events during development can shape the rest of an individual's life. During my time as a student, my PhD advisor, Dr. Leonard Hamilton, and postdoctoral advisor, Dr. Frank Bronson, profoundly shaped my development as a scientist. The idea that minute differences in fetal hormones could lead to profound differences in an individual's life history was developed while I was a postdoctoral fellow with Dr. Bronson. It was a review article I wrote in 1989 covering over a decade of research revealing the exquisite sensitivity of fetuses to infinitesimally small changes in their hormones that led Dr. Theo Colborn (author of *Our Stolen Future*) to contact me in 1990. Theo said that reading about these experimental findings triggered an "ah ha" moment that led her to predict that very small exposures to environmental pollutants were disrupting the endocrine control systems in wildlife, and thus potentially also in humans. Theo and I met a short time later, and I began a life-changing journey. I joined Theo, and initially a relatively small band of close colleagues/friends who were willing to keep conducting research in spite of continuous personal attacks by chemical companies and their surrogates (Pete Myers, Ana Soto, Lou Guillette, Shanna Swan; my Italian colleagues, Stefano Parmigiani and Paola Palanza; Japanese colleagues, Taisen Iguchi, Koji Arizono, Chisato Mori; and my main collaborator at the University of Missouri, Wade Welshons) as well as many others since that early time during the 1990s, and created the field of endocrine disrupting chemicals (EDCs). Of course, along the way I had fantastic students (including Professors Susan Nagel and Monica Montano, who made critical discoveries while conducting their thesis research and afterwards; their intelligence, integrity, long hours in the lab, and love of science made this journey a lot of fun. Throughout this journey my wife Kathi has been there to help guide me through the mine field that EDC research put all of us into. This has been a family adventure, and our daughter Jillian has helped spread the message, that you will find by reading this book, to her generation. The book is needed because the FDA and EPA have failed to protect us and the environment in which we live. It is thus up to each of us, individually, to acquire the knowledge needed to avoid the myriad of contaminants that are allowed to invade our lives. My aim, along with my dedicated physician colleague, Dr. Aly Cohen, is to help you achieve this goal.

Index

Boxes, figures, and tables are indicated by b, f, and t following the page number.